The Complete
Self-Healing Collection of
Natural Herbal Remedies
Inspired by Barbara O'Neill

*Everything You Need to Know to Restore Your
Body's Ability to Heal Itself*

Clara Whitfield

'able of Contents

Part 1:
Barbara O'Neill's Holistic Health Overview

Chapter 1: Barbara O'Neill's Approach to Healing – A Holistic View of Health

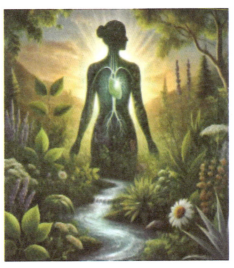

1.1 Introduction to Holistic Healing

Holistic healing is founded on the principle that the body is a self-cleansing, self-repairing organism with the inherent ability to heal itself when given the proper support. This concept is central to understanding the body as an interconnected set of systems that, when in balance, has the power to overcome illness and maintain health. The body's natural mechanisms—like the immune system, detoxification pathways, and regenerative processes—are always at work to repair damage, remove toxins, and restore homeostasis. However, for these processes to function optimally, the body requires the right environment, nourishment, and lifestyle practices.

This fundamental concept of self-healing challenges the conventional approach, which focuses on managing symptoms instead of addressing the root cause of disease. Holistic healing emphasizes creating the right conditions for the body to thrive, allowing its natural healing processes to unfold.

The self-cleansing nature of the body is seen in its ability to detoxify and eliminate waste through organs such as the liver, kidneys, and skin. These detoxification processes remove harmful substances that could lead to disease. Similarly, the body's self-repair mechanisms allow for tissue regeneration and cell renewal. When the body is given adequate rest, proper nutrition, and a toxin-free environment, these processes work more efficiently.

Barbara O'Neill's Journey from Conventional Medicine to Holistic Approaches

Barbara O'Neill's journey into holistic healing was shaped by her personal experiences and dissatisfaction with the limitations of conventional medicine. Initially trained within the traditional medical system, O'Neill became aware of the shortcomings of an approach that primarily focused on treating symptoms rather than addressing underlying causes. This realization led her to explore alternative healing methods that emphasize the body's natural ability to heal itself.

Her personal health challenges and observations of patients dealing with chronic conditions inspired her to seek a more comprehensive approach to health. Through her research and experience, O'Neill discovered that many chronic illnesses could be managed, and even reversed, through lifestyle changes, detoxification, and natural therapies. This journey from conventional to holistic healing allowed her to develop a deeper understanding of how nutrition, the environment, and emotional well-being play integral roles in overall health.

Understanding Health Beyond Symptoms

While conventional medicine often treats symptoms as isolated issues, the holistic approach views symptoms as signals from the body, indicating imbalances that need to be addressed. For example, recurring headaches may not be an isolated condition but rather a sign of deeper issues such as poor diet, dehydration, or chronic stress. By addressing these underlying causes, the symptoms can be resolved, and overall health improved.

Lifestyle changes play a crucial role in this approach. For instance, diet is foundational to maintaining health. Processed foods, refined sugars, and unhealthy fats burden the body, leading to inflammation, digestive issues, and eventually chronic disease. By shifting to a whole-food, plant-based diet rich in nutrients, individuals can support the body's detoxification processes, reduce inflammation, and promote healing. Incorporating regular physical activity, adequate rest, and stress management techniques into daily life can help restore balance and enhance the body's self-healing abilities.

Environmental factors also have a significant impact on health. Exposure to toxins in the air, water, and household products can overwhelm the body's detoxification systems, leading to a buildup of harmful substances that contribute to illness. By creating a clean, toxin-free living environment and avoiding exposure to harmful chemicals, individuals can support their body's natural ability to cleanse and repair itself.

1.2 Components of Holistic Health

There are several critical components of the holistic lifestyle, and this book is broken down to detail what needs to be done to encourage your body's natural healing and regenerative processes:

- The Importance of Preventative Care
    o Nutrition as Preventative Medicine
    o Practical Steps for Preventative Care
    o Healing Foods as Fuel for the Body
- Harnessing the Body's Self-Healing Mechanisms
    o Immune System Support
    o Cell Repair and Regeneration
    o Detoxification Pathways
    o How Stress and Toxins Inhibit Healing

Chapter 2: The Body's Self-Healing Mechanisms – How to Tap into Natural Resilience

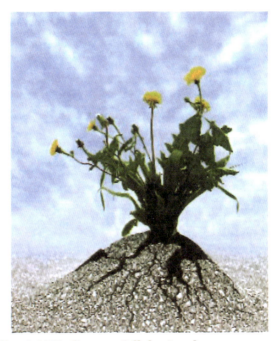

2.1 Understanding Self-Healing at a Cellular Level

Cells are the fundamental building blocks of life, and their ability to heal and regenerate is essential for maintaining overall health and vitality. Self-healing at the cellular level depends on providing the body with optimal conditions, including proper nutrition, hydration, and rest. Each of these factors plays a crucial role in enabling cells to repair themselves, regenerate, and continue functioning efficiently.

The Role of Nutrition in Cellular Healing

Proper nutrition is at the core of the body's ability to self-heal at a cellular level. Every cell in the body requires a steady supply of nutrients to carry out essential functions, from energy production to DNA repair. Nutrient-dense foods provide the vitamins, minerals, and antioxidants necessary to support cellular processes, enabling cells to repair damage caused by oxidative stress and environmental factors.

Cells rely on essential nutrients such as vitamins A, C, and E, which are powerful antioxidants that protect against free radical damage. These vitamins help neutralize harmful molecules that can damage cellular structures, such as the cell membrane and DNA. Vitamin C, in particular, plays a crucial role in collagen production, which is essential for the repair of connective tissues. It also aids in the absorption of iron, which supports oxygen transport to cells, ensuring that they receive the energy they need to function and regenerate.

Minerals such as magnesium, zinc, and selenium are equally important for cellular health. Magnesium, for example, is involved in over 300 enzymatic reactions in the body, including those that regulate DNA repair and protein synthesis. Zinc plays a vital role in maintaining the structural integrity of cells and is crucial for immune function, which supports the body's natural defense against infections that can damage cells. Selenium, a potent antioxidant, helps protect cells from oxidative damage and supports the immune system.

Hydration and Its Impact on Cellular Function

Hydration is another critical factor in the self-healing process at the cellular level. Water is essential for nearly every bodily function, and cells require adequate hydration to maintain their structural integrity and perform their roles effectively. Without sufficient hydration, cellular processes slow down, impairing the body's ability to repair damage and maintain overall health.

Barbara O'Neill emphasizes the importance of maintaining proper hydration to support cellular healing. Drinking enough water throughout the day helps keep cells hydrated, allowing them to function optimally. It also aids in regulating body temperature, lubricating joints, and supporting the digestive system, all of which contribute to the overall health of cells.

Rest and Cellular Regeneration

Rest and sleep are fundamental to the process of cellular healing and regeneration. During periods of rest, particularly deep sleep, the body enters a state of repair where cells work to restore damage caused by daily stress, physical exertion, and environmental toxins. When the body is deprived of adequate rest, cellular repair processes are compromised. This can lead to the accumulation of damaged cells and hinder the body's ability to maintain homeostasis, leading to premature aging and an increased risk of illness.

Deep sleep, in particular, is crucial for brain health and cognitive function. During this stage of rest, the brain undergoes its own detoxification process, removing waste products that have accumulated throughout the day. This supports not only brain function but also the overall health of the nervous system, which plays a vital role in communicating signals for healing and regeneration to other parts of the body.

The Role of DNA Repair in Maintaining Health

At the core of cellular regeneration is the process of DNA repair. DNA carries the genetic instructions that guide every function in the body, and when DNA is damaged, it can lead to cellular dysfunction and disease. DNA damage can occur due to a variety of factors, including exposure to toxins, radiation, and oxidative stress. However, the body has built-in mechanisms to repair damaged DNA and maintain cellular integrity.

Essential minerals like zinc and magnesium support the enzymes responsible for DNA repair. These minerals ensure that damaged sections of DNA are identified and repaired, preventing mutations that could lead to the development of chronic diseases or cancer. Additionally, antioxidants such as vitamin C and selenium protect DNA from oxidative damage, further supporting the body's ability to maintain healthy, functional cells.

2.2 The Power of Detoxification in Self-Healing

Barbara O'Neill emphasizes that detoxification is a fundamental aspect of self-healing. The body's ability to cleanse itself is crucial for maintaining optimal health, and key detox organs, such as the liver, kidneys, and lymphatic system, play an essential role in this process. Supporting these detox pathways with natural remedies like dandelion, turmeric, and milk thistle can enhance the body's ability to eliminate toxins and promote overall well-being.

The Role of the Liver in Detoxification

The liver is the body's primary detoxification organ, responsible for filtering toxins from the blood and breaking down harmful substances so they can be safely eliminated. It processes everything from environmental toxins to chemicals found in food, medications, and alcohol. When the liver becomes overburdened due to exposure to these substances, its detoxifying capacity is diminished, which can lead to a buildup of toxins in the body and a range of health issues.

Supporting liver function is essential for effective detoxification. Dandelion root is particularly effective in this regard. Dandelion is known for its ability to stimulate bile production, which helps the liver break down fats and remove waste products. It also acts as a natural diuretic, assisting the body in eliminating toxins through urine. Regular consumption of dandelion root tea or supplements can help promote liver health and ensure that it operates efficiently as a detoxifying organ.

Milk thistle is another potent herb that supports liver detoxification. It contains silymarin, a compound that has been shown to protect liver cells from damage and promote their regeneration. By shielding the liver from harmful toxins and supporting its ability to repair itself, milk thistle enhances the overall detoxification process. Including milk thistle in a detox regimen can improve liver function and reduce the toxic burden on the body.

Kidney Function in Detoxification

The kidneys are responsible for filtering waste products from the blood and regulating the body's fluid balance. They play a crucial role in removing water-soluble toxins through urine. When kidney function is compromised, toxins can accumulate, leading to a range of health problems, including fatigue, headaches, and poor digestion.

To support kidney health, it is important to stay hydrated, as water is essential for kidney function. In addition to hydration, certain herbs, such as dandelion and nettle, can further promote kidney detoxification. Dandelion's diuretic properties help the kidneys eliminate excess fluids and waste more effectively, while nettle works to reduce inflammation in the kidneys, enhancing their ability to filter toxins.

Turmeric, commonly known for its anti-inflammatory properties, also plays a supportive role in kidney health. By reducing inflammation in the body, turmeric helps protect the kidneys from oxidative stress and damage caused by toxins. Regular use of turmeric in food or as a supplement can contribute to improved kidney function, allowing the body to efficiently detoxify.

The Importance of the Lymphatic System

The lymphatic system is often overlooked in discussions about detoxification, but it plays a vital role in the body's ability to cleanse itself. The lymphatic system is responsible for transporting waste and toxins from tissues to the bloodstream, where they can be filtered and eliminated by the liver and kidneys. It also supports immune function by helping to remove bacteria, viruses, and other harmful substances from the body.

Unlike the circulatory system, the lymphatic system does not have a pump, such as the heart, to move lymph fluid. Instead, it relies on muscle movement and deep breathing to circulate lymph throughout the body. Therefore, physical activity, including stretching, yoga, and even walking, is essential to keeping the lymphatic system functioning properly.

Dry brushing is another effective way to stimulate the lymphatic system. This practice involves using a natural bristle brush to gently brush the skin in the direction of the heart, which encourages the movement of lymph fluid and supports the elimination of toxins. Regular dry brushing can help improve lymphatic drainage and enhance overall detoxification.

Supporting Detox Pathways with Natural Remedies

To optimize the body's detoxification processes, Barbara O'Neill advocates the use of natural remedies like dandelion, turmeric, and milk thistle. These herbs work synergistically to support the liver, kidneys, and lymphatic system, enhancing the body's ability to cleanse itself and promote healing.

Dandelion, as previously mentioned, stimulates bile production and acts as a diuretic, supporting both liver and kidney detoxification. Turmeric, with its powerful anti-inflammatory and antioxidant properties, protects the body's organs from toxin-induced damage and improves overall detoxification efficiency. Milk thistle offers specific protection to the liver, helping it regenerate and function optimally in processing toxins.

2.3 Identifying Obstacles to Healing

In today's modern world, there are several obstacles that can hinder the body's natural ability to heal. These obstacles often stem from lifestyle choices and environmental factors that disrupt the body's internal balance, making it difficult to maintain good health. Addressing these barriers is essential to restoring the body's innate healing capabilities and promoting overall well-being.

Poor Diet

One of the most significant obstacles to healing is a poor diet. Diets high in processed foods, refined sugars, and unhealthy fats create a toxic internal environment that leads to inflammation, weight gain, and various chronic diseases. These foods are often stripped of essential nutrients, leaving the body deficient in the vitamins and minerals needed to function properly. Over time, this can weaken the immune system and reduce the body's ability to repair itself.

Chronic Stress

Chronic stress is another major barrier to healing. When the body is under constant stress, it produces excessive amounts of cortisol, the hormone responsible for managing the body's stress response. While cortisol is necessary in short bursts for handling acute stress, prolonged elevations in cortisol levels can lead to a host of health problems, including weakened immune function, poor digestion, and hormonal imbalances. Chronic stress also contributes to inflammation, which can exacerbate existing health conditions and impede the body's ability to heal itself.

Environmental Toxins

Exposure to environmental toxins is another significant obstacle that can prevent the body from healing. Toxins can be found in many everyday products, such as household cleaners, personal care items, and processed foods. Over time, these toxins accumulate in the body and place a heavy burden on the liver, kidneys, and other detoxification organs. When these organs become overworked, the body's ability to eliminate waste and toxins is compromised, leading to a weakened immune system and an increased risk of disease.

Lack of Movement

A sedentary lifestyle is another common obstacle to healing. Lack of physical movement can lead to poor circulation, reduced lymphatic function, and increased inflammation, all of which impair the body's ability to heal. Regular movement is essential for maintaining healthy circulation, which ensures that oxygen and nutrients are delivered to tissues and that waste products are removed efficiently. Without adequate movement, the body's detoxification systems, including the lymphatic system, become sluggish, allowing toxins to accumulate and contribute to illness.

Chapter 3: The Impact of Whole-Food, Plant-Based Nutrition on Overall Health

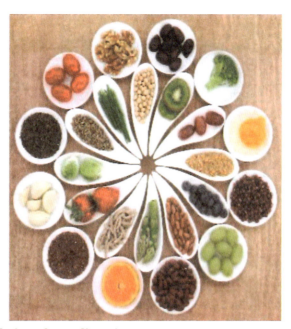

3.1 The Foundation of a Healing Diet

The foundation of a healing diet is rooted in the consumption of whole, nutrient-dense foods grown in mineral-rich soils. Barbara O'Neill emphasizes that the quality of the food we consume plays a critical role in maintaining the body's nutritional integrity and supporting its ability to heal. A focus on fresh, plant-based foods that are minimally processed ensures that the body receives the essential nutrients it needs to function optimally and repair itself.

Food quality begins with the soil in which it is grown. Mineral-rich soils are essential for producing plants that are high in vital nutrients such as vitamins, minerals, and antioxidants. These nutrients are not only necessary for overall health but are particularly important in aiding the body's natural healing processes. When plants are grown in depleted soils that lack adequate minerals, the food produced contains significantly fewer nutrients, which can compromise the body's ability to maintain health and recover from illness.

Soil health is critical because it affects the entire ecosystem of food production. Plants grown in healthy soils have stronger root systems and are more resilient to pests and diseases, reducing the need for chemical fertilizers and pesticides. The result is cleaner, more nutrient-dense produce that supports the body's detoxification and healing processes. Barbara O'Neill emphasizes that when we consume food grown in nutrient-rich soils, we are giving our bodies the best possible foundation for healing.

3.2 Whole-Food Nutrition and Disease Prevention

The link between a nutrient-dense, whole-food diet and the prevention of chronic diseases such as cancer, heart disease, and diabetes is well established. Whole foods, particularly those that are plant-based, provide essential vitamins, minerals, and antioxidants that help protect the body from the damaging effects of oxidative stress and inflammation, two primary contributors to chronic disease development.

Whole-Food Nutrition for Disease Prevention

A whole-food diet focuses on consuming foods in their most natural state, unprocessed and free from artificial additives. This includes fruits, vegetables, legumes, whole grains, nuts, and seeds, which are rich in nutrients that the body needs for optimal function. Diets high in processed foods, sugars, and unhealthy fats contribute to inflammation and oxidative damage, which can lead to the development of diseases such as cancer, cardiovascular issues, and metabolic disorders like diabetes.

One of the key benefits of a whole-food diet is its ability to reduce inflammation, which is a common denominator in many chronic diseases. Whole plant foods are rich in fiber, which helps maintain healthy digestion, regulate blood sugar levels, and support heart health. Furthermore, these foods are packed with antioxidants, which neutralize free radicals that damage cells and contribute to the onset of diseases such as cancer. By protecting cells from this damage, a whole-food diet helps maintain cellular integrity and reduce the risk of mutations that can lead to cancerous growths.

Plant-Based Diet and Immune Function

A plant-based diet, in particular, offers significant advantages in supporting the immune system. By supplying the body with a broad spectrum of phytonutrients, vitamins, and minerals, such a diet ensures that the immune system has the resources it needs to function optimally. Immune function relies heavily on the intake of certain vitamins, such as vitamin C, which is abundant in fruits and vegetables. This vitamin enhances the production of white blood cells, which are the body's primary defense against infections and abnormal cells.

Whole, plant-based foods also provide essential fatty acids, such as omega-3s, which are known to reduce inflammation and improve heart health. These healthy fats are found in foods like flaxseeds, chia seeds, and walnuts. Additionally, plant-based diets are low in saturated fats and cholesterol, further protecting cardiovascular health and reducing the risk of heart disease, one of the leading causes of death worldwide.

Supporting Cell Repair and Longevity

Whole, plant-based foods play a critical role in promoting cell repair and longevity. Foods rich in antioxidants, such as leafy greens, berries, and cruciferous vegetables, help the body repair damaged cells and support the regeneration of healthy tissue. The fiber found in whole foods also aids in the elimination of toxins from the body, reducing the burden on the liver and other detoxification organs.

Barbara O'Neill emphasizes that a diet rich in whole, plant-based foods can significantly enhance the body's ability to heal and regenerate at the cellular level. This not only helps prevent the onset of chronic diseases but also promotes long-term vitality. By focusing on foods that nourish the body and provide the building blocks for cellular repair, individuals can improve their overall health, strengthen their immune system, and reduce the risk of developing serious diseases over time.

Incorporating a variety of colorful fruits and vegetables, whole grains, and plant-based proteins into daily meals ensures that the body receives a wide range of nutrients necessary for maintaining health and preventing disease

Chapter 4: Nutrient-Dense Foods for Optimal Body Function

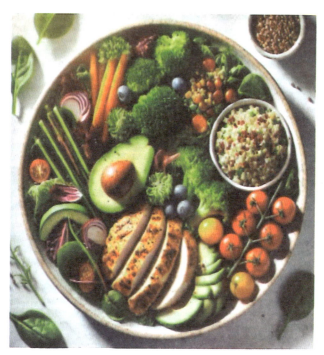

2.1 Protein: The Building Block of Healing

Protein plays a pivotal role in the body's ability to repair, regulate, and maintain essential functions. It is a fundamental component in processes such as DNA repair, enzyme production, and energy regulation. Without sufficient protein, the body would struggle to regenerate cells, manage energy efficiently, and sustain overall health.

Protein and DNA Repair

Proteins are involved in nearly every cellular process, including the repair of DNA. DNA damage occurs regularly due to exposure to environmental factors like toxins, UV light, or even as a result of normal metabolic activity. To protect the body from the harmful effects of damaged DNA, specific proteins act as repair agents, ensuring the integrity of genetic material. These repair proteins work continuously to correct mutations and prevent diseases that can arise from genetic errors, such as cancer or immune dysfunction.

The body's ability to heal wounds, restore damaged tissues, and fight off infections is largely dependent on the presence of these protein-based repair systems. Without the necessary building blocks provided by protein, the efficiency of DNA repair mechanisms is compromised.

Enzyme Production and Energy Regulation

Proteins are also the building blocks of enzymes, which are critical for almost every biochemical reaction in the body. Enzymes facilitate the digestion and absorption of nutrients, enabling the body to utilize vitamins, minerals, and other compounds necessary for health. They also regulate energy production by breaking down carbohydrates, fats, and proteins, converting them into usable energy.

When the body lacks sufficient protein, enzyme production can become impaired, leading to issues such as poor digestion, fatigue, and sluggish metabolism. Energy regulation relies heavily on a steady supply of enzymes, and thus, adequate protein intake ensures that energy levels remain stable, supporting overall vitality and endurance.

Vegetarian Sources of Protein

For individuals following a plant-based diet, there are numerous sources of high-quality protein. Barbara O'Neill highlights the importance of seeds, grains, legumes, nuts, and edible seeds as excellent sources of vegetarian protein. These plant-based foods provide all the essential amino acids required for the body's various functions, making them complete sources of protein.

Seeds such as chia, flax, and pumpkin seeds are rich in protein and essential fatty acids. They are easily incorporated into a variety of meals, offering a nutrient-dense option for maintaining adequate protein levels.

Grains like quinoa and amaranth are unique in the plant world because they contain all nine essential amino acids. These grains are not only high in protein but also rich in fiber, supporting both digestive health and sustained energy.

Legumes, including lentils, chickpeas, and black beans, are staples in plant-based diets. They are high in protein, fiber, and a range of micronutrients that support overall health. Legumes are particularly effective in promoting muscle repair and recovery, making them ideal for active individuals or those recovering from injury.

Nuts, such as almonds, walnuts, and cashews, provide healthy fats along with protein, making them a powerful combination for energy and brain health. They are also easy to snack on or add to meals, ensuring that protein needs are met throughout the day.

4.2 Fats for Cellular Health

Fats play an essential role in the overall health and functioning of the human body. One of the key reasons fats are so important is that they make up a substantial portion of every cell membrane, with approximately 50% of the cell membrane structure composed of fat. This fat is crucial for maintaining the integrity and flexibility of cells, allowing them to communicate and function properly.

The Role of Unsaturated Fats

Unsaturated fats, particularly those found in nuts, seeds, and oils, are vital for several bodily functions. These fats are essential for hormone production, brain function, and joint lubrication. Hormones, which regulate numerous processes in the body, rely on fats as key building blocks. For instance, certain hormones, such as estrogen and testosterone, are synthesized from cholesterol, a type of fat. Without an adequate intake of healthy fats, the body may struggle to produce the necessary hormones, leading to imbalances that affect overall health.

In terms of brain function, the brain itself is composed of approximately 60% fat, which makes healthy fat consumption critical for cognitive processes. Omega-3 fatty acids, found in flaxseeds, chia seeds, and fish oils, are particularly beneficial for maintaining brain health and improving cognitive function. These fats help protect neurons, facilitate communication between brain cells, and reduce inflammation, which is linked to neurodegenerative diseases.

Additionally, unsaturated fats contribute to joint lubrication, ensuring smooth movement and reducing friction between bones. Omega-3 and omega-6 fatty acids help maintain the integrity of joint tissue, which can alleviate discomfort and improve mobility, especially in individuals suffering from arthritis or other joint-related conditions.

Misconceptions About Fat and the Impact of Fat Avoidance

There has long been a misconception that consuming fat leads to weight gain and various health problems, prompting many people to adopt low-fat diets. However, this approach can have unintended consequences. When people reduce their fat intake, they often replace it with carbohydrates, particularly refined sugars and processed foods. This shift can lead to a spike in blood sugar levels, followed by insulin resistance and weight gain, especially around the abdominal area.

Barbara O'Neill explains that fats are not the enemy; rather, they are a crucial macronutrient that supports many essential bodily functions. By avoiding fats, individuals may experience cravings for quick energy sources, which often results in the overconsumption of carbohydrates. These refined carbohydrates can lead to rapid spikes and crashes in energy levels, increased fat storage, and higher risks of developing metabolic disorders like type 2 diabetes.

Moreover, fat-free or low-fat processed foods are frequently laden with sugar or artificial additives to compensate for the loss of flavor and texture that fats provide. This can further contribute to health problems such as inflammation, digestive issues, and poor nutrient absorption.

To maintain optimal cellular health, it is important to include healthy unsaturated fats from natural sources in the diet. Incorporating a balance of fats from nuts, seeds, olive oil, and avocados provides the body with the necessary components to support cellular structure, hormone production, and overall well-being.

4.3 Carbohydrates: A Balanced Approach

Carbohydrates are an essential component of the diet, but they must be consumed with care to maintain health and prevent disease. A mindful approach to carbohydrates involves distinguishing between refined sugars and processed grains, which can harm the body, and complex carbohydrates, which provide the necessary energy for daily functions.

The Impact of Refined Carbohydrates

Refined carbohydrates, including processed sugars and grains, are found in many modern diets. These include white bread, pastries, sugary snacks, and sodas. Refined carbs are rapidly broken down into glucose, leading to sharp spikes in blood sugar levels. While these foods provide quick energy, they lack the nutritional value found in whole grains and other complex carbohydrates. Over time, consuming large amounts of refined carbs can disrupt the body's metabolic balance and contribute to weight gain.

Refined carbohydrates feed harmful pathogens in the body, which can increase the risk of infections and contribute to inflammation. The excessive intake of sugar promotes the growth of yeast and harmful bacteria in the gut, which can disturb the balance of the microbiome. This disruption weakens the immune system and makes the body more susceptible to chronic conditions.

Barbara O'Neill highlights the link between a high intake of refined carbohydrates and the development of diseases such as diabetes. When the body is constantly exposed to refined sugars, the pancreas is forced to produce more insulin to manage the rapid influx of glucose. Over time, this can lead to insulin resistance, where cells no longer respond properly to insulin, resulting in chronically high blood sugar levels. This condition is a precursor to type 2 diabetes, a disease that affects millions worldwide. Additionally, the excess glucose in the bloodstream is often stored as fat, leading to weight gain, particularly around the abdominal area.

The Benefits of Complex Carbohydrates

In contrast to refined sugars, complex carbohydrates are digested more slowly, providing a steady source of energy without causing significant fluctuations in blood sugar levels. Foods such as whole grains, legumes, vegetables, and fruits are rich in fiber, which not only supports digestion but also helps regulate blood sugar by slowing the absorption of glucose.

Complex carbohydrates also promote a healthy gut environment by supporting beneficial bacteria in the digestive tract. Fiber from these foods acts as a prebiotic, nourishing the good bacteria that play a crucial role in immune function, digestion, and even mental health. A balanced diet rich in complex carbs can reduce inflammation and protect against conditions such as obesity and heart disease.

Maintaining a balanced approach to carbohydrates involves prioritizing whole, unprocessed foods over refined options. By focusing on nutrient-dense complex carbohydrates, individuals can maintain stable energy levels, support metabolic health, and reduce the risk of developing chronic diseases such as diabetes. This mindful consumption of carbohydrates is key to overall health and well-being.

Chapter 5: Detoxifying the Body with a Clean Diet – Avoiding Processed Foods and Sugar

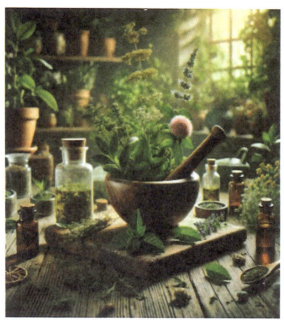

5.1 The Harmful Effects of Sugar and Processed Foods

Excessive consumption of sugar and processed foods has detrimental effects on overall health. One of the most significant risks associated with sugar is its role in feeding harmful microorganisms in the body, including fungi, yeasts, and even cancer cells. Eliminating sugar from the diet is crucial for reducing inflammation and preventing chronic diseases, as sugar fuels these microorganisms and creates an environment in which they can thrive.

Sugar and Harmful Microorganisms

Sugar is known to feed harmful microorganisms such as Candida, a type of yeast that naturally occurs in the body but can grow out of control when sugar is abundant in the diet. This overgrowth leads to infections, digestive issues, and can severely weaken the immune system. Additionally, sugar promotes the growth of fungi and other harmful organisms, further exacerbating health problems related to immune function and chronic inflammation.

Cancer cells, too, are known to feed on sugar. Elevated blood glucose levels provide a direct source of energy for cancer cells, allowing them to grow and multiply more rapidly. By eliminating sugar from the diet, the body becomes less hospitable to these harmful cells, reducing the risk of cancer progression. Reducing sugar intake also lowers insulin levels, which is beneficial for preventing conditions such as insulin resistance and type 2 diabetes.

Barbara O'Neill highlights the importance of addressing sugar consumption to combat the overgrowth of harmful microorganisms in the body. Inflammatory processes are often triggered by the presence of these organisms, and chronic inflammation is a well-known precursor to many diseases, including cancer, heart disease, and autoimmune disorders.

Processed Foods and Nutrient Deficiencies

Processed foods are another significant contributor to poor health. These foods are stripped of essential nutrients during production, leaving behind "empty calories" that provide little to no nutritional value. Regular consumption of processed foods can lead to nutrient deficiencies, as the body fails to receive the vitamins, minerals, and antioxidants needed to maintain optimal health.

In addition to being devoid of nutrients, processed foods often contain harmful additives, preservatives, and artificial ingredients that can build up in the body over time. This toxic build-up places a burden on the liver, which is responsible for detoxifying the body. When the liver becomes overburdened with toxins from processed foods, its ability to function efficiently is compromised, leading to further health problems.

Moreover, processed foods tend to be high in refined carbohydrates and unhealthy fats, both of which contribute to inflammation in the body. This chronic, low-grade inflammation is a major factor in the development of many diseases, including cardiovascular disease, diabetes, and obesity. Over time, the continued intake of processed foods weakens the body's natural defenses and creates an environment conducive to the development of chronic conditions.

Reducing Inflammation and Preventing Disease

By eliminating sugar and processed foods from the diet, it is possible to reduce inflammation and lower the risk of chronic diseases. Replacing these harmful substances with whole, nutrient-dense foods supports the body's natural healing processes and promotes long-term health. A diet rich in vegetables, fruits, whole grains, and healthy fats provides the essential nutrients needed to combat inflammation and protect against disease.

5.2 Natural Detoxifying Foods

Certain foods are well-known for their natural detoxifying properties, playing a critical role in helping the body eliminate toxins and maintain overall health. Leafy greens, garlic, onions, and fibrous vegetables are particularly effective in supporting the body's detoxification processes, especially the liver, which is the primary organ responsible for filtering toxins from the bloodstream.

Leafy Greens: Nature's Detoxifiers

Leafy green vegetables such as spinach, kale, and collard greens are essential for promoting detoxification in the body. These vegetables are rich in chlorophyll, a green pigment that helps detoxify the tissues by binding to toxins and heavy metals and aiding their elimination from the body. Chlorophyll also supports oxygenation of the blood, which is important for maintaining healthy cellular function.

Green vegetables also play a significant role in maintaining an alkaline environment in the body. An alkaline diet helps to neutralize excess acidity, which can be caused by poor dietary habits, stress, and exposure to environmental toxins. By incorporating more leafy greens into the diet, the body's pH balance can be improved, reducing inflammation and enhancing the detoxification process. Furthermore, these greens are loaded with essential vitamins and minerals, including vitamins A, C, and K, all of which support liver health and overall detoxification.

Garlic: A Powerful Detox Agent

Garlic is renowned for its detoxifying properties, particularly its ability to support liver function. It contains sulfur compounds, which activate enzymes in the liver responsible for flushing out toxins. Garlic also contains a compound called allicin, which has strong antioxidant and anti-inflammatory properties. These properties help protect the liver from oxidative stress, which can occur when the liver is overburdened by toxins.

Garlic also promotes the production of glutathione, one of the body's most important antioxidants, which aids in detoxification. By enhancing the liver's natural detoxifying capacity, garlic helps the body eliminate harmful substances more effectively. Additionally, garlic's antimicrobial properties contribute to maintaining a healthy gut, which is crucial for proper detoxification since the gut plays a major role in the elimination of waste products.

Onions: Supporting Liver Health

Onions, like garlic, are part of the allium family and share many of its detoxifying benefits. They are rich in sulfur-containing compounds that aid in liver detoxification by promoting the activity of detoxifying enzymes.

Onions also contain quercetin, a powerful antioxidant that helps reduce inflammation and supports the immune system.

Incorporating onions into the diet can help protect the liver from damage and enhance its ability to process and eliminate toxins. Onions are also rich in prebiotics, which support gut health by feeding beneficial bacteria. A healthy gut is essential for effective detoxification, as it helps to ensure that waste is properly eliminated from the body.

Fibrous Vegetables: Promoting Gut Health and Detoxification

Fibrous vegetables such as broccoli, Brussels sprouts, and carrots are also highly effective in promoting detoxification. These vegetables are rich in both soluble and insoluble fiber, which aid in the removal of toxins by supporting healthy digestion and regular bowel movements. Fiber binds to toxins in the digestive tract and helps to transport them out of the body, preventing them from being reabsorbed.

Broccoli and Brussels sprouts, in particular, are known for their high levels of sulforaphane, a compound that supports the liver's detoxification pathways and enhances the elimination of harmful substances. These cruciferous vegetables also contain compounds that help neutralize toxins, making them easier for the body to excrete.

Incorporating these fibrous vegetables into the diet not only supports detoxification but also promotes overall digestive health. A healthy digestive system is key to maintaining a toxin-free body, as it ensures that waste products are efficiently eliminated.

Chapter 6: Meal Planning and Dietary Choices for Enhanced Vitality and Healing

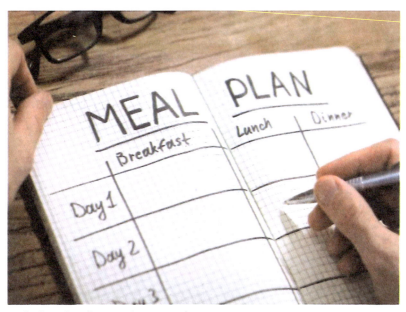

6.1 Meal Planning for Nutrient Density

Effective meal planning is essential for ensuring that each meal provides the body with the nutrients necessary for optimal health, healing, and longevity. By focusing on a balance of proteins, healthy fats, and fibrous vegetables, meals can be designed to support the body's natural healing processes and promote sustained energy throughout the day. Barbara O'Neill's dietary principles emphasize nutrient density and a holistic approach to meal preparation, which ensures that each meal serves as a tool for enhancing vitality.

Combining Proteins, Healthy Fats, and Fibrous Vegetables

One of the key aspects of nutrient-dense meal planning is the combination of proteins, healthy fats, and fiber-rich vegetables in every meal. Proteins are crucial for cell repair, muscle growth, and immune function. They should be derived from high-quality sources such as legumes, nuts, seeds, and plant-based proteins, as well as clean, organic animal proteins where appropriate. These protein sources provide the building blocks needed for healing and regeneration.

Healthy fats are another important component, as they support brain health, hormone balance, and the absorption of fat-soluble vitamins (A, D, E, and K). Fats from sources like avocados, nuts, seeds, olive oil, and coconut oil should be included in every meal. These fats not only provide long-lasting energy but also support the body's anti-inflammatory pathways, which are essential for preventing chronic disease.

Fibrous vegetables, such as leafy greens, cruciferous vegetables, and root vegetables, are essential for providing vitamins, minerals, and dietary fiber. Fiber supports digestion, helps regulate blood sugar levels, and promotes the elimination of toxins. Additionally, fibrous vegetables are low in calories but rich in micronutrients, making them a perfect addition to every meal to ensure nutrient density without excess calories.

Practical Tips for Meal Planning

To create nutrient-dense meals on a regular basis, it's essential to plan meals ahead of time. Barbara O'Neill advocates for meal planning as a way to stay consistent with healthy eating habits and ensure that meals are both satisfying and nourishing. A few practical tips for meal planning include:

Prepare in Batches: Cooking in larger quantities allows for easy access to nutrient-dense meals throughout the week. Preparing staples like roasted vegetables, cooked grains, or lean proteins in advance ensures that quick, balanced meals are always available.

Focus on Variety: Incorporate a wide range of vegetables, proteins, and fats in the meal plan to ensure diverse nutrient intake. Eating a rainbow of vegetables not only provides different vitamins and minerals but also keeps meals interesting and flavorful.

Balance Macronutrients: Each meal should have a balance of protein, healthy fats, and fiber-rich vegetables. For example, a salad with mixed greens, avocado, grilled chicken, and a sprinkle of nuts provides a perfect balance of nutrients to keep energy levels steady and promote healing.

Incorporate Superfoods: Foods like chia seeds, flaxseeds, and seaweed are excellent sources of nutrients and can be easily added to salads, smoothies, or oatmeal to boost the nutritional profile of meals.

6.2 The Role of Meal Timing in Digestion and Health

Meal timing plays a critical role in optimizing digestion, reducing toxic load, and improving overall energy levels. By allowing the digestive system adequate rest between meals, the body can perform essential functions like detoxification and cellular repair, which are key to maintaining good health.

Resting the Digestive System

The process of digestion requires significant energy and resources from the body. When meals are eaten too frequently, the digestive system is forced to work continuously, leaving little time for essential functions such as repair and detoxification. Barbara O'Neill explains that allowing the digestive system proper rest between meals, typically a gap of 4 to 5 hours, can significantly improve digestive efficiency. This period of rest gives the stomach and intestines time to fully process and absorb nutrients before being tasked with another meal.

When the body is given this rest, it can more effectively detoxify itself by clearing out residual waste and toxins from the digestive tract. This prevents the buildup of toxic substances that could otherwise lead to inflammation, bloating, and digestive discomfort. Furthermore, this rest period allows the digestive organs to recover, ensuring that they function optimally with the next meal.

Meal Timing and Energy Levels

Spacing meals properly and incorporating periods of fasting can significantly improve energy levels throughout the day. When meals are consumed too frequently, the body is continuously expending energy on digestion. By allowing time between meals, energy can be redirected toward other vital processes, such as physical activity and mental focus.

Moreover, intermittent fasting can improve energy efficiency by encouraging the body to use stored fat for fuel rather than constantly relying on glucose from frequent meals. This metabolic shift promotes sustained energy and prevents the energy crashes often associated with irregular or excessive eating patterns.

6.3 Incorporating Superfoods for Maximum Health

Certain superfoods play a crucial role in promoting optimal health due to their nutrient density and powerful health benefits. Among the superfoods that Barbara O'Neill recommends are stinging nettle, aloe vera, flaxseed, and chlorophyll-rich plants like wheatgrass and spirulina. These foods can easily be incorporated into daily meals through smoothies, salads, and juices, providing sustained energy and enhancing overall body function.

Stinging Nettle

Stinging nettle is a nutrient-rich plant known for its detoxifying and anti-inflammatory properties. It contains high levels of vitamins A, C, and K, as well as minerals like iron and magnesium, which support the immune system and overall vitality. Nettle is particularly useful for reducing inflammation and supporting kidney function by promoting detoxification through the urinary tract.

Stinging nettle can be easily integrated into the diet by adding it to smoothies or as an herbal tea. The leaves can also be used in soups or salads, providing a mild, earthy flavor that complements a variety of dishes. By incorporating stinging nettle into daily meals, individuals can benefit from its ability to cleanse the body and support healthy circulation.

Aloe Vera

Aloe vera is widely recognized for its soothing and healing properties, particularly for digestive health. It contains compounds that aid in reducing inflammation and promoting tissue repair, making it a valuable superfood for gut health. Aloe vera also contains antioxidants, enzymes, and essential vitamins that support skin health and immune function.

To incorporate aloe vera into meals, it can be added to smoothies or juices for a refreshing, hydrating boost. The gel extracted from the aloe vera plant has a subtle taste, making it an easy addition to beverages without overpowering other flavors. Regular consumption of aloe vera helps support digestive health by soothing the lining of the gut, making it beneficial for individuals with digestive issues.

Flaxseed

Flaxseed is a highly nutritious superfood rich in omega-3 fatty acids, fiber, and lignans, which are powerful antioxidants. These nutrients contribute to cardiovascular health, improved digestion, and hormone balance. The high fiber content in flaxseeds supports digestive health by promoting regular bowel movements, while the omega-3s are essential for reducing inflammation and supporting brain health.

Flaxseed can be incorporated into daily meals by adding it to smoothies, oatmeal, or baked goods. Ground flaxseed is particularly easy to mix into various dishes and provides a nutty flavor that enhances both sweet and savory recipes. By adding flaxseed to the diet, individuals can support heart health, improve digestion, and promote balanced hormone levels.

Wheatgrass and Spirulina

Wheatgrass and spirulina are chlorophyll-rich plants that are packed with nutrients essential for detoxification and energy production. Wheatgrass is rich in vitamins A, C, and E, as well as minerals like calcium and iron. Spirulina, a type of blue-green algae, is known for its high protein content and abundance of antioxidants, which protect the body from oxidative stress and support immune function.

These superfoods are often consumed in powdered or liquid form, making them ideal for adding to smoothies and juices. Wheatgrass can also be juiced on its own for a concentrated shot of nutrients, while spirulina can be mixed into water or smoothies for a powerful nutrient boost. Both wheatgrass and spirulina enhance detoxification processes and provide the body with sustained energy, making them valuable additions to a daily health routine.

Part 2:
The Role of
Microorganisms in
Health

Chapter 1: Understanding Microorganisms in the Human Body

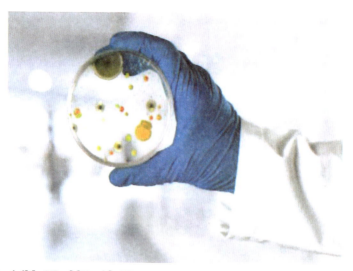

1.1 The Invisible World Inside Us

The human body is host to trillions of microorganisms, a vital component of our biology, which outnumber human cells. This "invisible world" of bacteria, viruses, fungi, and other microbes plays an essential role in maintaining overall health and wellness. These microorganisms inhabit various parts of the body, but the GI tract houses the largest concentration. Their presence in the gut has profound effects on digestion, immunity, and even mental health.

The Role of Microorganisms in the Gut

The gastrointestinal (GI) tract is home to a diverse ecosystem of microorganisms, commonly referred to as the gut microbiome. This collection of microbes works symbiotically with the human body to aid in the digestion of food, absorption of nutrients, and the protection against harmful pathogens. The gut microbiome plays a crucial role in nutrient absorption, particularly in breaking down complex carbohydrates, fiber, and other difficult-to-digest compounds that human enzymes cannot process on their own.

One of the most critical functions of gut microorganisms is the production and absorption of B vitamins. These vitamins, including B12, B6, and folate, are vital for energy production, brain function, and the maintenance of healthy red blood cells. Without the gut microbiota's assistance in synthesizing and absorbing these nutrients, the body would struggle to maintain optimal health. This highlights the importance of maintaining a balanced and healthy gut microbiome, as disruptions can lead to deficiencies in essential vitamins and minerals.

Nutrient Absorption and Microbial Balance

Maintaining the balance between beneficial and harmful microorganisms is key to ensuring proper nutrient absorption. When the gut microbiome is healthy, beneficial bacteria thrive and outcompete harmful pathogens, helping to optimize digestive processes. However, imbalances in this delicate ecosystem, often referred to as dysbiosis, can disrupt digestion and nutrient absorption. Dysbiosis can result from factors such as poor diet, antibiotic use, stress, and lack of sleep, all of which can lead to the overgrowth of harmful bacteria or yeast.

When dysbiosis occurs, the body's ability to absorb essential nutrients, including B vitamins, becomes compromised. This can lead to deficiencies that manifest in symptoms such as fatigue, weakened immunity, and cognitive difficulties. Additionally, an unhealthy gut can contribute to the development of chronic conditions such as irritable bowel syndrome (IBS), inflammatory bowel disease (IBD), and metabolic disorders.

A balanced microbiome supports the immune system, as the majority of the body's immune cells are located in the gut. It also plays a role in mental health through the gut-brain axis, the communication network that links the gut and the brain, influencing mood and cognitive function.

Supporting a Healthy Microbiome

To promote a healthy and diverse gut microbiome, it is essential to adopt lifestyle practices that nurture beneficial microorganisms. A diet rich in fiber, particularly from fruits, vegetables, and whole grains, is fundamental. Fiber serves as a prebiotic, feeding the beneficial bacteria and helping them flourish. Fermented foods such as sauerkraut, kimchi, and yogurt are also beneficial, as they contain probiotics—live beneficial bacteria that can help repopulate the gut microbiome.

Barbara O'Neill underscores the importance of the gut microbiome in nutrient absorption, particularly for essential vitamins like B vitamins. She emphasizes that maintaining a healthy gut is not only critical for digestion but also for overall health, including immunity and mental well-being. By focusing on nurturing the microorganisms within, individuals can improve their nutrient absorption, prevent deficiencies, and support their overall health.

1.2 Microorganisms as Nutrient Processors

The human gut is home to trillions of microorganisms that play a crucial role in breaking down complex nutrients and transforming them into forms that the body can easily absorb. These microorganisms, particularly beneficial bacteria such as **Lactobacillus acidophilus** and **Bifidobacterium bifidum**, are essential for maintaining both a healthy digestive system and a robust immune defense.

Lactobacillus Acidophilus: The Digestive Supporter

Lactobacillus acidophilus is one of the most well-known and researched strains of beneficial bacteria, often found in the human intestines and fermented foods like yogurt. This microorganism plays a critical role in breaking down lactose, the sugar found in milk, into lactic acid. This process not only aids individuals who are lactose intolerant but also helps maintain a balanced gut environment by lowering the pH, which discourages the growth of harmful bacteria.

Lactobacillus acidophilus also contributes to the breakdown of complex carbohydrates and fibers, which are otherwise difficult for the body to digest. By breaking down these substances into simpler sugars and fatty acids, it supports the body's ability to absorb essential nutrients. This bacterium also helps in the synthesis of vitamins, such as vitamin K and certain B vitamins, which are vital for energy production and overall well-being.

Moreover, the presence of Lactobacillus acidophilus in the gut enhances the production of short-chain fatty acids, such as butyrate, which are beneficial for colon health. Butyrate serves as an energy source for colon cells, promoting a healthy gut lining and preventing conditions such as leaky gut syndrome, where harmful substances can pass through the gut wall into the bloodstream.

Bifidobacterium Bifidum: The Immune Enhancer

Bifidobacterium bifidum is another essential bacterium that resides in the intestines, particularly in the colon. It is instrumental in digesting dietary fibers, breaking them down into simpler compounds that the body can absorb. This process is crucial for maximizing nutrient absorption, as fibers, when broken down properly, provide vital fuel for the body.

This bacterium also plays a significant role in maintaining immune system health. Bifidobacterium bifidum helps to strengthen the gut barrier, which is the body's first line of defense against harmful pathogens. It lowers the risk of infections and inflammation by keeping the stomach lining robust and preventing toxic substances and harmful bacteria from entering the circulation.

In addition, Bifidobacterium bifidum has been found to enhance the body's immune responses by stimulating the production of certain antibodies, which are critical for recognizing and neutralizing pathogens. This bacterium also supports the immune system by reducing inflammation within the gut, creating a balanced environment where beneficial microorganisms can thrive, and harmful bacteria are kept in check.

1.3 The Double Role of Microorganisms: Helpers and Harmers

Microorganisms play a critical role in maintaining health, with some functioning as helpful organisms that support various bodily processes, while others can become harmful when the natural balance is disrupted. The delicate balance between saprophytes and parasites within the body is essential for maintaining health, as it prevents the overgrowth of harmful pathogens such as fungi and bacteria that can cause infections and other health issues.

Saprophytes: The Helpers

Saprophytes are microorganisms that feed on dead or decaying organic matter. They are vital in breaking down dead cells and waste material, facilitating decomposition and recycling nutrients back into the environment. In the human body, saprophytes exist primarily within the gut and on the skin, where they assist in keeping the internal environment clean and functioning smoothly. Their presence prevents the accumulation of dead organic material that could otherwise provide a breeding ground for harmful microorganisms.

The role of saprophytes extends to supporting the immune system. By keeping the body's internal and external environments clean, saprophytes help reduce the likelihood of infections caused by pathogenic organisms. They play a crucial role in maintaining the microbial balance within the gut, which is key to supporting digestion and nutrient absorption. A healthy population of saprophytes ensures that the gut flora remains in balance, allowing the body to better defend itself against external threats.

However, when this balance is disrupted, saprophytes may not function effectively, leaving space for harmful organisms to proliferate. This imbalance can occur due to various factors such as poor diet, excessive use of antibiotics, or chronic stress, all of which can weaken the immune system and the natural microbial defense mechanisms.

Parasites and Pathogens: The Harmers

Parasites, unlike saprophytes, feed on living tissues, often causing harm to their hosts. While the body naturally harbors certain parasites without negative effects, an overgrowth or infection of pathogenic parasites can lead to significant health issues. Pathogenic bacteria and fungi are the primary culprits in this category, with some of the most common infections being athlete's foot, ringworm, and internal fungal infections.

When the balance between saprophytes and parasites is disrupted, pathogens can begin to overgrow. For instance, in the case of athlete's foot, the fungus that causes the infection is naturally present on the skin. However, under conditions of moisture, warmth, and poor hygiene, this fungus can multiply uncontrollably, leading to infection. Similarly, ringworm is caused by a fungus that thrives on the surface of the skin, particularly in areas that remain damp or are frequently exposed to contaminated surfaces.

In addition to external infections, internal fungal infections can also arise when the natural microbial balance is disturbed. Candida, a type of yeast that normally exists in small amounts within the digestive tract, can become pathogenic under certain conditions. When the balance of gut flora is compromised, such as after antibiotic use, Candida can overgrow, leading to fungal infections that affect not only the digestive system but also other parts of the body.

Disruption of Balance and Health Implications

The body's ability to maintain a balance between helpful microorganisms and harmful pathogens is crucial to overall health. When this balance is disturbed, infections and diseases can arise, potentially leading to more severe health issues. Barbara O'Neill highlights the importance of maintaining this equilibrium through proper nutrition, lifestyle choices, and hygiene practices. A healthy diet rich in nutrients supports the immune system, making it more capable of controlling pathogenic organisms.

When the immune system is weakened, or when the environment allows harmful microorganisms to flourish, the risk of infection increases. For instance, warm, moist environments provide ideal conditions for fungi to multiply, as seen in cases of athlete's foot and ringworm. Similarly, an overgrowth of yeast in the gut due to a disrupted microbial balance can lead to systemic fungal infections that compromise the body's ability to function optimally.

Maintaining this balance involves supporting the body's natural defenses, particularly the skin and the gut, which are the first lines of defense against pathogenic organisms. Proper hygiene, the use of antifungal remedies when necessary, and a diet that promotes a healthy gut flora can all help prevent the overgrowth of harmful fungi and bacteria.

Chapter 2: The Balance Between Good and Bad Microbes

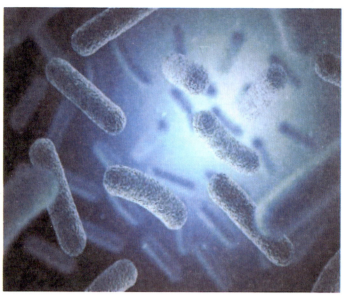

2.1 The Importance of Balance

The human body thrives on a delicate balance of microorganisms that play an essential role in maintaining health and protecting against harmful pathogens. Beneficial microorganisms, including bacteria, yeast, and fungi, work synergistically to create a healthy internal environment. When this balance is maintained, it supports proper digestion, nutrient assimilation, and protection against harmful microbes. However, when this balance is disrupted, it can lead to a variety of health issues, including infections and digestive problems.

Beneficial Microorganisms and Pathogen Protection

Beneficial microorganisms serve as the body's first line of defense against harmful pathogens. By colonizing the skin, mucous membranes, and the gut, they create a protective barrier that prevents harmful microbes from taking hold. These microorganisms compete with pathogens for resources and space, effectively crowding out harmful bacteria, viruses, and fungi. This competition limits the growth of harmful organisms and reduces the risk of infections.

In addition to outcompeting pathogens, beneficial microorganisms produce substances that inhibit the growth of harmful microbes. Certain strains of bacteria, for example, produce antimicrobial compounds that can directly neutralize or kill harmful organisms. These beneficial bacteria also help to modulate the immune system, enhancing its ability to recognize and respond to potential threats without overreacting and causing inflammation.

A well-balanced microbiome not only protects against external invaders but also helps regulate the body's inflammatory response. Chronic inflammation is a key contributor to many diseases, and by supporting a healthy microbiome, the body can better manage inflammation and reduce the risk of inflammatory conditions.

The Role of Bacteria in Digestion

Bacteria play a crucial role in the digestive process, aiding in the breakdown of complex carbohydrates, fibers, and proteins that the body would otherwise struggle to digest. This breakdown process is essential for the proper absorption of nutrients, as it enables the body to extract vitamins, minerals, and other beneficial compounds from food.

In particular, certain strains of bacteria in the gut produce enzymes that help break down dietary fibers into short-chain fatty acids (SCFAs), which are essential for gut health. These SCFAs not only provide energy for the cells lining the gut but also have anti-inflammatory properties that protect the gut lining from damage. A healthy gut microbiome supports regular bowel movements and prevents issues like constipation, bloating, and indigestion.

When the balance of bacteria in the gut is disrupted—whether due to poor diet, stress, or the use of antibiotics—digestion can be impaired, leading to nutrient deficiencies and digestive discomfort. Re-establishing a healthy balance of bacteria through diet and, if necessary, probiotics, can help restore proper digestion and improve overall health.

Yeast and Fungi: Their Protective and Digestive Roles

While often associated with infections, certain yeasts and fungi also play beneficial roles in maintaining health. For example, Saccharomyces boulardii, a type of beneficial yeast, helps to maintain gut integrity and protect against harmful pathogens. It works by promoting the growth of beneficial bacteria and preventing the colonization of harmful organisms, such as Candida and pathogenic strains of E. coli.

Yeast also contributes to the digestive process by helping to break down food and absorb nutrients. In a balanced microbiome, beneficial yeast helps to prevent the overgrowth of harmful fungi, such as Candida albicans, which can cause infections when allowed to proliferate unchecked. Maintaining a proper balance of yeast and bacteria is essential for preventing fungal overgrowth and promoting a healthy digestive environment.

Certain fungi, such as those belonging to the genus Aspergillus, also aid in the fermentation process, which is crucial for breaking down complex food molecules. This process not only enhances nutrient availability but also promotes the production of beneficial compounds that support gut health and immune function.

2.2 The Impact of Modern Lifestyle on Microbial Balance

The modern lifestyle, characterized by high stress, processed foods, and the overuse of antibiotics, has a profound impact on the balance of beneficial bacteria within the human microbiome. This delicate ecosystem of microbes plays a crucial role in maintaining health by supporting digestion, bolstering the immune system, and preventing the overgrowth of harmful pathogens. However, factors such as refined sugar, alcohol consumption, and environmental stressors can disrupt this balance, leading to the proliferation of harmful microbes like *Candida albicans*.

Antibiotics and Microbial Disruption

One of the most significant contributors to microbial imbalance is the overuse of antibiotics. While antibiotics are essential for treating bacterial infections, they often have the unintended consequence of wiping out both harmful and beneficial bacteria. This creates an opportunity for opportunistic pathogens, such as *Candida albicans*, to thrive. *Candida*, a type of yeast, normally exists in small amounts in the body without causing harm. However, when beneficial bacteria are reduced, *Candida* can grow unchecked, leading to issues such as yeast infections, digestive problems, and even systemic fungal infections.

Barbara O'Neill emphasizes the importance of being cautious with antibiotic use. While necessary in some cases, antibiotics should not be relied upon for every minor illness, as they can weaken the body's natural defenses by disrupting the balance of the microbiome. The beneficial bacteria in the gut play a critical role in immune function, producing short-chain fatty acids that help regulate inflammation and protect against harmful invaders. When these beneficial microbes are diminished, the immune system is compromised, making the body more susceptible to infections and chronic inflammation.

Stress and Its Effect on the Microbiome

Chronic stress is another factor that significantly impacts microbial balance. Stress triggers the release of cortisol, a hormone that, when elevated over long periods, can suppress the immune system and alter the gut environment. Extended periods of stress alter the intestinal lining's permeability, which is commonly known as "leaky gut," allowing germs and dangerous substances to enter the circulation. This increases the risk of systemic infections and inflammation, further disrupting the delicate microbial ecosystem.

Moreover, stress has been shown to reduce the diversity of beneficial bacteria in the gut. A diverse microbiome is essential for maintaining health, as different species of bacteria perform various functions, including producing vitamins, breaking down fiber, and protecting against pathogens. Reduced bacterial diversity can lead to an imbalance, making the gut more hospitable to harmful organisms like *Candida albicans*. Stress management techniques such as meditation, deep breathing, and adequate sleep are critical for maintaining a healthy microbiome and preventing the overgrowth of harmful microbes.

The Role of Refined Sugar in Microbial Imbalance

Refined sugar is another major disruptor of microbial balance. Diets high in processed foods and sugar provide fuel for harmful microbes, particularly yeast like *Candida*. Sugars, especially refined carbohydrates, feed *Candida*, allowing it to proliferate and outcompete beneficial bacteria. This imbalance can result in a range of health issues, including digestive problems, fatigue, skin rashes, and recurrent yeast infections.

A diet high in sugar also contributes to systemic inflammation, which further weakens the immune system. Inflammatory conditions such as obesity, diabetes, and heart disease have been linked to dysbiosis, an imbalance of the microbiome, caused in part by the consumption of refined sugars. Reducing sugar intake and focusing on whole, unprocessed foods that are rich in fiber can help restore balance to the microbiome, as fiber feeds beneficial bacteria and promotes their growth.

Alcohol and Fungal Overgrowth

Alcohol consumption also plays a role in disrupting microbial balance. Alcohol is not only a toxin that the liver must work hard to process, but it also disrupts the gut lining and can lead to an overgrowth of harmful bacteria and yeast. In particular, alcohol can exacerbate *Candida albicans* overgrowth by damaging the intestinal barrier and weakening the immune response.

In addition to its direct impact on the gut, alcohol contributes to dehydration, which affects the body's ability to maintain a healthy balance of microbes. Dehydration can reduce the production of mucus in the gut, which serves as a protective layer against harmful pathogens. Without this protective barrier, harmful microbes can take hold more easily, leading to infections and other health problems.

Environmental Factors and the Microbiome

Environmental factors, including exposure to chemicals, pesticides, and pollutants, further disrupt the balance of the microbiome. These toxins can damage the gut lining and kill beneficial bacteria, creating an environment where harmful microbes can flourish. Additionally, many modern-day personal care products and cleaning agents contain chemicals that, when absorbed through the skin or ingested, negatively impact microbial health.

To combat the impact of these environmental factors, Barbara O'Neill recommends reducing exposure to toxins by choosing organic foods, using natural cleaning products, and avoiding unnecessary antibiotics. Supporting the body's detoxification processes through adequate hydration, a fiber-rich diet, and the use of detoxifying herbs can help the body eliminate harmful substances and restore microbial balance.

2.3 The Domino Effect of Microbial Imbalance

Microbial balance in the body is crucial for maintaining overall health. When the balance between beneficial and harmful microorganisms is disrupted, the overgrowth of harmful microbes can lead to a cascade of health problems. This imbalance, also known as dysbiosis, can cause inflammation, digestive issues, and overwhelm the immune system, triggering a domino effect that affects various bodily systems.

The Role of the Gut in Microbial Balance

Known as the microbiome, the gut is home to a wide variety of bacteria. These microbes, including bacteria, yeast, and fungi, play essential roles in digestion, nutrient absorption, and immune regulation. When the microbiome is balanced, beneficial bacteria help to keep harmful microbes in check. Poor nutrition, stress, antibiotic use, and exposure to environmental pollutants, on the other hand, can upset this equilibrium and cause an overabundance of harmful bacteria.

When harmful microbes dominate the gut environment, they can damage the gut lining, leading to a condition known as "leaky gut." The gut lining normally acts as a barrier, preventing harmful substances from entering the bloodstream. However, when the integrity of this barrier is compromised, harmful microbes, toxins, and undigested food particles can pass through the gut lining into the bloodstream. This triggers an immune response, as the body recognizes these foreign invaders as threats and mounts an inflammatory reaction.

Inflammation and Chronic Health Issues

Inflammation is the body's natural response to injury or infection, but when it becomes chronic, it can lead to a wide range of health problems. The overgrowth of harmful microbes in the gut can cause constant low-grade inflammation, which may not only affect the digestive system but also lead to systemic inflammation throughout the body.

Chronic inflammation resulting from microbial imbalance has been linked to various health conditions, including autoimmune diseases. Autoimmune diseases occur when the immune system mistakenly attacks the body's own tissues, and microbial imbalance can play a significant role in triggering this response. When harmful microbes and toxins enter the bloodstream through a compromised gut lining, the immune system becomes hyperactive, leading to the development of autoimmune conditions such as rheumatoid arthritis, lupus, and inflammatory bowel disease.

In addition to autoimmune diseases, chronic inflammation caused by microbial imbalance has been associated with other chronic conditions, including cardiovascular disease, diabetes, and even neurodegenerative disorders. The ongoing inflammatory response can damage tissues and organs over time, leading to long-term health consequences.

Immune System Overload

The immune system is constantly working to defend the body against harmful pathogens. However, when there is an overgrowth of harmful microbes, the immune system can become overwhelmed. The constant presence of pathogenic microorganisms, combined with the passage of toxins into the bloodstream, forces the immune system to remain in a heightened state of activity.

This immune overload can lead to immune system dysfunction, where the body is no longer able to distinguish between harmful invaders and its own tissues. As a result, the immune system may start attacking healthy tissues, further contributing to autoimmune diseases and chronic inflammation. Additionally, an overloaded immune system becomes less effective at protecting the body from actual pathogens, making individuals more susceptible to infections and illnesses.

Restoring Microbial Balance

Restoring microbial balance is essential for reducing inflammation, supporting the immune system, and preventing the development of chronic health issues. One of the most effective ways to rebalance the microbiome is through dietary changes. A diet rich in fiber, fermented foods, and prebiotics can promote the growth of beneficial bacteria, while reducing the intake of processed foods and sugars can help suppress the overgrowth of harmful microbes.

Probiotic supplements, which contain live beneficial bacteria, can also help restore balance in the gut. These supplements can repopulate the gut with healthy bacteria, crowding out harmful microbes and supporting the gut's natural barrier function.

Part 3:
Nature's Garbage Collectors

—

The Role of Fungi and Bacteria in Healing

Chapter 1: How Microorganisms Act as "Clean-Up" Agents in the Body

1.1 The Essential Role of Microorganisms in Health

Microorganisms play an indispensable role in maintaining the body's health, as they contribute to a wide range of essential functions that are necessary for survival and well-being. According to Barbara O'Neill, microorganisms, including bacteria and fungi, are critical to several processes such as detoxification, nutrient absorption, and the breakdown of cellular waste. These microorganisms, particularly those residing in the gut microbiome, are responsible for keeping the body in a state of balance and supporting its natural healing mechanisms.

Microorganisms as "Nature's Garbage Collectors"

Barbara O'Neill describes microorganisms as "nature's garbage collectors" due to their ability to clean up cellular debris, toxins, and waste products that accumulate in the body over time. This role is essential for maintaining homeostasis and preventing the buildup of harmful substances that could impair health. In the gut, beneficial bacteria and fungi work together to break down indigestible compounds, neutralize toxins, and promote tissue repair. By doing so, they help to support the body's detoxification pathways and ensure that waste products are efficiently processed and eliminated.

Without these microorganisms, the body would struggle to detoxify harmful substances, which could lead to an overload of toxins and the development of various chronic diseases. Microorganisms help to protect the body from such conditions by enhancing its ability to remove potentially harmful compounds and repair damaged tissues.

Microorganisms and the Body's Symbiotic Relationship

The human body is home to trillions of microorganisms that live in symbiosis with their host, providing a variety of health benefits. In the gut, beneficial bacteria and fungi assist in breaking down complex carbohydrates, proteins, and fats, transforming them into essential nutrients that the body can absorb and utilize. These microorganisms also play a crucial role in regulating immune function, protecting the body from infections, and promoting overall resilience.

Barbara O'Neill explains that maintaining a healthy balance of these microorganisms is crucial for optimal health. When the balance of bacteria and fungi in the body is disrupted—whether due to poor diet, stress, or the overuse of antibiotics—it can lead to a range of health problems, including digestive disorders, inflammation, and impaired detoxification. A diverse and balanced microbiome, on the other hand, helps to support the body's natural defenses and improve its capacity to heal.

Fungi: A Lesser-Known Ally

While bacteria in the gut microbiome receive much attention, fungi also play a significant role in maintaining health. Fungi, such as yeasts, are an integral part of the microbiome and contribute to various processes, including fermentation and the breakdown of complex plant fibers. Certain species of fungi help to convert dietary fibers into short-chain fatty acids, which are vital for gut health and contribute to the regulation of immune function.

However, when the balance of fungi in the microbiome is disturbed, it can lead to fungal overgrowth, which can disrupt the gut environment and promote inflammation. One of the most well-known examples of this is Candida, a type of yeast that can cause infections when it grows out of control. Barbara O'Neill emphasizes the importance of managing fungal overgrowth through proper diet and lifestyle choices. By maintaining a healthy gut environment, beneficial fungi can thrive and contribute to the body's overall well-being.

1.2 The Role of Bacteria in Detoxification

The process of detoxification is critical for eliminating harmful substances from the body, and the bacteria in the gut play an essential role in this process. The gut microbiome is involved in breaking down toxins, chemicals, and other harmful compounds that enter the body through food, air, and the environment. By aiding in the detoxification process, beneficial bacteria help prevent these harmful substances from entering the bloodstream and causing systemic damage.

The Role of Short-Chain Fatty Acids in Detoxification

Short-chain fatty acids (SCFAs) are another critical component of gut health and detoxification. SCFAs are produced when beneficial bacteria ferment dietary fibers in the colon, and they play an important role in maintaining the integrity of the gut lining. A healthy gut lining is essential for preventing the entry of toxins into the bloodstream and promoting efficient waste elimination.

Barbara O'Neill emphasizes that consuming a diet rich in fiber supports the production of SCFAs, which in turn enhances the detoxification capabilities of the gut. Foods such as whole grains, fruits, vegetables, and legumes are excellent sources of fiber that promote the growth of beneficial bacteria and improve gut health. By fostering the production of SCFAs, individuals can strengthen their gut barrier and support the body's detoxification processes.

Chapter 2: The Natural Transformation of Fungi and Bacteria in Response to Cell Damage

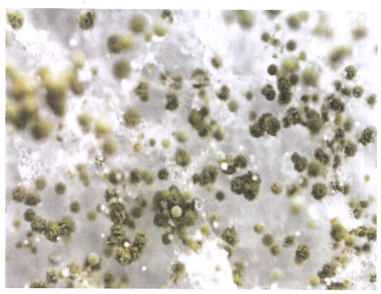

2.1 The Body's Response to Cellular Damage

When the body encounters cellular damage—whether from injury, illness, or environmental stressors—it initiates a highly organized healing process to restore function and structure. Barbara O'Neill emphasizes the role of microorganisms, such as fungi and bacteria, in this complex biological response. These microorganisms, often overlooked, play an essential part in cleaning up damaged tissue, ensuring that the area is prepared for regeneration and healing.

The healing process begins when cells are injured or die, and the body mobilizes its natural repair mechanisms. In this state, the immune system identifies the damaged cells and sends signals to recruit microorganisms like fungi and bacteria. These microorganisms act as a cleaning crew, breaking down dead cells and waste materials that the body needs to remove. This process is crucial for clearing the debris from the damaged area, which can include dead cells, toxins, and other waste byproducts that result from inflammation or infection.

Fungi, in particular, have an ability to break down more resilient structures that may be resistant to bacterial digestion alone. Fungi produce enzymes that decompose tough, fibrous materials in dead cells, helping to remove debris that could otherwise linger and contribute to chronic inflammation. By aiding in the decomposition of these tough materials, fungi assist in preventing the accumulation of waste that could block the healing process. This detoxification process also minimizes the risk of secondary infections by reducing the presence of harmful waste.

Once fungi have begun the breakdown of dead cells and other materials, bacteria step in to complete the cleaning process. These bacteria can metabolize and digest the remnants left by fungi, ensuring that the area is fully cleared and ready for the next stage of healing: tissue regeneration. This cooperative effort between fungi and bacteria ensures that the body efficiently removes harmful substances, preventing chronic inflammation and encouraging faster recovery.

Cellular Cleanup and Detoxification

This microbial action is particularly important in areas of the body where waste products can accumulate, such as in wounds or inflamed tissues. Without the presence of fungi and bacteria to clear out the debris, toxins could build up, creating an environment that fosters further disease or inflammation. The body's natural healing response relies on this cleanup process to keep tissues free from debris and harmful substances.

The removal of dead cells and toxins through the action of fungi and bacteria also reduces the burden on the immune system. When these microorganisms handle waste removal, the immune system can focus on promoting new cell growth and managing the inflammation that accompanies injury. This collaborative process leads to a smoother, more efficient healing experience, reducing the risk of complications.

Fungi's Role in Tissue Regeneration

Fungi have a unique ability to produce enzymes that break down dead or damaged cells, but they also play an indirect role in tissue regeneration. By clearing out old or damaged tissue, fungi create space for new, healthy cells to take their place. This cleansing function is especially important in chronic conditions where damaged cells may accumulate, preventing healing.

In addition to their role in clearing dead cells, fungi also interact with the immune system, helping to modulate the body's response to injury. In some cases, certain fungal species can stimulate immune cells to enhance their function, further promoting tissue repair and regeneration. This interaction underscores the importance of fungi in both cleaning up cellular damage and facilitating the body's natural healing mechanisms.

2.2 Symbiosis of Fungi and Bacteria in Healing

Barbara O'Neill highlights the symbiotic relationship between fungi and bacteria in the healing process. These microorganisms, while distinct in their functions, often work together to create an optimal environment for tissue repair and regeneration. Fungi, in particular, have the ability to break down tough materials, such as dead tissue and environmental toxins, which bacteria alone may not be able to handle.

In many instances, fungi act as the first responders, initiating the breakdown of complex organic materials. For example, when cells die and leave behind fibrous tissue or other tough substances, fungi can enzymatically break these down into simpler molecules. Once these materials have been sufficiently decomposed, bacteria step in to complete the process, further breaking down the byproducts and converting them into useful compounds. This collaboration between fungi and bacteria ensures that the damaged area is thoroughly cleaned and prepared for healing.

A prime example of this symbiosis is found in the gut, where fungi like yeast help break down complex carbohydrates that the body cannot digest on its own. Bacteria in the gut then take over, fermenting the remaining material and producing nutrients, such as short-chain fatty acids, that are essential for maintaining gut health and supporting the body's immune response. This cooperative interaction between fungi and bacteria not only aids in digestion but also enhances the body's overall ability to heal itself by promoting a healthy microbiome.

This symbiotic relationship between fungi and bacteria is crucial not only in localized tissue repair but also in maintaining the overall health of the body. By working together to remove dead cells, toxins, and other waste materials, these microorganisms help prevent chronic inflammation, promote tissue regeneration, and support the immune system's ability to respond to future damage.

Chapter 3: The Connection Between Environmental Changes and Microbial Activity

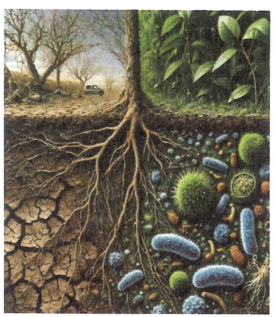

3.1 Environmental Impact on Microbial Behavior

The internal environment of the human body plays a significant role in determining the behavior of microorganisms, including beneficial bacteria and fungi. Barbara O'Neill explains that when the body maintains an optimal balance—achieved through proper diet, pH regulation, and toxin management—microbes perform essential functions, such as detoxification and cellular repair. However, when the body's environment is disrupted by factors like poor dietary choices, toxin overload, or chronic stress, the behavior of these microorganisms can shift, leading to imbalances that may contribute to illness.

The Role of pH Levels

One of the key factors influencing microbial behavior is the body's pH level. A balanced pH is crucial for the optimal functioning of beneficial bacteria and fungi. The ideal pH for most beneficial microbes in the gut is slightly acidic, which helps to keep harmful pathogens in check while allowing healthy bacteria to thrive. When the body's pH becomes too alkaline or too acidic due to poor diet, stress, or toxin exposure, the delicate balance of the microbiome can be disrupted.

For instance, an overly acidic environment may promote the overgrowth of harmful bacteria and fungi, such as Candida, which thrives in acidic conditions. This imbalance can lead to various health issues, including digestive problems, infections, and chronic inflammation. On the other hand, an environment that is too alkaline may inhibit the activity of beneficial microbes, reducing their ability to perform essential functions like breaking down food, absorbing nutrients, and eliminating toxins.

Maintaining a balanced pH through diet is essential. Consuming alkaline-forming foods, such as leafy greens, vegetables, and fruits, helps to neutralize excess acidity in the body, thereby supporting the healthy function of the microbiome. Additionally, staying hydrated and reducing the intake of highly acidic foods like processed meats, refined sugars, and alcohol further promotes a balanced pH, creating a more favorable environment for beneficial microorganisms.

Temperature and Microbial Behavior

The body's internal temperature also influences the activity of microorganisms. Beneficial bacteria and fungi thrive at normal body temperature, allowing them to efficiently perform tasks such as digestion, detoxification, and immune support. However, when the body's temperature fluctuates—due to fever, illness, or extreme environmental conditions—microbial activity can become disrupted. For example, a persistent fever may reduce the population of beneficial bacteria while allowing harmful pathogens to proliferate, leading to infections or weakened immune function.

Supporting the body's natural temperature regulation is crucial for maintaining microbial health. This can be achieved by keeping the immune system strong through a healthy diet and lifestyle. Herbs like ginger and garlic, known for their warming properties, can help regulate body temperature and support microbial health during colder months. On the other hand, cooling foods and practices, such as staying hydrated and avoiding excess heat exposure, can help maintain balance during warmer seasons.

Nutrient Availability

The availability of nutrients plays a central role in determining the behavior of microorganisms. Beneficial bacteria and fungi rely on a consistent supply of nutrients to perform their detoxifying and healing roles. Barbara O'Neill emphasizes the importance of clean, nutrient-dense eating to support microbial health. When the body is deprived of essential nutrients, the efficiency of these microbes diminishes, weakening the body's ability to detoxify and repair itself.

A diet rich in vitamins, minerals, and antioxidants helps feed beneficial microbes, allowing them to thrive. Conversely, a diet high in processed foods, refined sugars, and unhealthy fats starves these beneficial microorganisms, leading to imbalances that can contribute to the overgrowth of harmful bacteria and fungi. Ensuring that the body receives a steady supply of whole, unprocessed foods supports microbial diversity and enhances the body's natural defense mechanisms.

Toxin Overload and Microbial Disruption

Toxin overload is another factor that can disrupt the delicate balance of the microbiome. Exposure to environmental toxins, such as pesticides, heavy metals, and chemicals in processed foods, can overwhelm the body's detoxification systems, creating an unfavorable environment for beneficial microbes. When the liver, kidneys, and other detoxification organs become overburdened, harmful bacteria and fungi can take advantage of this weakened state, leading to dysbiosis and a range of health problems, including fatigue, brain fog, and chronic digestive issues.

Barbara O'Neill advises reducing toxin exposure by consuming organic produce, avoiding processed foods, and incorporating detoxifying herbs like milk thistle and dandelion into the diet. These practices help to reduce the toxic load on the body, allowing beneficial microbes to function optimally. Detoxification is an ongoing process, and by maintaining a clean internal environment, the body's microbial population remains balanced, supporting overall health and wellness.

3.2 Supporting Microbial Health Through Diet

Supporting microbial health begins with the food we consume. Barbara O'Neill advocates for a diet rich in prebiotic and probiotic foods to nourish beneficial bacteria and fungi in the gut. Prebiotics, found in fiber-rich foods such as bananas, garlic, and onions, act as food for beneficial microbes, ensuring they have the resources they need to thrive. By providing the gut with ample prebiotics, the growth and activity of healthy microorganisms are supported, enhancing their ability to detoxify the body and promote healing.

Prebiotic Foods: Fuel for Beneficial Microbes

Prebiotics are non-digestible fibers that stimulate the growth of beneficial bacteria in the gut. Foods like bananas, garlic, onions, asparagus, and leeks are rich in prebiotics and help maintain a healthy microbiome by providing nourishment for gut bacteria. These fibers pass through the digestive system intact, reaching the colon where they are fermented by beneficial microbes. This fermentation process produces short-chain fatty acids (SCFAs), which are critical for gut health, immune function, and reducing inflammation throughout the body.

Incorporating prebiotic foods into the daily diet is essential for maintaining a balanced microbiome. By regularly consuming fiber-rich foods, individuals can enhance the activity of beneficial microbes, improve digestion, and support the body's detoxification processes. Prebiotics also play a role in preventing the overgrowth of harmful bacteria and fungi, ensuring that the microbiome remains in harmony.

Probiotic Foods: Introducing Beneficial Bacteria

Probiotic foods introduce beneficial bacteria directly into the gut. Fermented foods, such as sauerkraut, kimchi, kefir, and yogurt, are excellent sources of probiotics that support microbial diversity. These foods contain live cultures that help restore and maintain a healthy balance of gut bacteria, particularly after disruptions caused by illness, antibiotic use, or poor diet.

Consuming probiotic foods regularly helps to populate the gut with beneficial microbes, which play a critical role in digestion, nutrient absorption, and immune defense. Barbara O'Neill emphasizes the importance of including fermented foods in the diet to replenish beneficial bacteria and support the body's natural detoxification and healing processes. By promoting a diverse and thriving microbiome, probiotics aid in reducing inflammation, improving digestion, and enhancing overall well-being.

Balancing Beneficial Bacteria and Fungi

The balance between beneficial bacteria and fungi in the gut is crucial for optimal health. While bacteria often receive the most attention in discussions about gut health, fungi also play an important role in maintaining the balance of the microbiome. When beneficial fungi are supported through proper diet and a clean internal environment, they contribute to the breakdown of waste products and assist in detoxification.

A diet rich in prebiotics and probiotics helps to maintain the balance between bacteria and fungi, preventing the overgrowth of harmful species like Candida. By fostering a balanced microbiome, the body's natural defense systems are strengthened, and the risk of developing fungal infections, digestive disorders, and inflammatory conditions is reduced.

Chapter 4: Natural Remedies for Supporting Microbial Health and Detoxification

Maintaining a healthy balance of microorganisms in the body is essential for overall wellness, particularly for digestion and immunity. At the same time, detoxification is vital for ensuring that harmful substances and toxins do not accumulate in the body, disrupting the natural balance of beneficial microbes. There are several natural remedies, including herbs, that can support microbial health and aid in detoxification. These remedies can be incorporated into daily routines, ensuring that the body remains balanced and clean.

1. Garlic

Garlic is one of the most effective herbs for supporting microbial health due to its potent antibacterial, antifungal, and antiviral properties. It is especially useful for combating harmful bacteria and yeast overgrowth in the gut, such as Candida. To use garlic for microbial health, it is best consumed raw for maximum potency.

How to use: Crush or finely chop one clove of garlic and consume it raw. If the taste is too strong, you can mix it with a small amount of honey or olive oil.

When: Take in the morning on an empty stomach for best results.

How often: Daily or 3-4 times a week for maintenance.

2. Ginger

Ginger is known for its anti-inflammatory and antimicrobial properties, making it a great addition to any detoxification routine. It helps improve digestion and aids in flushing out toxins from the body by stimulating circulation and promoting sweating.

How to use: Fresh ginger can be grated and added to hot water to make tea or incorporated into meals like soups and stews.

When: Drink ginger tea after meals to support digestion or first thing in the morning for detoxification.

How often: Daily, especially during a detox program or if you have digestive concerns.

3. Dandelion Root

Dandelion root is a powerful herb for liver detoxification, helping to eliminate toxins and supporting bile production, which is crucial for digesting fats. It also acts as a diuretic, promoting the removal of waste through urine.

How to use: Dandelion root can be taken as a tea or in tincture form. To make tea, steep 1-2 teaspoons of dried root in boiling water for 10-15 minutes.

When: Drink the tea in the morning or afternoon to support liver function.

How often: 2-3 times a week, or more frequently during a dedicated detox period.

4. Echinacea

Echinacea is a well-known immune booster with antimicrobial effects that help fight off infections. It is especially effective in promoting microbial health by stimulating the body's natural defenses.

How to use: Echinacea is available in tea, tincture, or capsule form. For a quick boost, take 1-2 droppers of tincture in water or tea.

When: Take at the first sign of infection or when feeling run down.

How often: Once or twice a day for up to a week during periods of illness or microbial imbalance.

5. Milk Thistle

Milk thistle is another excellent herb for liver detoxification. Its active compound, silymarin, helps regenerate liver cells and protect against toxins, ensuring the body can efficiently eliminate waste.

How to use: Milk thistle can be consumed as a tea or in capsule form. For ten minutes, steep one teaspoon of crushed seeds in boiling water to prepare tea.

When: Drink milk thistle tea in the evening or after meals to support liver function.

How often: 3-4 times a week during detox periods or for ongoing liver support.

6. Turmeric

Turmeric contains curcumin, which has powerful anti-inflammatory and antimicrobial properties. It supports detoxification by stimulating bile production and aiding in the removal of harmful bacteria.

How to use: Add 1 teaspoon of turmeric powder to warm water or milk to create a "golden milk" drink. It can also be incorporated into meals.

When: Drink in the evening to promote relaxation and detoxification overnight.

How often: Daily, especially during periods of detox or microbial imbalance.

7. Aloe Vera

Aloe vera is known for its soothing properties, particularly for the digestive system. It can help balance gut flora and promote healthy bowel movements, aiding in detoxification.

How to use: Aloe vera gel can be consumed in small amounts (1-2 tablespoons) mixed with water or juice.

When: Take first thing in the morning or before bed.

How often: Daily for a week, especially during digestive issues or a cleanse.

8. Clove

Clove has strong antimicrobial properties, making it effective in killing harmful bacteria and parasites. It can also support gut health and detoxification through its digestive-enhancing properties.

How to use: Clove can be brewed into tea or taken in capsule form.

When: Drink clove tea after meals to aid digestion and kill harmful microbes.

How often: 2-3 times a week during detoxification or microbial imbalance.

9. Fennel

Fennel is excellent for promoting digestive health and flushing out toxins. It acts as a natural diuretic, encouraging the elimination of waste and reducing bloating.

How to use: Fennel seeds can be chewed after meals or made into a tea by steeping 1 teaspoon of seeds in hot water.

When: Take after meals to support digestion.

How often: Daily, especially after heavy meals or during a cleanse.

10. Green Tea

Green tea is rich in antioxidants and catechins, which support detoxification and the elimination of toxins from the liver. It also promotes a healthy microbial balance in the gut.

How to use: Drink 1-2 cups of green tea per day.

When: Best consumed in the morning or early afternoon to avoid disrupting sleep.

How often: Daily as part of an overall health routine.

11. Lemon Balm

Lemon balm is a calming herb that helps reduce stress, which can negatively affect microbial health. It also supports digestion and detoxification by calming the nervous system.

How to use: Drink lemon balm tea by steeping 1-2 teaspoons of dried leaves in hot water for 10 minutes.

When: Best consumed in the evening to promote relaxation and digestion.

How often: Daily, especially during stressful periods.

12. Peppermint

Peppermint is excellent for supporting digestion and soothing the GI tract. It also has antimicrobial properties that help maintain a healthy microbial balance.

How to use: Peppermint tea is the most common form, made by steeping fresh or dried leaves in hot water for 5-10 minutes.

When: Drink after meals to aid digestion and promote microbial health.

How often: Daily or as needed.

13. Cilantro

Cilantro is particularly useful for detoxifying heavy metals from the body, such as mercury and lead. It helps flush toxins from the liver and tissues, promoting overall detoxification.

How to use: Incorporate fresh cilantro into drinks, smoothies, and salads.

When: Best consumed in the morning or as part of a detox smoothie.

How often: Several times a week during detoxification.

14. Oregano Oil

Oregano oil has strong antimicrobial and antiviral properties, making it effective for fighting infections and supporting microbial balance.

How to use: Take oregano oil in capsule form or diluted in water (1-2 drops).

When: Use during periods of microbial imbalance or infection.

How often: Up to twice a day for short-term use, no longer than 2 weeks.

15. Psyllium Husk

Psyllium husk is a natural source of fiber that helps detoxify the colon by promoting regular bowel movements and removing toxins from the digestive tract.

How to use: Mix 1 tablespoon of psyllium husk with water or juice and drink immediately.

When: Take first thing in the morning or before bed.

How often: Daily for up to a week during a cleanse.

16. Triphala

Triphala is an Ayurvedic remedy consisting of three fruits that support detoxification and digestion. It helps cleanse the colon and supports liver function.

How to use: Take Triphala in powder or capsule form, typically 500mg-1g.

When: Best taken before bed to support detoxification during sleep.

How often: Daily for up to 2 weeks during a detox program.

17. Activated Charcoal

Activated charcoal binds to toxins and chemicals in the body, helping to eliminate them through the digestive system. It is particularly effective for detoxifying the gut and preventing reabsorption of toxins.

How to use: Take 500-1,000 mg of activated charcoal with a full glass of water.

When: Use during detoxification or if experiencing digestive issues from toxin exposure.

How often: Occasionally, as needed during detox periods.

18. Burdock Root

Burdock root is known for its blood-purifying properties and ability to support liver detoxification. It helps remove toxins from the blood and promotes healthy skin by reducing inflammation.

How to use: Burdock root can be taken as tea or in tincture form.

When: Drink burdock root tea in the evening for detox support.

How often: 2-3 times a day

Part 4:
Anti-Candida Strategies for Fungal Overgrowth

Chapter 1: Understanding Fungal Infections – Candida and Its Effects on the Body

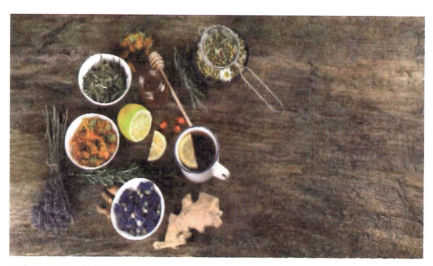

1.1 What Is Candida?

Candida is a type of yeast that exists naturally within the human body. It is primarily found in small quantities in areas such as the mouth, gut, and skin. Under normal conditions, Candida is harmless and coexists with other microorganisms that make up the body's microbiome. However, when there is an imbalance, Candida can grow uncontrollably, leading to what is commonly referred to as Candida overgrowth or candidiasis.

Causes of Candida Overgrowth

Candida overgrowth is often triggered by several factors that disrupt the body's natural balance. One of the primary causes is a poor diet, particularly one high in refined sugars, processed foods, and carbohydrates. These foods provide fuel for Candida, allowing it to proliferate rapidly in the digestive tract. Excessive consumption of sugar creates an environment in which Candida thrives, feeding off the sugars and producing toxins that can weaken the immune system.

Additionally, a weakened immune system can make it easier for Candida to grow. This can be due to chronic stress, poor nutrition, or conditions that suppress immune function. The body's immune system typically controls the growth of Candida, but when compromised, it loses the ability to keep the yeast population in balance. Hormonal imbalances, particularly during pregnancy or menopause, can also trigger Candida overgrowth due to changes in the body's internal environment.

Symptoms of Candida Overgrowth

Candida overgrowth can manifest in a variety of symptoms that affect multiple systems in the body. One of the most common signs is digestive discomfort, including bloating, gas, constipation, or diarrhea. This is because Candida overgrowth often occurs in the gut, disrupting normal digestive processes and causing inflammation in the GI tract.

Fatigue is another frequent symptom associated with Candida overgrowth. When the body is constantly fighting an infection, energy levels are depleted, leading to persistent tiredness. This fatigue can be chronic and difficult to relieve, even with rest.

Skin rashes and irritation are other signs of Candida overgrowth, particularly in areas that are warm and moist, such as the armpits, groin, or under the breasts. These rashes can appear as red, itchy patches and may be accompanied by discomfort.

Recurrent infections, particularly yeast infections in women or oral thrush, are further indicators of Candida imbalance. These infections can be persistent and difficult to treat with conventional methods, as the underlying cause of Candida overgrowth may not be addressed.

Other symptoms may include brain fog, difficulty concentrating, joint pain, and mood swings, all of which can result from the systemic impact of Candida toxins spreading throughout the body.

1.2 How Candida Affects the Body

Candida, a type of yeast commonly found in the human body, can become problematic when it overgrows, leading to a variety of health issues. Barbara O'Neill explains how Candida overgrowth releases toxins into the bloodstream, compromising immune function and causing a condition known as "leaky gut." This imbalance can lead to inflammation, digestive issues, and an increased susceptibility to infections.

Leaky Gut and Immune Function

One of the most significant impacts of Candida overgrowth is its ability to weaken the gut lining. The intestinal walls serve as a barrier, regulating the passage of nutrients into the bloodstream while keeping harmful substances out. However, when Candida multiplies excessively, it produces toxic byproducts that weaken the gut lining, leading to increased permeability. This condition is commonly referred to as "leaky gut."

With a permeable gut lining, undigested food particles, toxins, and harmful bacteria can pass through the intestinal walls into the bloodstream, triggering immune responses. This creates a cycle of inflammation as the body tries to combat these foreign invaders. The immune system becomes overwhelmed, and as a result, overall immune function is compromised, making the body more susceptible to infections. Chronic inflammation can also contribute to various health problems, such as autoimmune disorders and allergic reactions, as the body mistakenly targets its own tissues.

Inflammation and Candida Toxins

Candida overgrowth introduces a range of toxins into the body, further fueling inflammation. These toxins, including acetaldehyde and other byproducts of Candida metabolism, can circulate in the bloodstream and affect multiple systems within the body. Acetaldehyde, for instance, is known to cause oxidative stress, which damages cells and tissues. This contributes to feelings of fatigue, brain fog, and general malaise, common symptoms in individuals struggling with Candida overgrowth.

The presence of Candida-related toxins in the bloodstream also leads to inflammation in various organs, including the liver and kidneys, which are responsible for detoxifying the body. The constant burden placed on these detoxification systems can lead to impaired function, making it harder for the body to eliminate waste and fight off infections. Over time, the accumulation of toxins and chronic inflammation can have far-reaching effects on overall health.

Candida and Dietary Triggers

Candida thrives on sugars and processed foods, which exacerbate its overgrowth. Sugars provide the perfect environment for Candida to multiply, and a diet rich in refined carbohydrates and sugary foods encourages its proliferation. This creates a vicious cycle, as Candida overgrowth leads to cravings for more sugar, further fueling its growth.

Barbara O'Neill emphasizes the importance of dietary changes in combating Candida. One of the key steps in addressing Candida overgrowth is to eliminate sugars, refined carbohydrates, and processed foods from the diet. This starves the yeast, limiting its ability to multiply. In addition to cutting out these foods, it is crucial to incorporate whole, nutrient-dense foods that support the body's natural detoxification processes and strengthen the immune system.

A diet rich in fresh vegetables, leafy greens, and healthy fats provides the body with the nutrients it needs to repair the gut lining, reduce inflammation, and restore balance to the digestive system. By avoiding foods that feed Candida and focusing on those that promote gut health, it is possible to regain control over the infection and support the body's healing process.

The Role of Probiotics

Restoring a healthy balance of gut flora is another essential aspect of managing Candida overgrowth. Probiotics, which are beneficial bacteria, play a key role in maintaining a healthy gut microbiome. When the balance of good bacteria in the gut is disrupted, Candida is more likely to thrive. Introducing probiotics through fermented foods or supplements helps to repopulate the gut with healthy bacteria that can outcompete Candida and restore balance to the digestive system.

Incorporating probiotic-rich foods such as yogurt, sauerkraut, and kefir into the diet can help strengthen the gut lining, reduce inflammation, and improve digestion. By promoting the growth of beneficial bacteria, probiotics can help reduce Candida's hold on the gut and support the body's overall immune function.

Detoxification and Candida Management

Detoxification plays a crucial role in managing Candida overgrowth. As Candida dies off during treatment, it releases even more toxins into the bloodstream, a phenomenon known as "die-off" or the Herxheimer reaction. This can lead to temporary worsening of symptoms, including headaches, fatigue, and digestive discomfort. Supporting the body's detoxification pathways is essential to minimize the effects of Candida die-off and prevent further strain on the liver and kidneys.

Barbara O'Neill recommends herbal remedies and natural detox strategies to support the body during this process. Herbs such as milk thistle and dandelion root are particularly effective in supporting liver function and aiding in the elimination of toxins. Additionally, staying well-hydrated and consuming foods that support liver and kidney health can help the body cope with the increased toxic load during Candida treatment.

In summary, Candida overgrowth can significantly impact the body's health by compromising the gut lining, disrupting immune function, and increasing inflammation. By addressing dietary triggers, incorporating probiotics, and supporting detoxification, it is possible to reduce Candida's hold on the body and restore balance to the gut and immune system.

Chapter 2: Key Antifungal Herbs and Natural Remedies

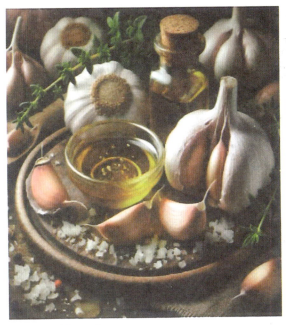

2.1 Garlic – A Potent Antifungal

Garlic has long been recognized as one of nature's most potent antifungal agents, with a reputation for combating infections and boosting the immune system. According to Barbara O'Neill, garlic is particularly effective against fungal infections, especially those caused by Candida. This is due to its active compound, allicin, which has strong antifungal, antibacterial, and antiviral properties. Allicin is released when garlic is crushed or chopped, activating its defense mechanism to fight off pathogens, making it a powerful tool in treating fungal overgrowth both internally and externally.

2.2 Oregano Oil

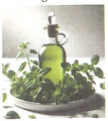

Oregano oil is another powerful natural antifungal that has gained attention for its ability to fight Candida overgrowth and other fungal infections. According to Barbara O'Neill, oregano oil contains two key compounds, carvacrol and thymol, both of which have potent antifungal and antimicrobial properties. These compounds disrupt the integrity of fungal cell membranes, effectively killing the fungus and preventing its spread.

2.3 Pau D'Arco for Immune Support

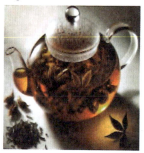

Pau D'Arco is a powerful herb that has been traditionally used for its antifungal and immune-supporting properties. It is often recommended by Barbara O'Neill for its effectiveness in combating fungal infections such as Candida, as well as for boosting the body's resilience against reinfections. This herb, derived from the inner bark of the Pau D'Arco tree, has been a staple in natural medicine for centuries, particularly for its ability to address fungal overgrowth and support overall immune health.

Antifungal Properties of Pau D'Arco

One of the primary reasons Pau D'Arco is so effective in treating fungal infections is due to its rich content of active compounds, including lapachol and beta-lapachone. These compounds have demonstrated potent antifungal effects, specifically in inhibiting the growth of Candida and other pathogenic fungi. Candida overgrowth is a common problem for many individuals, particularly those with compromised immune systems or poor gut health. Pau D'Arco helps to eliminate these fungal pathogens by disrupting their cellular processes, making it more difficult for the fungi to replicate and thrive.

Candida infections, if left untreated, can lead to a variety of symptoms, including digestive issues, fatigue, and skin problems. By incorporating Pau D'Arco into a treatment plan, individuals can help reduce the fungal load in their body and restore balance to their gut microbiome. Barbara O'Neill often discusses the importance of maintaining a healthy gut as the foundation of overall well-being, and Pau D'Arco plays a key role in achieving that balance by keeping fungal populations in check.

How to Use Pau D'Arco

Pau D'Arco can be consumed in various forms, with Pau D'Arco tea being one of the most popular methods. The tea can be brewed from the inner bark of the tree and consumed regularly to help clear up Candida infections and support overall immune health. For those who prefer not to drink tea, Pau D'Arco is also available in supplement form, making it easy to incorporate into a daily wellness routine.

When using Pau D'Arco, it is important to follow recommended dosages and consult with a healthcare professional, particularly if using it for chronic infections. Barbara O'Neill emphasizes the importance of natural remedies being part of a holistic approach, incorporating proper diet, hydration, and lifestyle adjustments alongside herbal treatments for optimal results.

2.4 Olive Leaf Extract

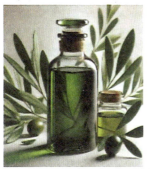

Olive leaf extract is another powerful herb frequently discussed by Barbara O'Neill for its antifungal and immune-boosting properties. Derived from the leaves of the olive tree, olive leaf extract contains a compound called oleuropein, which has been extensively studied for its ability to inhibit the growth of fungi, particularly Candida. In addition to its antifungal effects, oleuropein also possesses strong antiviral, anti-inflammatory, and antioxidant properties, making olive leaf extract a versatile remedy for supporting overall health.

Antifungal Benefits of Olive Leaf Extract

Candida overgrowth can lead to a host of health problems, including digestive disturbances, skin issues, and fatigue. Olive leaf extract works by targeting the cell walls of Candida fungi, disrupting their structure and making it difficult for them to reproduce. This makes olive leaf extract an excellent choice for those seeking to cleanse their body of fungal overgrowth naturally.

In addition to fighting Candida, olive leaf extract has been shown to be effective against other types of fungi, including those that cause athlete's foot and fungal nail infections. The broad-spectrum antifungal properties of olive leaf extract make it a valuable tool for addressing a variety of fungal-related health concerns. When taken consistently, olive leaf extract helps to reduce fungal populations in the body, restoring balance and preventing the overgrowth of harmful fungi.

Detoxifying the Body with Olive Leaf Extract

Olive leaf extract is often used as part of a detox protocol, particularly for those dealing with chronic Candida infections. By cleansing the body of fungal overgrowth, olive leaf extract helps to reduce the toxic burden on the liver and other organs involved in detoxification. This allows the body to function more efficiently and reduces the likelihood of reinfection.

The detoxifying properties of olive leaf extract are further enhanced by its ability to support the immune system. By improving immune function, olive leaf extract helps the body fight off infections more effectively, preventing the recurrence of fungal overgrowth. This makes it a key component in any detox plan aimed at eliminating Candida and other fungal pathogens from the body.

How to Use Olive Leaf Extract

Olive leaf extract is available in various forms, including capsules, tinctures, and powders. It can be taken as a supplement on its own or combined with other antifungal herbs as part of a comprehensive detox program. For individuals looking to address fungal overgrowth, it is important to use olive leaf extract consistently over a period of time to achieve the best results.

When using olive leaf extract for detoxification, it is crucial to support the body with plenty of water and a clean diet to help flush out toxins released by the dying fungi. This process, known as a Herxheimer reaction or "die-off" effect, can sometimes cause temporary symptoms such as headaches or fatigue as the body eliminates toxins. Staying well-hydrated and supporting the liver and kidneys with detoxifying herbs can help minimize these symptoms and ensure a smoother detox process.

Chapter 3: Dietary Changes to Starve Fungus

3.1 Eliminating Sugars and Processed Foods

Candida overgrowth is a common issue in those with an imbalanced gut, and one of the key elements in addressing this problem is dietary modification. According to Barbara O'Neill, one of the most important factors in managing Candida is eliminating the sugars and processed foods that fuel the growth of this fungus. Candida thrives on sugar, and without restricting its food source, it becomes challenging to control or eradicate the infection.

Vegetables and Their Role in Candida Treatment

Non-starchy vegetables play a significant role in Candida treatment. Foods like leafy greens, cruciferous vegetables (broccoli, cauliflower, and cabbage), and garlic are especially beneficial due to their antifungal properties. These vegetables help support the body's detoxification processes, reducing inflammation and aiding the immune system in combating the overgrowth of yeast. Garlic, in particular, contains allicin, a compound known for its antifungal and immune-boosting properties, making it a valuable addition to any Candida-fighting diet.

Barbara emphasizes the importance of avoiding starchy vegetables such as potatoes and corn, as they can raise blood sugar levels and feed Candida. Sticking to low-glycemic vegetables ensures that the body maintains stable blood sugar levels, reducing the fuel available for Candida to thrive.

Healthy Fats and Proteins

In addition to vegetables, healthy fats and proteins form the foundation of a Candida-fighting diet. Healthy fats such as those found in avocados, olive oil, and coconut oil are essential for providing energy and helping the body absorb fat-soluble vitamins. Coconut oil, in particular, contains caprylic acid, which has antifungal properties that help kill off Candida. Incorporating coconut oil into the diet, whether through cooking or as part of meals, can be a powerful tool in combating Candida overgrowth.

Proteins are also crucial for maintaining strength and repairing the body's tissues during Candida treatment. Lean meats, fish, eggs, and plant-based proteins like legumes and seeds provide the necessary building blocks for healing without raising blood sugar levels. Maintaining adequate protein intake ensures that the body has the resources it needs to support the immune system and keep Candida at bay.

Reducing Fruits During Initial Candida Treatment

While fruits are typically considered healthy, many are high in natural sugars that can feed Candida. Barbara O'Neill advises that during the initial stages of Candida treatment, it is best to reduce or avoid fruits, particularly those with a high sugar content like bananas, grapes, and mangoes. These fruits, while nutritious, can provide the sugar Candida needs to grow. By temporarily reducing fruit intake, the body can more effectively starve the fungus and prevent its spread.

Once the Candida is under control, low-sugar fruits such as berries and green apples can be gradually reintroduced. These fruits have a lower glycemic index and are less likely to spike blood sugar levels, allowing the body to maintain control over Candida without compromising nutritional intake.

3.2 Avoiding Yeast and Fermented Foods

In addition to eliminating sugars, it is essential to avoid yeast and fermented foods that can exacerbate Candida overgrowth. Many fermented foods contain yeasts or sugars that can feed Candida and worsen the infection, making recovery more difficult.

Yeast-Containing Foods to Avoid

Barbara recommends avoiding foods that contain yeast, such as bread, beer, and certain condiments like soy sauce and vinegar-based dressings. Bread, especially, is a common source of yeast, and its consumption can lead to an imbalance in gut flora, making it harder for the body to control Candida. Beer and other yeast-fermented alcoholic beverages can also exacerbate Candida, as they introduce additional yeast into the digestive system. By avoiding these foods, the body can begin to restore balance to the gut and reduce the burden of yeast on the system.

Additionally, processed foods that contain hidden sources of yeast or sugar, such as packaged snacks, sauces, and dressings, should also be avoided. These processed items often contain ingredients that can feed Candida without being immediately obvious, such as high-fructose corn syrup, malt, or certain additives that contribute to yeast growth.

Fermented Foods and Candida Overgrowth

Fermented foods, while generally beneficial for gut health, can be problematic for those dealing with Candida overgrowth. Foods like sauerkraut, kefir, and kombucha contain natural yeasts that, while normally helpful in maintaining a healthy gut flora, can contribute to the overgrowth of Candida in those already dealing with an infection. During Candida treatment, it is best to avoid these fermented foods until the overgrowth is under control.

Once the body has achieved balance and the infection is no longer an issue, Barbara suggests gradually reintroducing fermented foods like sauerkraut or kefir. These foods contain beneficial probiotics that can help restore and maintain a healthy gut microbiome. However, it is essential to wait until the Candida overgrowth has been managed before incorporating these foods, as introducing them too early may cause setbacks in the treatment process.

3.3 Supporting Gut Health with Probiotics

Probiotics are essential in maintaining and restoring gut health, particularly when it comes to controlling the growth of Candida and other harmful microorganisms. The balance of the gut microbiome, which consists of trillions of microorganisms, can be easily disrupted by factors such as poor diet, stress, and the overuse of antibiotics. This imbalance often leads to an overgrowth of Candida, a yeast that can cause digestive discomfort, fatigue, and other health issues.

Probiotic Supplements

In addition to probiotic-rich foods, probiotic supplements can also be effective in restoring gut health. Barbara O'Neill suggests that individuals suffering from Candida overgrowth may benefit from taking high-quality probiotic supplements that contain multiple strains of beneficial bacteria. These supplements help rebuild the gut's bacterial population, especially after antibiotic use or periods of poor diet.

Probiotic supplements are particularly useful when it is challenging to obtain enough beneficial bacteria from food alone. Choosing a supplement with a variety of strains, such as Lactobacillus and Bifidobacterium, ensures that different areas of the gut receive the support they need. These bacteria work together to enhance digestion, boost immunity, and prevent the overgrowth of harmful microorganisms.

Chapter 4: Long-Term Strategies for Maintaining Fungal Balance and Preventing Reinfection

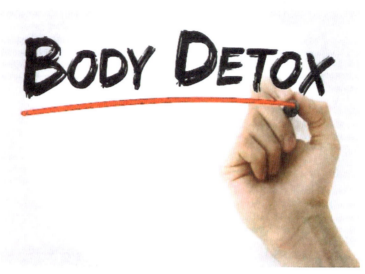

4.1 Regular Detoxification

Detoxification is a fundamental aspect of maintaining overall health and preventing the recurrence of fungal infections, such as those caused by Candida. Barbara O'Neill emphasizes the need for regular detoxification to rid the body of toxins and fungal elements that can compromise health over time. By focusing on key organs such as the liver, colon, and kidneys, the body can more effectively eliminate harmful substances and restore balance.

There are three primary components to detox:

- Liver
- Colon
- Kidnesy

4.2 Boosting the Immune System

A strong immune system is the body's best defense against fungal overgrowth, particularly Candida infections. Barbara O'Neill emphasizes the importance of bolstering the immune system to prevent the return of Candida and other fungal infections. This can be achieved through a combination of nutrient-rich foods and immune-boosting herbs.

Herbal Remedies for Immune Support

Herbal remedies also play a significant role in boosting the immune system and preventing Candida overgrowth. **Echinacea** is a well-known herb that helps stimulate the immune system by increasing the activity of white blood cells. By enhancing the body's natural defenses, echinacea helps the immune system identify and eliminate fungal elements more effectively.

Astragalus is another powerful immune-boosting herb. It has been used in traditional medicine for centuries to strengthen the body's resistance to infection. Astragalus works by enhancing the immune system's response to pathogens, making it particularly useful in preventing the recurrence of fungal infections like Candida.

Reishi mushroom is a potent adaptogen that helps modulate the immune system, ensuring it responds appropriately to infections without becoming overactive. Reishi is also known for its antifungal properties, making it an excellent addition to a regimen designed to prevent fungal overgrowth. By supporting overall immune health, reishi mushroom helps create an environment that is less hospitable to Candida and other fungi.

Lifestyle Practices for Immune Health

In addition to diet and herbs, lifestyle practices that reduce stress and promote relaxation can further support the immune system. Chronic stress is known to weaken immune function, making the body more susceptible to infections. Practicing stress-reducing techniques such as meditation, yoga, and deep breathing can help regulate the body's stress response and promote better immune function.

Chapter 5: 18 Natural Remedies for Candida Overgrowth

Candida overgrowth is a common fungal issue that can cause a wide range of health problems, from digestive disturbances to fatigue and skin infections. To combat this, it is important to use natural remedies that work synergistically to reduce Candida populations while supporting overall health. Below are 18 effective remedies for Candida overgrowth, building on the 9 remedies found in Barbara O'Neill's work.

The appendix provides more details for each remedy.

1. Garlic Infusion

2. Oregano Oil Capsules

3. Pau D'Arco Tea

4. Olive Leaf Extract

5. Coconut Oil

6. Turmeric-Ginger Tea

7. Apple Cider Vinegar

8. Cinnamon Bark Tea

9. Probiotic Supplement

10. Aloe Vera Juice

11. Clove Oil

12. Black Walnut Extract

13. Berberine

14. Calendula Tea

15. Lemon Balm

16. Caprylic Acid

17. Grapefruit Seed Extract

18. Neem Oil

Part 5:
Immune System Strengthening with Herbal Remedies

Chapter 1: Boosting the Immune System Naturally – Key Strategies

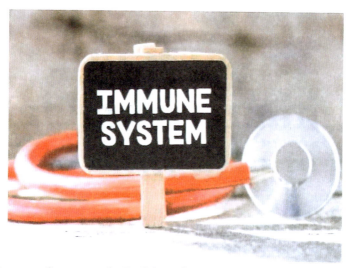

1.1 The Immune System as the Body's Defense Mechanism

The immune system serves as the body's primary defense against infections, bacteria, and viruses. It operates through a complex network of cells, tissues, and organs that work together to identify and neutralize harmful invaders, such as pathogens, toxins, and foreign substances. When functioning optimally, the immune system protects the body from both acute infections and chronic illnesses, ensuring overall health and vitality.

The Immune System's Role in Protecting Against Infections

The immune system is designed to detect and eliminate harmful microorganisms that threaten the body. It does this through two main components: the innate immune system and the adaptive immune system. The innate immune system is the body's first line of defense, providing a rapid response to infections by recognizing general markers of harmful invaders. This includes cells like macrophages that consume and eliminate infections, this also refers to physical barriers like the skin and mucous membranes.

The adaptive immune system, on the other hand, provides a more specialized and targeted defense. It consists of lymphocytes, including T cells and B cells, which have the ability to recognize specific pathogens the body has encountered before. This aspect of the immune system is responsible for long-term immunity, allowing the body to respond more effectively to recurring infections.

By maintaining a strong immune system, the body is better equipped to fight off infections such as colds, flu, and other viral or bacterial threats. When the immune system is compromised, either through poor diet, lack of sleep, or chronic stress, the body becomes more susceptible to these infections, and the ability to recover quickly is diminished.

Signs of a Weakened Immune System

Common signs of a weakened immune system include frequent colds, fatigue, and slow wound healing. When the immune system is compromised, the body becomes less efficient at fighting off infections, leading to frequent bouts of illness. Fatigue is another indicator, as the body uses more energy to compensate for the reduced immune function. Additionally, slow wound healing is a sign that the body's repair processes are impaired, which is often a result of weakened immunity.

1.2 Factors that Weaken the Immune System

Several key factors contribute to the weakening of the immune system, making the body more susceptible to infections and slower to recover from illnesses. These include stress, poor diet, environmental toxins, and lack of sleep. Together, these elements can disrupt the body's natural defense mechanisms and compromise immune function.

Stress and the Immune System

Poor Diet and Immune Health

Environmental Toxins and Immunity

Lack of Sleep and Immune Health

1.3 Key Lifestyle Changes to Boost Immunity

Maintaining a strong immune system is essential for preventing illness and promoting overall well-being. Certain lifestyle changes can significantly enhance immune function by providing the body with the necessary tools to fight off infections and stay resilient against external stressors.

Proper Nutrition and Hydration

Nutrition plays a foundational role in boosting immunity. A diet rich in whole, nutrient-dense foods like fruits, vegetables, whole grains, and lean proteins provides the essential vitamins and minerals that support immune function. Specifically, vitamins C and D, along with zinc, are known to strengthen the immune system. Vitamin C, found in citrus fruits, bell peppers, and broccoli, helps stimulate the production of white blood cells, which are crucial for fighting infections. Vitamin D, often synthesized through sunlight exposure, is vital for immune cell function and can be obtained through foods like fatty fish and fortified products.

Regular Exercise and Sleep

Incorporating regular physical activity into daily life is another key lifestyle change that supports immune health. Exercise helps to improve circulation, allowing immune cells to move more freely throughout the body. Moderate, consistent exercise has been shown to enhance the activity of immune cells, making it easier for the body to detect and eliminate harmful pathogens. Activities such as walking, cycling, swimming, or yoga can be integrated into a daily routine to promote overall health and immunity.

Adequate sleep is critical for maintaining immune function. During sleep, the body undergoes repair and regeneration processes, including the production of immune cells like cytokines, which play a crucial role in combating infections and inflammation. Chronic sleep deprivation can lower the body's defenses, making it more susceptible to illness. Aiming for 7-9 hours of restorative sleep each night is essential for supporting immune health.

Mindful Stress Management

Taking time to relax and engage in activities that promote mental well-being is essential for maintaining strong immunity. Simple practices such as spending time in nature, journaling, or practicing gratitude can help manage stress levels and promote a healthier immune response.

Detoxification for Immune Support

Detoxification is another important aspect of enhancing immune function. The accumulation of toxins from environmental pollutants, processed foods, and stress can weaken the immune system over time. Supporting the body's natural detoxification pathways through proper nutrition, hydration, and specific herbs can help remove these toxins and reduce the burden on the immune system.

Chapter 2: Immune-Boosting Herbs – Echinacea, Garlic, Elderberry, and More

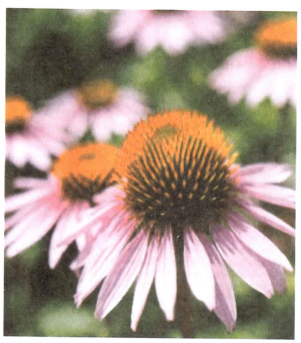

2.1 Echinacea: The Immune System Powerhouse

Echinacea is widely recognized for its ability to support the immune system, particularly by enhancing the body's natural defenses. This herb has long been used to combat infections, colds, and flu, making it a cornerstone of natural remedies for immune support. One of the key ways Echinacea boosts the immune system is by stimulating the production and activity of white blood cells, which are essential for fighting off infections and pathogens.

How Echinacea Enhances the Immune System

Echinacea stimulates the immune system by increasing the number and activity of white blood cells, particularly phagocytes, which are responsible for engulfing and destroying harmful pathogens like bacteria and viruses. This action helps the body respond more rapidly and effectively to infections, thereby reducing the severity and duration of illness. Echinacea has also been shown to increase the production of cytokines, which are signaling molecules that help regulate the immune response.

In addition to its effects on white blood cell production, Echinacea also has anti-inflammatory properties that help to reduce the overall burden on the immune system. By lowering inflammation, Echinacea enables the body to focus its efforts on fighting infections rather than dealing with systemic inflammation. This dual action of boosting immune activity while reducing inflammation makes Echinacea particularly effective in preventing and treating common respiratory infections, such as colds and the flu.

Best Ways to Use Echinacea

There are several effective ways to incorporate Echinacea into a daily routine for immune support, including teas, tinctures, and supplements. Each method has its own benefits, and the choice often depends on personal preference and convenience.

Echinacea Tincture: Tinctures are another highly effective way to use Echinacea. A tincture is a concentrated extract of the herb, usually made with alcohol, that can be taken by the dropper full. Tinctures are often more potent than teas, making them a good option for those seeking a stronger immune boost. Tinctures are also convenient, as they can be added to water or juice for easy consumption. Barbara O'Neill recommends taking Echinacea tincture at the onset of symptoms to give the immune system an immediate boost.

Echinacea Supplements: For those who prefer a more convenient method, Echinacea is available in capsule or tablet form. Supplements are an easy way to ensure a consistent daily dose of Echinacea, especially during times of increased exposure to illness, such as during the winter months or when traveling. When selecting a supplement, it is important to choose a high-quality product that contains a standardized amount of active compounds to ensure efficacy.

2.2 Garlic: Nature's Antibiotic

Garlic is renowned for its potent antimicrobial and antiviral properties, making it a powerful natural remedy for boosting the immune system and fighting infections. Often referred to as "nature's antibiotic," garlic has been used for centuries in various cultures to prevent and treat illness, particularly during cold and flu seasons. Its active compound, allicin, is responsible for much of its healing power, providing broad-spectrum antimicrobial effects that can help the body defend against bacterial, viral, and fungal infections.

Antimicrobial and Antiviral Properties

Garlic's ability to fight infections stems from its high concentration of sulfur-containing compounds, the most notable of which is allicin. When garlic is crushed or chopped, allicin is released, producing powerful antimicrobial and antiviral effects. These properties make garlic an effective natural remedy for a variety of health conditions, including respiratory infections, digestive issues, and even skin conditions caused by bacteria or fungi.

Allicin has been shown to inhibit the growth of harmful bacteria and viruses, making it particularly effective in combating colds, flu, and other viral infections. Additionally, garlic's antifungal properties make it useful in treating conditions like candida overgrowth. The immune system benefits from garlic's capacity to reduce the load of pathogens in the body, which allows the body's natural defenses to work more efficiently.

Garlic also has anti-inflammatory properties that can help reduce inflammation in the body, further supporting immune function. Chronic inflammation can weaken the immune system and lead to the development of more serious conditions, but incorporating garlic into the diet can help modulate the body's inflammatory response and protect against long-term health issues.

Medicinal Forms of Garlic

In addition to its culinary uses, garlic can also be consumed in more concentrated medicinal forms, such as garlic oil, tinctures, or extracts. Garlic oil is often used topically to treat skin infections or ear infections due to its antimicrobial properties. For instance, a few drops of garlic oil in the ear can help reduce the symptoms of an ear infection, particularly when combined with other natural remedies.

Garlic extracts or supplements, available in capsule form, are another convenient way to take advantage of garlic's healing properties without having to consume large amounts of raw garlic. These supplements often concentrate the active compounds, making them an effective option for those looking to target specific health issues like chronic infections, cardiovascular health, or immune support.

2.3 Elderberry: The Antiviral Wonder

Elderberry is renowned for its potent antiviral properties, making it a powerful ally in fighting viral infections such as the flu, colds, and sinus infections. This small, dark berry contains a wealth of nutrients and compounds that enhance the body's immune response, particularly through its ability to boost cytokine production. Cytokines are proteins that play a crucial role in immune system communication, signaling the body to mount an effective defense against invading pathogens.

Boosting Immunity with Elderberry

One of the key ways elderberry supports the immune system is by increasing the production of cytokines. When the body detects a virus, cytokines act as messengers, instructing immune cells to respond and fight off the infection. Elderberry has been shown to stimulate this process, leading to a more robust and faster immune response. This makes elderberry particularly effective in the early stages of a viral infection, as it can help reduce the severity and duration of symptoms.

Additionally, elderberry is rich in flavonoids, which are antioxidants that help reduce inflammation and oxidative stress, both of which can weaken the immune system. By neutralizing free radicals and reducing inflammation, elderberry enhances the body's overall immune resilience, allowing it to better fend off viral threats.

How to Use Elderberry

Elderberry can be consumed in various forms, including syrups, teas, and tinctures, each offering different benefits and methods of application. One of the most popular ways to use elderberry is in syrup form, which can be taken daily as a preventative measure during cold and flu season or at the onset of symptoms to reduce the duration of illness.

2.4 Other Immune-Boosting Herbs

Herbs have been used for centuries to support the immune system, providing natural ways to protect against infections and illnesses. These immune-boosting herbs can be especially helpful during times of stress, seasonal changes, or when there is a risk of respiratory infections. Here are six potent herbs that strengthen the immune system and support overall health.

Astragalus: Strengthening Immune Resilience

Astragalus is a well-known herb in traditional Chinese medicine, praised for its ability to strengthen the immune system and enhance resistance to infections, particularly respiratory illnesses. It works by stimulating the production of white blood cells, which are the body's primary defense against pathogens. Astragalus also supports the body's ability to manage stress, which in turn helps maintain a strong immune system.

This herb is especially beneficial during cold and flu season as a preventative measure. By enhancing the immune response, astragalus helps the body fight off infections before they take hold, making it an excellent herb for long-term immune health.

Andrographis: A Potent Antiviral

Andrographis is known for its powerful antiviral properties, making it an effective herb for reducing the severity of cold and flu symptoms. It has been traditionally used in Ayurvedic and Chinese medicine to treat infections and fevers. Andrographis works by inhibiting the replication of viruses and supporting the immune system's natural defenses.

During cold and flu season, andrographis can help shorten the duration of illness and reduce symptoms such as sore throat, fever, and fatigue. Its ability to bolster the immune response makes it a valuable tool in both the prevention and treatment of viral infections.

Ginger: Anti-Inflammatory and Immune-Supporting

Ginger is a well-known anti-inflammatory and antioxidant that plays a significant role in immune health. Its warming properties enhance circulation, helping the body to eliminate toxins more effectively. By improving blood flow, ginger ensures that immune cells can quickly reach areas of the body where they are needed most during an infection.

Ginger's ability to reduce inflammation also supports the immune system by lowering the body's overall inflammatory load. This is particularly important in preventing chronic inflammation, which can weaken immune function over time. Incorporating ginger into the diet or as a tea can help maintain strong immune health year-round.

Turmeric: The Power of Curcumin

Turmeric, and more specifically its active compound curcumin, is highly regarded for its anti-inflammatory and immune-supporting properties. Curcumin helps modulate the body's immune response by reducing excessive inflammation, which is often a contributing factor in both chronic and acute illnesses.

Turmeric is particularly useful in supporting the body's defense against pathogens by enhancing the activity of immune cells. By reducing inflammation and promoting a balanced immune response, turmeric helps the body fight infections more effectively. Including turmeric in the diet or as a supplement can be an excellent way to support immune health, especially during times of heightened risk for infections.

Licorice Root: Immune-Boosting and Respiratory Relief

Licorice root is another herb that supports the immune system while also providing relief for respiratory infections. It contains compounds that stimulate the production of immune cells and fight off viruses. Additionally, licorice root's anti-inflammatory properties help soothe inflamed airways, making it particularly beneficial for respiratory infections like colds, bronchitis, and sore throats.

Licorice root also acts as an expectorant, helping to loosen mucus and clear the respiratory passages, which can be particularly helpful during a cold or flu. Its dual action of boosting immunity and alleviating respiratory symptoms makes it a valuable herb during illness.

Olive Leaf: Antioxidant Protection Against Viruses

Olive leaf contains powerful antioxidants and antiviral compounds that help fight off infections and strengthen the body's natural defenses. Its primary active compound, oleuropein, has been shown to inhibit the replication of viruses, making it particularly effective against viral infections.

Olive leaf supports the immune system by reducing oxidative stress and protecting the body's cells from damage caused by free radicals. This antioxidant effect not only enhances immune function but also helps prevent chronic diseases associated with inflammation and oxidative damage. Olive leaf can be consumed as a tea, extract, or supplement to boost immunity and protect against infections.

Chapter 3: Herbal Teas, Tinctures, and Foods to Enhance Immunity

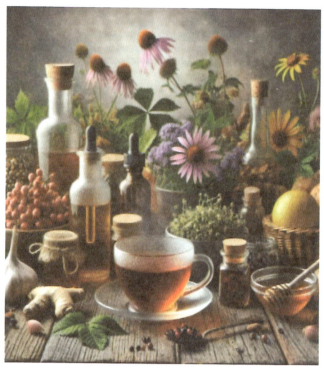

3.1 Herbal Teas for Immune Health

Herbal teas are a natural and effective way to support the immune system and promote overall well-being, particularly during times when the body is more vulnerable to infections. A combination of immune-boosting herbs such as echinacea, elderberry, and ginger can be used to create simple yet potent teas that help the body fend off illness, soothe sore throats, and reduce inflammation. These herbs not only strengthen the immune system but also offer additional benefits such as antioxidant and anti-inflammatory properties, making them a valuable part of a daily routine for immune support.

Echinacea Tea

Echinacea is widely known for its ability to stimulate the immune system. It works by increasing the activity of white blood cells, which are essential for fighting off infections. Echinacea can be particularly effective when used at the onset of illness, as it helps to reduce the severity and duration of symptoms.

To make an echinacea tea, simply steep dried echinacea roots or leaves in boiling water for 10-15 minutes. Adding a touch of honey not only enhances the flavor but also provides additional soothing properties, particularly for sore throats. Drinking this tea regularly during cold and flu season can help strengthen the body's defenses and reduce the likelihood of getting sick.

Elderberry Tea

Elderberry is another powerful herb known for its immune-boosting properties. It is rich in antioxidants, particularly flavonoids, which help protect the body from oxidative stress and support immune function. Elderberry is also known to reduce the severity of cold and flu symptoms by inhibiting the replication of viruses.

Elderberry tea is made by simmering dried elderberries in water for about 10-15 minutes. The berries release their beneficial compounds into the water, creating a rich, flavorful tea. Elderberry tea can be sweetened with honey or combined with other herbs like echinacea or ginger for a more comprehensive immune-boosting blend.

Ginger Tea

Ginger is renowned for its warming and anti-inflammatory properties, making it an excellent herb for immune health. It stimulates circulation and promotes sweating, which can help the body expel toxins. Additionally, ginger is effective in soothing sore throats and reducing inflammation, which are common symptoms of colds and flu.

Simmer fresh ginger in water for around ten minutes after slicing it thinly to prepare ginger tea. The result is a spicy, warming tea that can be enjoyed on its own or with the addition of lemon and honey. This combination is particularly soothing for sore throats and can help reduce coughing and inflammation.

Immune-Strengthening Tea Recipes

A combination of these herbs can be used to create powerful immune-boosting teas. One simple recipe involves combining equal parts dried echinacea, elderberries, and ginger in a teapot or strainer. Pour boiling water over the mixture and allow it to steep for 10-15 minutes. This tea can be consumed daily during cold and flu season or at the first sign of illness to help the body recover more quickly.

For added benefits, herbs such as peppermint or chamomile can be included in the mix to provide additional soothing and anti-inflammatory effects. Chamomile, for example, is known for its calming properties and can help promote relaxation, which is crucial for immune function during illness.

3.2 Immune-Boosting Tinctures

Tinctures are a powerful and effective way to harness the medicinal properties of herbs, and alcohol-based tinctures are particularly beneficial for concentrating these properties. Herbs such as garlic, echinacea, and astragalus have been widely recognized for their immune-boosting abilities, and using tinctures allows these herbs to be easily absorbed by the body for both prevention and early treatment of illness. Barbara O'Neill recommends the use of tinctures as a natural approach to fortifying the immune system, especially during times of increased vulnerability to infections.

Garlic Tincture

Garlic is known for its potent antimicrobial and antiviral properties, making it an excellent herb for immune support. When garlic is made into a tincture, its active compounds, particularly allicin, become concentrated and more readily available to the body. Allicin is responsible for garlic's ability to combat harmful pathogens, including bacteria and viruses.

A garlic tincture is simple to make. Finely chopped or crushed garlic cloves are placed in a jar and covered with alcohol, usually vodka or another high-proof alcohol. The mixture is left to steep for a few weeks, allowing the alcohol to extract the beneficial compounds from the garlic. Once the tincture is ready, it can be taken in small doses, typically a few drops diluted in water or tea, to prevent illness or support the body during the early stages of a cold or flu.

Garlic tincture not only supports the immune system but also helps improve circulation and reduce inflammation. It is particularly useful during the winter months when the body is more susceptible to respiratory infections and the immune system requires extra support.

Echinacea Tincture

Echinacea is one of the most well-known herbs for immune support, especially for its ability to stimulate white blood cell production and enhance lymphatic function. Echinacea tinctures are commonly used as both a preventive measure and a treatment during the early stages of illness. The herb is particularly effective when taken at the onset of a cold or flu, as it helps to reduce the severity and duration of symptoms.

To create an echinacea tincture, the root, leaves, or flowers of the echinacea plant are soaked in alcohol, much like the garlic tincture. After steeping for several weeks, the mixture is strained, and the resulting liquid can be used in small doses to stimulate the immune system. Echinacea tincture is effective in fighting off upper respiratory infections, reducing inflammation, and enhancing the body's ability to fend off viral attacks.

When using echinacea tincture, it is important to take it at the first sign of illness for maximum effectiveness. It can be taken in small doses throughout the day, either diluted in water or directly under the tongue, to boost the body's immune response.

Astragalus Tincture

Astragalus is another powerful herb known for its immune-boosting properties. Unlike echinacea, which is best used at the onset of illness, astragalus is particularly effective for long-term immune support and prevention. It helps strengthen the body's natural defenses by enhancing the function of the immune system and improving the body's resistance to stress and infection.

An astragalus tincture is made by soaking the dried root of the astragalus plant in alcohol, similar to the process for garlic and echinacea tinctures. This tincture can be taken daily as a preventive measure, especially during cold and flu season or when the immune system is under stress. Astragalus works by supporting the production of immune cells and improving the body's ability to respond to infections.

The tincture can be used in small doses over an extended period to maintain immune health and prevent illness. It is particularly useful for individuals who are prone to frequent infections or those looking to build long-term immune resilience.

How to Use Immune-Boosting Tinctures Effectively

When illness strikes, tinctures such as garlic and echinacea can be used more frequently, typically a few drops every few hours, to support the body's fight against infection. Tinctures are best taken diluted in water or herbal tea to make them more palatable. They can also be combined with other immune-boosting practices, such as maintaining a healthy diet rich in vitamins and minerals, to provide comprehensive support for the immune system.

3.3 Nutrient-Rich Foods to Support the Immune System

Supporting the immune system through diet is essential for maintaining overall health. Nutrient-dense foods, rich in vitamins and antioxidants, play a crucial role in fortifying the body's defenses against illness. Incorporating a variety of whole foods such as berries, citrus fruits, leafy greens, and cruciferous vegetables can ensure that the immune system functions optimally, providing the nutrients needed for repair, protection, and regeneration.

Berries and Citrus Fruits: Vitamin C Powerhouses

Berries and citrus fruits are well-known for their high vitamin C content, which is vital for immune health. As a potent antioxidant, vitamin C guards against the oxidative harm that free radicals can bring to cells. It also enhances the production of white blood cells, which are crucial for fighting infections. Berries, such as blueberries, strawberries, and raspberries, not only provide vitamin C but are also rich in other antioxidants that support cellular health and immune function.

Citrus fruits like oranges, lemons, and grapefruits are particularly beneficial during cold and flu season. Their high vitamin C content helps reduce the severity and duration of illnesses by supporting the body's natural defenses. Additionally, vitamin C aids in the absorption of iron from plant-based sources, further supporting immune health by improving oxygen transport throughout the body.

Leafy Greens: A Nutritional Foundation

Leafy greens such as spinach, kale, and Swiss chard are packed with essential nutrients that support the immune system. These greens are rich in vitamins A, C, and K, as well as folate and iron, all of which contribute to maintaining strong immune defenses. Vitamin A, in particular, helps to maintain the health of the skin and mucous membranes, which are the body's first line of defense against pathogens.

Spinach and kale are also high in antioxidants, which help neutralize harmful free radicals in the body. The chlorophyll found in these greens supports detoxification, aiding the liver in eliminating toxins and waste, which can otherwise weaken the immune system. Including leafy greens in the daily diet ensures that the body is equipped with the necessary nutrients to ward off infections and recover quickly from illness.

Cruciferous Vegetables: Detoxifying and Immune-Boosting

Cruciferous vegetables, such as broccoli, cauliflower, Brussels sprouts, and cabbage, are known for their immune-boosting and detoxifying properties. These vegetables are rich in sulfur-containing compounds called glucosinolates, which help support the liver's detoxification processes. By aiding the liver in removing toxins from the body, cruciferous vegetables help reduce the burden on the immune system, allowing it to function more effectively.

Broccoli, in particular, is an excellent source of vitamins C and E, both of which are important for immune health. Vitamin E is a powerful antioxidant that helps protect cells from damage, while vitamin C boosts the immune response by supporting the production of white blood cells. Regular consumption of cruciferous vegetables ensures that the body receives a wide range of nutrients necessary for maintaining a strong and resilient immune system.

The Role of Zinc and Essential Minerals

Zinc is a key mineral for immune function, playing a critical role in the development and activation of immune cells. A diet rich in zinc helps to support the immune system's ability to fight off infections. Foods such as pumpkin seeds, lentils, chickpeas, and quinoa are excellent plant-based sources of zinc. Ensuring adequate zinc intake is especially important during times of stress or illness, as the body's need for this mineral increases during these periods.

In addition to zinc, other essential minerals such as selenium, magnesium, and iron play supportive roles in immune health. Selenium, found in foods like Brazil nuts and sunflower seeds, helps regulate the immune response and reduce inflammation. Magnesium, which is abundant in nuts, seeds, and leafy greens, supports a healthy immune system by helping to maintain normal muscle and nerve function.

Chapter 4: Natural Methods to Combat Infections and Support Long-Term Immune Health

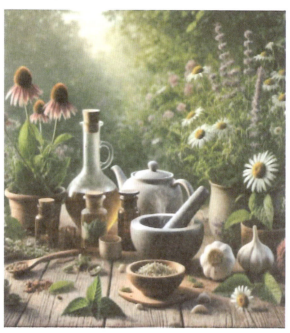

4.1 How Herbal Remedies Help Fight Infections

Herbal remedies have been used for centuries to support the body in combating infections and illnesses. When used at the first signs of sickness, herbs can help prevent the progression of infection by boosting the immune system and addressing the root cause of the illness. Many natural remedies contain powerful antimicrobial and antiviral properties, which can help the body fend off pathogens before they become overwhelming.

Using Herbs at the Onset of Illness

When illness first strikes, the body's immune system works to neutralize invading pathogens. By introducing herbal remedies early on, the immune response can be strengthened, reducing the severity and duration of the illness. Some of the most effective herbs for this purpose include garlic, elderberry, and echinacea, all of which possess immune-boosting and antimicrobial properties.

Treating Common Infections Naturally

For common infections like colds, the flu, and sinus infections, a combination of garlic, elderberry, and echinacea can provide a natural and effective treatment plan. When these herbs are used in conjunction with each other, they can address different aspects of the immune response and help the body fight off infection from multiple angles.

In the case of a cold, garlic can be consumed raw or in the form of a tea to fight the bacteria or viruses responsible for the infection. Elderberry syrup or tincture can be taken to reduce the severity of symptoms and support the immune system's ability to clear the virus. Echinacea can be used in tea or supplement form to further enhance the body's immune response, particularly in the upper respiratory tract.

For the flu, elderberry's antiviral properties are especially valuable. Taking elderberry syrup or capsules at the first sign of flu symptoms can help reduce the duration of the illness. Garlic can also be incorporated into the treatment plan to fight the flu virus, while echinacea can help strengthen the immune system and prevent secondary infections from taking hold.

Sinus infections, which are often caused by bacteria or viruses, can also be treated naturally using these herbs. Garlic's antimicrobial properties can help fight the infection at its source, while echinacea can reduce inflammation in the sinuses and support the immune system in clearing the infection. Elderberry can be taken to boost the body's overall immune response and reduce the severity of symptoms.

4.2 Strengthening the Immune System Over Time

A key principle in building long-term immune resilience is consistency. The immune system is a complex network that requires ongoing support to function optimally, and this support must come from daily habits rather than occasional interventions. Immune-boosting herbs, a healthy diet, and effective stress management all play significant roles in maintaining immune strength, but their benefits are only fully realized when practiced consistently over time.

Herbs such as echinacea, elderberry, and garlic are well-known for their immune-boosting properties. White blood cells are vital for warding off illnesses, and these herbs aid in promoting their development. When incorporated regularly into one's routine, either through teas, tinctures, or supplements, they can provide sustained support to the immune system. It's not enough to use these herbs sporadically—consistent use ensures that the immune system is always prepared to defend the body against pathogens.

In addition to herbs, a nutrient-dense diet is essential for immune function. Whole foods such as fruits, vegetables, nuts, and seeds are rich in vitamins, minerals, and antioxidants that the immune system needs to function efficiently. Vitamin C from citrus fruits, for example, plays a critical role in strengthening the immune response, while zinc found in nuts and seeds helps to improve the function of immune cells. A consistent intake of these nutrients ensures that the body has the resources it needs to protect against illness. Furthermore, reducing processed foods and sugars is equally important, as these can weaken the immune response and contribute to inflammation, which hinders immune function over time.

Stress management is another crucial aspect of building long-term immune resilience. Chronic stress can have a profound negative impact on the immune system, as it leads to the release of cortisol, a hormone that suppresses immune function when present in high levels over extended periods. Incorporating daily stress-reduction techniques such as meditation, deep breathing exercises, and time spent in nature can help lower cortisol levels, allowing the immune system to remain robust. Consistency in managing stress not only supports the immune system but also promotes overall physical and emotional well-being.

4.3 Preventing Chronic Immune Weakness

Chronic immune weakness is a growing concern in today's society, often exacerbated by the overuse of antibiotics, medications, and the cumulative effects of stress and toxins. To maintain a resilient immune system, it is essential to understand how lifestyle factors, such as the use of herbs, regular exercise, and proper nutrition, can support immune function. Additionally, detoxification plays a crucial role in preventing the immune system from becoming overwhelmed.

Herbs as Natural Immune Support

Many herbs have long been recognized for their immune-boosting properties. Echinacea, for example, is well known for its ability to stimulate the immune system and increase the production of white blood cells, which are crucial in defending the body against infections. Other herbs such as garlic, astragalus, and ginger have natural antimicrobial and anti-inflammatory properties, helping to fend off pathogens while reducing inflammation that can otherwise compromise the immune system's efficiency.

Using these herbs as part of a daily regimen can help to prevent chronic immune burnout, particularly in individuals who may have previously relied heavily on antibiotics. Antibiotics, while sometimes necessary, often kill not only harmful bacteria but also the beneficial bacteria that play a key role in maintaining a healthy immune response. By turning to herbs as a preventive measure or first line of defense, the immune system can be supported in a more natural and sustainable way, reducing the need for conventional medications that can weaken the body's natural defenses over time.

Exercise and Its Impact on Immune Health

Exercise is another vital component in preventing chronic immune weakness. Regular physical activity helps to stimulate the circulation of immune cells, allowing them to move more freely through the body and perform their protective functions more efficiently. Moderate exercise, such as walking, swimming, or yoga, has been shown to enhance the body's immune response by increasing the production of natural killer cells and other immune components.

However, it's important to note that while moderate exercise boosts immunity, excessive or intense exercise can have the opposite effect, leading to a temporary suppression of the immune system. Striking the right balance is key to maintaining a strong, resilient immune system. Incorporating regular, moderate exercise into daily routines is one of the most effective ways to keep the immune system active without overwhelming it.

Nutrition: Fuel for the Immune System

Proper nutrition is foundational to immune health, providing the body with the essential vitamins, minerals, and antioxidants it needs to function optimally. Nutrient-rich foods, particularly those high in vitamins C and D, zinc, and selenium, play a critical role in strengthening the immune response. A diet rich in whole foods— such as fruits, vegetables, nuts, seeds, and legumes—helps to provide these necessary nutrients while minimizing the intake of processed foods, sugars, and additives that can burden the immune system.

Eating a balanced diet that supports gut health is also crucial, as a significant portion of the immune system resides in the gut. Probiotics from fermented foods like sauerkraut, kimchi, and kefir help maintain a healthy balance of gut bacteria, which in turn supports the immune system's ability to fight off infections and reduce inflammation.

The Role of Detoxification in Immune Support

Detoxification is essential in preventing the immune system from becoming overloaded by toxins and stress. The body's detox pathways—primarily through the liver, kidneys, lymphatic system, and skin—help to eliminate waste and reduce the toxic burden that can impair immune function. Regular detoxification practices, such as drinking purified water, consuming detoxifying herbs like dandelion and milk thistle, and eating fiber-rich foods, assist in flushing out toxins and reducing inflammation that can lead to immune fatigue.

Chapter 5: 17 Specific Natural Remedies for Immune Health

Supporting immune health through natural remedies is a key approach in holistic medicine. A combination of herbs, lifestyle adjustments, and nutrition can provide the body with the necessary tools to strengthen the immune system and maintain overall health. Here are 18 specific natural remedies that can be used to bolster immune function.

The appendix provides more details for each remedy.

1. Echinacea

2. Elderberry

3. Garlic

4. Ginger

5. Astragalus

6. Turmeric

7. Oregano Oil

8. Vitamin C

9. Zinc

10. Probiotics

11. Honey

12. Lemon Balm

13. Reishi Mushroom

14. Green Tea

15. Licorice Root

16. Thyme

17. Eucalyptus

Part 6:
Stress Management and Mental Health with Natural Remedies

Chapter 1: The Connection Between Stress and Overall Health

1.1 Understanding the Impact of Chronic Stress on the Body

Chronic stress is often described as a silent contributor to numerous health problems, affecting both physical and mental well-being. When the body is exposed to prolonged periods of stress, various systems become compromised, leading to conditions such as weakened immune function, hormonal imbalances, and digestive issues. Stress, in this way, disrupts the body's natural balance and can have far-reaching effects on overall health.

As covered in previous chapters, stress has several negative effects on the body:

- Weakened Immune Function
- Hormonal Imbalances
- Digestive Issues
- Inflammation and Long-Term Health Problems

1.2 The Stress Response: Fight or Flight

The body's stress response, commonly known as the "fight or flight" response, is a natural reaction to perceived danger or threats. This mechanism is essential for survival, as it prepares the body to either confront or flee from a dangerous situation. When the body perceives stress, the adrenal glands release hormones such as adrenaline and cortisol, which increase heart rate, raise blood pressure, and sharpen mental focus. However, when this response becomes prolonged due to chronic stress, it can overwhelm the adrenal glands and lead to a state of burnout.

Prolonged activation of the stress response, without adequate periods of recovery, places significant strain on the adrenal glands. The adrenal glands, located just above the kidneys, are responsible for producing cortisol, the hormone that helps regulate the body's stress response. When the body experiences chronic stress, the adrenal glands are forced to continuously produce cortisol, which can eventually lead to adrenal fatigue or burnout. In this state, the adrenal glands become exhausted, resulting in a range of physical and emotional symptoms, including extreme fatigue, difficulty concentrating, and weakened immune function.

Unaddressed emotional stress can manifest physically in a variety of ways. Headaches, insomnia, and fatigue are among the most common symptoms that arise when stress is prolonged. Stress-induced headaches are often caused by muscle tension in the neck and shoulders, which constricts blood flow to the brain and triggers pain. Insomnia is another common consequence of chronic stress, as elevated cortisol levels interfere with the production of melatonin, the hormone responsible for regulating sleep. Without adequate sleep, the body cannot repair and regenerate, further exacerbating stress and leading to exhaustion. Fatigue, both physical and mental, becomes a constant companion, as the body struggles to keep up with the demands of daily life while coping with chronic stress.

1.3 Breaking the Cycle of Chronic Stress

Breaking the cycle of chronic stress is crucial for restoring balance and preventing more serious health issues. Recognizing the signs of chronic stress is the first step in managing it proactively. These signs may include persistent feelings of overwhelm, frequent irritability or mood swings, difficulty sleeping, and physical symptoms such as headaches, digestive problems, or muscle tension. Once the signs of chronic stress are identified, it is important to implement natural techniques to restore balance.

One of the key strategies for managing stress is to address it at its source by identifying and reducing stressors wherever possible. This may involve setting boundaries at work, delegating tasks, or practicing time management to create more balance in daily life. However, when certain stressors cannot be eliminated, it becomes essential to develop coping mechanisms that support the body in handling stress more effectively.

Relaxation techniques such as deep breathing, meditation, and progressive muscle relaxation are highly effective in reducing the physical symptoms of stress and calming the nervous system. The parasympathetic nerve system of the body, which reduces blood pressure and heart rate in reaction to stress, is activated, for instance, by deep breathing exercises. Regular practice of these techniques helps the body recover from stress more quickly and prevents the buildup of tension.

Another natural technique for managing chronic stress is incorporating physical activity into daily routines. Exercise not only helps release tension from the muscles but also boosts the production of endorphins, the body's natural mood enhancers. Activities such as walking, yoga, or swimming provide gentle, restorative exercise that helps alleviate the effects of stress without placing additional strain on the body. Physical activity also promotes better sleep, which is crucial for allowing the body to recover from stress and restore energy levels.

Barbara O'Neill suggests incorporating herbal remedies as part of a holistic approach to stress management. Adaptogenic herbs such as ashwagandha, rhodiola, and holy basil are known for their ability to help the body adapt to stress and reduce cortisol levels. These herbs work by supporting the adrenal glands, helping them function more efficiently under stress, and preventing the onset of adrenal fatigue. Drinking herbal teas made from these adaptogens, or taking them in supplement form, can help modulate the body's stress response and provide a sense of calm and balance.

Establishing a consistent routine that includes moments of relaxation and self-care is key to breaking the cycle of chronic stress. This might involve setting aside time each day for meditation, enjoying a relaxing bath, or engaging in a hobby that brings joy and fulfillment. Prioritizing sleep is also essential, as restorative sleep allows the body to recover from the day's stressors and prepare for the next.

Chapter 2: Managing Anxiety and Depression with Herbal Remedies

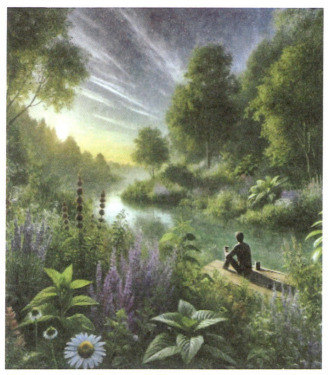

2.1 Anxiety and Depression: A Holistic Perspective

Barbara O'Neill views anxiety and depression as indicators that the body is signaling an imbalance, whether due to dietary factors, environmental influences, or lifestyle habits. Rather than seeing these mental health issues as purely psychological, the holistic approach suggests that physical health and emotional well-being are interconnected. When these signals emerge, it is a reminder that the body may require support on multiple levels—physically, mentally, and emotionally.

Diet and Mental Health

A core component of addressing anxiety and depression holistically involves evaluating and improving dietary habits. Nutritional deficiencies, particularly in essential vitamins and minerals, can profoundly affect brain function and mood. Diets high in processed foods, refined sugars, and unhealthy fats often exacerbate feelings of anxiety and depression. These types of foods lead to blood sugar imbalances, inflammation, and gut health disturbances, all of which can negatively affect mood.

The Role of Lifestyle in Mental Health

In addition to dietary improvements, lifestyle factors play a significant role in managing anxiety and depression. Regular physical activity is a powerful tool for improving mood, reducing stress, and boosting mental clarity. Exercise stimulates the release of endorphins, the body's natural "feel-good" chemicals, which help alleviate feelings of anxiety and depression. Activities like walking, yoga, and swimming can be particularly beneficial, as they promote both physical and mental relaxation without placing too much strain on the body.

Another essential lifestyle factor is ensuring adequate sleep. Sleep deprivation can lead to elevated cortisol levels and exacerbate symptoms of anxiety and depression. By prioritizing restful, restorative sleep, individuals can support their nervous system, balance hormones, and enhance emotional resilience.

Stress management is also crucial in addressing anxiety and depression. Chronic stress can trigger or worsen these mental health conditions by overwhelming the body and nervous system. Incorporating relaxation techniques such as meditation, deep breathing, or spending time in nature can help lower stress levels and promote a sense of calm. These practices activate the parasympathetic nervous system, which counteracts the stress response and supports emotional balance.

2.2 Ashwagandha: A Powerful Adaptogen

Ashwagandha is a powerful adaptogen, meaning it helps the body adapt to and manage stress more effectively. One of its key functions is lowering cortisol, the hormone that rises during times of stress. Elevated cortisol levels over prolonged periods can lead to various health problems, including anxiety, depression, weight gain, and weakened immunity. By helping to regulate cortisol levels, Ashwagandha provides a natural way to reduce the body's stress response.

Lowering Cortisol and Reducing Anxiety

Ashwagandha has been shown to be highly effective in reducing anxiety, particularly in individuals experiencing chronic stress. It functions by adjusting the hypothalamic-pituitary-adrenal (HPA) axis, which is in charge of regulating how the body reacts to stress. When this system is out of balance, cortisol levels remain elevated, which can lead to feelings of anxiety and overwhelm. By restoring balance to the HPA axis, Ashwagandha helps the body better manage stress and reduces anxiety symptoms.

In addition to its effects on cortisol, Ashwagandha has been found to improve mental clarity and focus. During periods of emotional stress, it is common for individuals to experience brain fog, difficulty concentrating, or memory problems. Ashwagandha supports cognitive function by promoting calm and reducing the mental fatigue that often accompanies prolonged stress. This makes it an excellent choice for those looking to enhance both mental and emotional resilience during challenging times.

How to Use Ashwagandha for Mental Health

Ashwagandha can be used in various forms, including capsules, powders, or tinctures, depending on personal preference. Many people choose to incorporate Ashwagandha powder into smoothies, teas, or warm milk to create a soothing, relaxing drink. Taken consistently, Ashwagandha can help reduce anxiety, improve mood, and promote a sense of well-being.

Barbara O'Neill suggests incorporating Ashwagandha into a holistic wellness routine that includes proper nutrition, regular physical activity, and relaxation practices. When used in combination with other lifestyle adjustments, Ashwagandha can provide long-term benefits for managing anxiety and depression.

2.3 Lemon Balm: Calming the Mind

Lemon balm (Melissa officinalis) has long been recognized for its soothing effects on the nervous system. Its calming properties make it an excellent herb for reducing anxiety, promoting relaxation, and helping to alleviate mild depression. Lemon balm contains active compounds that interact with the brain's neurotransmitters, particularly GABA (gamma-aminobutyric acid), which plays a role in reducing nervous tension and promoting a sense of calm. This natural herb has been traditionally used to help manage feelings of restlessness, agitation, and nervousness.

Lemon balm is particularly effective in cases of mild anxiety or when stress levels begin to interfere with daily life. It helps the body and mind relax without the sedative effects that other herbs may have, making it suitable for daytime use when focus and clarity are still needed. Barbara O'Neill recommends lemon balm for those who experience mild depression or anxiety, as it helps to gently uplift the mood and calm the racing thoughts that often accompany these conditions.

Recipes and Tips for Using Lemon Balm

Lemon balm is versatile and easy to incorporate into everyday routines, particularly in the form of teas and tinctures. A calming lemon balm tea can be made by steeping 1 to 2 teaspoons of dried lemon balm leaves in hot water for about 10 minutes. The tea can be enjoyed at any time of day to help reduce stress, but it is particularly effective when taken in the evening to help unwind before bed. The subtle lemon flavor makes it a refreshing yet soothing beverage that helps to ease tension.

Lemon balm tinctures are another option for those who prefer a more concentrated form of the herb. A tincture is typically made by soaking fresh lemon balm leaves in alcohol for several weeks, allowing the active compounds to infuse into the liquid. A few drops of lemon balm tincture can be added to water or taken directly under the tongue to quickly calm the mind and promote relaxation.

For those who enjoy cooking, lemon balm can also be added to salads, soups, or even used as a garnish for various dishes. The herb's mild lemony flavor pairs well with both savory and sweet foods, providing a subtle calming effect without overpowering the dish.

2.4 Valerian Root: Natural Sleep and Anxiety Support

Valerian root (Valeriana officinalis) has long been revered for its powerful effects on sleep and anxiety. Known as a natural sedative, valerian root is commonly used to promote better sleep quality and reduce symptoms of anxiety and tension. The active compounds in valerian, including valerenic acid and various volatile oils, interact with the brain's GABA receptors, much like lemon balm, to calm the nervous system and help the body relax.

Valerian root is particularly helpful for individuals who struggle with insomnia or find that stress and anxiety are interfering with their ability to fall asleep. It is known for its ability to improve both the duration and quality of sleep without causing the grogginess often associated with synthetic sleep aids. This makes valerian a popular choice for those seeking natural remedies for insomnia, particularly when sleep disturbances are linked to stress or nervous tension.

Using Valerian for Sleep and Stress Relief

Valerian root can be used in various forms, including teas, capsules, and tinctures, depending on the individual's needs and preferences. For those seeking a gentle approach to insomnia, valerian tea can be made by steeping 1 to 2 teaspoons of dried valerian root in hot water for 10 to 15 minutes. The tea is best consumed about 30 minutes to an hour before bedtime to allow the calming effects to take hold.

Some individuals may find the taste of valerian tea to be quite strong or earthy, which is why it is often blended with other herbs like chamomile or lemon balm to improve the flavor while still promoting relaxation. A popular bedtime blend may include valerian, lemon balm, and a touch of honey, creating a soothing tea that not only helps with sleep but also calms the mind after a stressful day.

Valerian tinctures provide a more concentrated dose of the herb and can be taken in a smaller volume than tea. Just a few drops of valerian tincture, taken directly under the tongue or added to water, can provide quick relief from anxiety or help prepare the body for sleep. This method is particularly useful for individuals who find it difficult to fall asleep due to racing thoughts or restlessness.

Valerian root capsules are another convenient option for those who prefer not to deal with the taste of the tea or tincture. Capsules are pre-measured, making it easy to take the correct dosage. However, it is essential to note that the effects of valerian root may vary from person to person, with some individuals experiencing immediate relief while others may require several days of regular use to notice its full benefits.

Considerations When Using Valerian

Although valerian root is a safe and effective natural remedy for most individuals, it is important to use it with care. Prolonged or excessive use of valerian can lead to grogginess or a slight "hangover" feeling the next morning for some people. For this reason, it is recommended to start with smaller doses and gradually increase if needed, paying attention to how the body responds.

Valerian is best used for short-term relief of sleep disturbances or anxiety, but it can also be incorporated into a long-term stress management plan when rotated with other calming herbs such as lemon balm or chamomile. Valerian is not typically recommended for pregnant or breastfeeding women, and anyone with underlying health conditions should consult a healthcare professional before using valerian root regularly.

Chapter 3: Breathing Exercises, Meditation, and Lifestyle Shifts for Mental Wellbeing

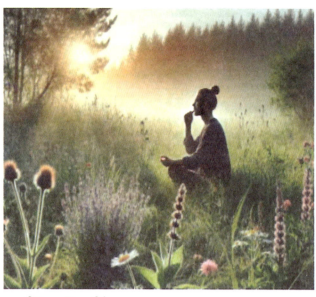

3.1 The Power of Deep Breathing

Deep, controlled breathing is one of the most effective ways to activate the parasympathetic nervous system, which is responsible for the body's "rest and digest" functions. This system works in contrast to the sympathetic nervous system, which governs the "fight or flight" response. When the body is under stress, the sympathetic nervous system is activated, causing an increase in heart rate, blood pressure, and cortisol levels. Deep breathing, however, triggers the parasympathetic nervous system, helping the body to relax and recover from stress.

By engaging in deep breathing exercises, individuals can lower their stress levels, reduce anxiety, and improve overall well-being. The slow, controlled inhalation and exhalation of deep breathing sends signals to the brain to calm down and shift away from a stress response. This practice also increases oxygen flow to the brain, enhancing mental clarity and promoting relaxation throughout the body.

Deep Breathing's Effect on Parasympathetic Nervous System Activation

When the parasympathetic nervous system is activated through deep breathing, the body experiences a number of physiological changes. Heart rate slows, blood pressure decreases, and cortisol levels — the stress hormone — are reduced. Additionally, deep breathing stimulates the vagus nerve, a key component of the parasympathetic system. The vagus nerve is responsible for regulating many of the body's internal organs, including the heart and digestive system.

Breathing deeply helps the body enter a state of homeostasis, where balance is restored, and stress is alleviated. Regular practice of deep breathing can help the body better manage acute stress, making it easier to return to a state of calm after a stressful event. This process is especially helpful for people who experience chronic stress, anxiety, or tension in their daily lives.

Barbara O'Neill's Recommended Breathing Exercises

Barbara O'Neill recommends several simple yet effective breathing exercises to calm the mind and reduce the physiological effects of stress. One of the most accessible techniques she suggests is **diaphragmatic breathing**, also known as belly breathing. In this method, the focus is on fully engaging the diaphragm, allowing the belly to expand with each inhale and contract with each exhale. This form of breathing ensures that the lungs are filled completely with air, maximizing oxygen intake.

To practice diaphragmatic breathing, sit or lie down in a comfortable position. Place one hand on the chest and the other on the abdomen. Inhale slowly through the nose, allowing the belly to rise as air fills the lungs. The hand on the chest should remain still, while the hand on the abdomen moves with each breath. Exhale slowly and completely, feeling the abdomen fall. Repeating this exercise for several minutes can significantly reduce stress and promote relaxation.

Another exercise O'Neill recommends is **4-7-8 breathing**, which involves inhaling for four counts, holding the breath for seven counts, and exhaling for eight counts. This technique is particularly effective for calming the nervous system before bedtime or during moments of high stress. The prolonged exhalation encourages the body to release tension and promotes a deeper sense of relaxation.

3.2 Meditation for Mental Clarity

Meditation is a powerful practice that not only reduces stress but also improves focus, creativity, and emotional resilience. By training the mind to stay present and focused, meditation helps to quiet the mental chatter that often leads to stress and anxiety. Regular meditation practice can lead to greater mental clarity, allowing individuals to think more clearly and make better decisions.

How Meditation Reduces Stress and Enhances Mental Function

Meditation works by encouraging mindfulness, which is the practice of being fully present in the current moment. When individuals meditate, they learn to observe their thoughts without judgment, which helps to create a sense of detachment from stressful or anxious thoughts. Over time, this practice can reduce the body's stress response, lower cortisol levels, and promote a sense of calm and well-being.

Moreover, meditation has been shown to increase gray matter in areas of the brain associated with emotional regulation and cognitive function. As a result, individuals who meditate regularly often report feeling more focused, creative, and emotionally resilient. The practice of meditation helps to rewire the brain, making it easier to manage stress, improve concentration, and enhance problem-solving abilities.

Simple Meditation Practices for Daily Life

Incorporating meditation into daily life doesn't require long sessions or complicated techniques. One of the simplest forms of meditation is **focused breathing meditation**, where individuals focus their attention solely on the breath. Sitting in a comfortable position, the individual closes their eyes and begins to observe the natural rhythm of their breathing. Each time the mind wanders, the individual gently brings their focus back to the breath. This practice helps to train the mind to stay present, which reduces stress and improves mental clarity.

Another effective meditation practice is **body scan meditation**, which involves focusing on different parts of the body to release tension and promote relaxation. To begin, lie down in a comfortable position and close your eyes. Start by focusing on the toes, noticing any sensations or tension. Gradually move your attention up through the legs, torso, arms, and head, consciously relaxing each area as you go. This practice not only reduces stress but also helps individuals become more aware of their body and any areas of tension that may need attention.

For those new to meditation, starting with just five to ten minutes a day can make a noticeable difference. Over time, as the practice becomes more comfortable, individuals can gradually increase the duration. The key to meditation is consistency, as regular practice helps to reinforce the benefits of mental clarity and emotional balance

3.3 Lifestyle Shifts for Managing Stress

Stress has become an inevitable part of modern life, but managing it effectively is key to maintaining overall health and well-being. Simple lifestyle changes can make a significant difference in how the body and mind cope with stress. Barbara O'Neill advocates for natural and practical solutions to manage stress, focusing on reconnecting with nature, regular physical activity, and reducing exposure to digital devices.

Reconnecting with Nature

One of the most effective ways to reduce stress is to spend time in nature. The calming effect of natural surroundings can help lower cortisol levels and improve mood. Taking time to walk in a park, hike in the mountains, or simply sit in a garden can significantly reduce the mental and emotional strain caused by daily life. Nature provides a space for relaxation and mindfulness, allowing the mind to reset and recover from stress.

Breathing in fresh air and being surrounded by greenery also supports the body's natural detoxification processes, aiding both physical and mental health. Exposure to natural light helps regulate circadian rhythms, which is essential for maintaining proper sleep cycles—another factor that directly impacts stress management. Spending time in nature encourages a slower pace, giving the body a chance to unwind and release tension that builds up during the day.

Reducing Exposure to Digital Devices

The constant use of digital devices can contribute to elevated stress levels. Prolonged exposure to screens, social media, and instant messaging creates mental clutter, which can overwhelm the mind and prevent it from properly unwinding. Additionally, blue light emitted by screens suppresses melatonin production, disrupting sleep and further exacerbating stress.

Limiting screen time, particularly before bed, is a crucial step in managing stress. Creating a digital detox routine—where time is spent away from devices—can help reduce mental fatigue and allow the brain to relax. Engaging in offline activities like reading, drawing, or spending time with loved ones can foster a sense of calm and promote better mental clarity.

Regular Physical Activity

Physical activity is one of the most effective ways to manage stress. Regular exercise not only improves physical health but also has a profound impact on mental well-being. When the body moves, endorphins—natural mood boosters—are released, helping to combat stress and anxiety. Barbara O'Neill recommends engaging in moderate forms of exercise such as yoga, walking, and stretching. These activities are gentle on the body while still providing the benefits of tension release and improved circulation.

Yoga is particularly beneficial for stress management because it combines physical movement with deep breathing and mindfulness. The practice encourages relaxation by helping the body release muscle tension and clear the mind of anxious thoughts. Yoga also promotes flexibility and strengthens the core muscles, which can reduce physical discomfort that may contribute to stress. The focus on deep, mindful breathing helps lower cortisol levels and brings the nervous system into a state of balance.

Walking is another simple yet powerful form of exercise that supports stress relief. Taking a walk, especially in nature, allows the mind to relax and process thoughts in a less pressured environment. Walking helps stimulate circulation, improves cardiovascular health, and promotes a sense of calm, making it an ideal daily practice for managing stress.

Stretching is also an excellent way to release muscle tension that builds up due to stress. Gentle stretching can be done throughout the day to relieve areas of tightness, particularly in the neck, shoulders, and lower back. Stretching not only improves flexibility but also increases blood flow to muscles, helping the body feel more relaxed and less tense.

Chapter 4: Enhancing Mental Clarity and Emotional Resilience Naturally

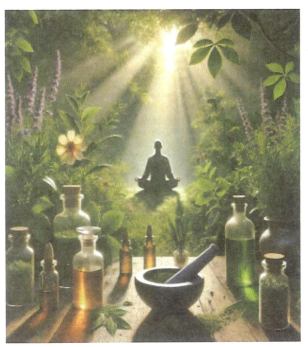

4.1 Improving Mental Clarity with Natural Remedies

Mental clarity and focus are often compromised by various factors such as stress, poor diet, and lack of sufficient sleep. Brain fog and mental fatigue, characterized by difficulty concentrating, forgetfulness, and a general feeling of mental sluggishness, are common complaints that many individuals face in today's fast-paced world. When the body and mind are consistently subjected to stressors, poor nutrition, or irregular sleep patterns, it is difficult to maintain cognitive function at an optimal level.

Barbara O'Neill emphasizes the importance of addressing the root causes of brain fog by targeting lifestyle habits and utilizing natural remedies to restore mental clarity. Improving one's diet, managing stress, and using specific herbs known for their cognitive-boosting properties are effective ways to combat mental fatigue and enhance focus.

The Role of Diet and Sleep in Mental Clarity

A poor diet lacking in essential nutrients can significantly affect brain function. Diets high in processed foods, sugars, and unhealthy fats deprive the brain of the vital nutrients it needs to function properly. Without the necessary vitamins, minerals, and antioxidants, the brain's capacity to concentrate and process information can decline. Incorporating nutrient-rich foods such as leafy greens, berries, nuts, and seeds into the diet can improve cognitive function. These foods are rich in antioxidants and essential fatty acids, which protect brain cells and support neurotransmitter function.

Sleep also plays a crucial role in mental clarity. Without sufficient rest, the brain cannot adequately process and store information. Consolidation of memories, emotional control, and cognitive processing all depend on sleep. Poor sleep patterns or insufficient sleep can lead to heightened stress, reduced cognitive function, and the development of brain fog.

Herbs to Enhance Focus and Combat Mental Fatigue

In addition to lifestyle changes, certain herbs are known to support brain health and improve focus. Adaptogenic herbs, in particular, help the body adapt to stress, which is often a major contributor to brain fog and mental fatigue. Herbs such as **rhodiola, ginseng,** and **ashwagandha** are well-known for their ability to increase energy, reduce stress, and improve mental clarity. These adaptogens work by regulating the body's stress response, promoting balance in the HPA axis, which controls how the body responds to stress.

Ginkgo biloba is another herb often used to enhance cognitive function. It improves circulation to the brain, allowing for better oxygenation of brain cells, which can lead to improved concentration and memory. This increased blood flow to the brain helps to combat mental fatigue and brain fog, making it easier to stay focused and alert throughout the day.

Bacopa monnieri, a traditional herb used in Ayurvedic medicine, is particularly beneficial for enhancing memory and reducing anxiety. It has been shown to improve cognitive performance by supporting neurotransmitter function and protecting the brain from oxidative damage. By incorporating these herbs into one's daily routine, it is possible to naturally enhance mental clarity and reduce the symptoms of brain fog.

4.2 Building Emotional Resilience

Emotional resilience is the ability to adapt to stress, adversity, and life's challenges with a positive mindset. It involves developing a set of mental and emotional tools that allow an individual to recover from setbacks and continue moving forward. Emotional resilience is crucial not only for maintaining mental health but also for protecting physical health, as chronic stress can negatively affect the body in multiple ways.

Strategies for Cultivating Emotional Resilience

One of the most effective ways to build emotional resilience is through **journaling**. Writing about one's thoughts and feelings allows for emotional processing and helps individuals gain clarity about their experiences. Journaling can also serve as a stress-relief technique, helping to externalize worries and reduce the mental load that often comes with stressful situations. By expressing emotions through writing, individuals can release built-up tension and gain insight into how they can approach challenges more effectively.

Another key practice for developing emotional resilience is **gratitude**. Focusing on what is going well, rather than solely on problems, can shift one's mindset and create a sense of emotional balance. Regularly practicing gratitude, whether through keeping a gratitude journal or simply taking a moment each day to reflect on positive experiences, can lead to a more optimistic outlook. Gratitude has been shown to improve mental well-being and reduce stress by helping individuals focus on positive aspects of their lives rather than dwelling on challenges.

Self-compassion is another powerful tool for building emotional resilience. Rather than being overly self-critical during times of difficulty, practicing self-compassion involves treating oneself with kindness and understanding. Acknowledging that setbacks and failures are a part of the human experience can help reduce feelings of frustration and disappointment. This shift in perspective allows for faster recovery from adversity and fosters emotional growth.

In addition to these mental practices, **physical movement** plays a significant role in building resilience. Exercise, particularly forms of movement that encourage mindfulness, such as yoga or tai chi, helps to release stress and tension from the body. Physical activity also promotes the release of endorphins, which are natural mood elevators, further supporting emotional well-being.

Developing emotional resilience takes time and practice, but with consistent effort, it is possible to navigate life's challenges with greater ease. By focusing on mental and emotional health, individuals can reduce the negative impact of stress on their bodies and minds, ultimately improving their overall well-being.

4.3 Nutrition's Role in Mental Wellbeing

Nutrition plays a crucial role in supporting mental health, brain function, and mood regulation. A balanced, nutrient-rich diet not only fuels the body but also provides the brain with the necessary components to function optimally. Certain nutrients have been shown to influence mood, mental clarity, and even stress levels, highlighting the profound connection between what we eat and how we feel.

Omega-3 Fatty Acids for Brain Health

Omega-3 fatty acids are essential for maintaining brain health and cognitive function. These healthy fats are integral components of brain cell membranes and are known to promote communication between brain cells. Omega-3s, particularly the types found in fatty fish like salmon, mackerel, and sardines, have been shown to reduce inflammation in the brain, which is linked to depression and other mood disorders.

Omega-3s also play a role in regulating neurotransmitters, such as serotonin and dopamine, which are responsible for mood regulation. By improving the fluidity of brain cell membranes, these fats enhance the functioning of these neurotransmitters, helping to alleviate symptoms of depression and anxiety.

Magnesium for Stress and Relaxation

Magnesium is another critical nutrient that supports mental wellbeing. Often referred to as the "relaxation mineral," magnesium helps regulate the body's stress response. It is involved in the regulation of the HPA axis, which controls the release of stress hormones like cortisol. When magnesium levels are adequate, the body is better equipped to manage stress and maintain a calm, balanced state.

In addition to reducing stress, magnesium also supports sleep, which is essential for mental clarity and mood stability. Foods rich in magnesium, such as leafy greens, nuts, seeds, and whole grains, are beneficial in promoting relaxation and reducing anxiety.

B-Vitamins for Energy and Mental Clarity

B-vitamins, particularly B6, B9 (folate), and B12, are essential for brain function and mental clarity. These vitamins are involved in the production of neurotransmitters, including serotonin and dopamine, which regulate mood and emotional wellbeing. Deficiencies in B-vitamins have been linked to mood disorders, including depression and anxiety.

B-vitamins also support energy production by helping the body convert food into usable energy, which is critical for mental clarity and focus. Foods rich in B-vitamins include whole grains, legumes, eggs, and leafy greens.

Chapter 5: 16 Natural Remedies for Stress Management and Mental Health

Managing stress and maintaining mental health through natural remedies is a holistic approach that incorporates the use of herbs, relaxation techniques, and lifestyle adjustments. Natural remedies can help regulate the body's stress response, reduce anxiety, and support overall emotional well-being. Below are 18 natural remedies that can aid in stress management and improve mental health.

The appendix provides more details for each remedy.

1. Valerian Root

2. Chamomile

3. Lavender

4. Passionflower

5. Ashwagandha

6. Rhodiola Rosea

7. Lemon Balm

8. Magnesium

9. Omega-3 Fatty Acids

10. Ginseng

11. B-Complex Vitamins

12. Holy Basil

13. Ashwagandha Tea

14. Rhodiola Rosea Capsules

15. Skullcap Tea

16. St. John's Wort Tincture

Part 7:
Physical Activity and Fitness for Holistic Health

Chapter 1: The Importance of Movement in Natural Healing

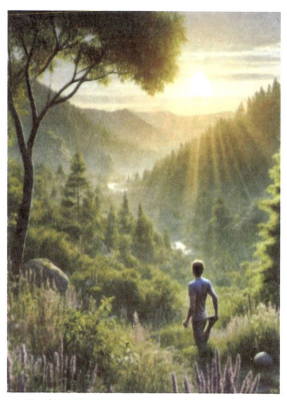

1.1 Movement as a Healing Force

Movement is one of the most powerful tools for maintaining and improving overall health. Regular physical activity is not solely about fitness but plays a vital role in the functioning of various bodily systems. According to Barbara O'Neill, movement supports circulation, digestion, and detoxification, ensuring the body's systems work in harmony and balance.

Circulation and Oxygen Delivery

One of the primary benefits of movement is its ability to improve circulation, which is critical for the delivery of oxygen and nutrients to every cell in the body. When circulation is optimized, blood flow increases, bringing with it essential nutrients and oxygen to the tissues and organs. This process allows cells to function at their best, supporting overall vitality.

Increased circulation also aids in the removal of waste products from the body. The lymphatic system, which plays a key role in detoxification, relies on physical movement to function effectively. Unlike the circulatory system, which has the heart to pump blood, the lymphatic system requires movement to propel lymph fluid through the body. Regular physical activity stimulates the flow of lymph, helping to flush out toxins, pathogens, and other unwanted materials.

Digestion and Gut Health

Movement also plays a significant role in supporting digestion. When the body is physically active, the muscles involved in digestion—particularly those in the abdomen—are stimulated, which helps food move more efficiently through the digestive tract. This enhanced motility can prevent issues such as constipation and bloating, which can arise when digestion is sluggish.

Physical activity promotes the production of digestive enzymes, which are crucial for breaking down food and absorbing nutrients. It also encourages the growth of healthy gut bacteria, which are essential for maintaining a balanced microbiome. A healthy gut microbiome not only aids

Detoxification

Detoxification is another critical process that is enhanced by regular movement. Physical activity encourages the body to eliminate toxins through multiple channels, including sweat, urine, and the lymphatic system. Sweating during exercise allows the skin, one of the body's primary detoxification organs, to release toxins that accumulate in the tissues.

Additionally, movement stimulates the kidneys and liver—organs responsible for filtering toxins out of the blood. By increasing circulation and fluid movement, the body is able to more effectively process and eliminate waste, reducing the toxic load that can contribute to various health problems.

Keeping the Body in Balance

Overall, movement helps maintain balance within the body by regulating various systems. Beyond the physical benefits of improved circulation, digestion, and detoxification, regular physical activity also has a profound effect on the nervous and endocrine systems, which play crucial roles in stress management and hormone regulation.

Additionally, regular movement supports musculoskeletal health by maintaining muscle tone, flexibility, and joint mobility. As people age, staying physically active becomes even more important to prevent the loss of muscle mass and joint stiffness, which can lead to injury or reduced mobility.

1.2 How Sedentary Lifestyles Lead to Health Problems

A sedentary lifestyle can have far-reaching consequences on overall health, contributing to a variety of chronic conditions, including heart disease, diabetes, and obesity. When the body is deprived of regular movement, essential physiological functions, such as circulation and joint mobility, become impaired, leading to both immediate discomfort and long-term health risks.

The Impact of Sedentary Lifestyles on Joint Health

One of the most immediate effects of a sedentary lifestyle is stiffness in the joints. Regular movement helps keep the joints lubricated and functional by promoting the production of synovial fluid, which cushions the joints and prevents friction between bones. Without adequate movement, the joints become stiff, and over time, this can lead to pain and a reduced range of motion.

A lack of physical activity also contributes to the weakening of the muscles that support the joints, further exacerbating joint pain and stiffness. In severe cases, prolonged inactivity can increase the risk of developing conditions such as arthritis or exacerbate existing joint problems. Regular, moderate exercise can help maintain joint flexibility and prevent the degeneration of cartilage, which is crucial for pain-free movement.

Poor Circulation and Its Health Implications

Another significant consequence of a sedentary lifestyle is poor circulation. When the body remains stationary for extended periods, blood flow becomes sluggish, particularly in the lower extremities. This can lead to a variety of health issues, ranging from swollen legs and varicose veins to more serious conditions like deep vein thrombosis (DVT), a potentially life-threatening condition caused by blood clots forming in the veins.

Increased Risk of Chronic Conditions

A sedentary lifestyle is closely linked to the development of several chronic conditions, including heart disease, diabetes, and obesity. Without regular physical activity, the body's metabolism slows down, leading to weight gain and fat accumulation, particularly around the abdomen. This visceral fat is not only unsightly but also dangerous, as it is associated with an increased risk of heart disease and type 2 diabetes.

Inactivity also leads to insulin resistance, a condition in which the body's cells become less responsive to insulin, resulting in elevated blood sugar levels. Over time, this can progress to type 2 diabetes, a condition that significantly increases the risk of other health complications, including kidney disease, nerve damage, and cardiovascular problems.

Obesity, which is often a result of both poor diet and inactivity, further compounds these health risks. Excess weight places additional strain on the joints, exacerbating conditions such as osteoarthritis, while also contributing to the development of sleep apnea, high cholesterol, and other metabolic disorders.

1.3 The Connection Between Physical Activity and Mental Wellbeing

Physical activity is a powerful tool for maintaining not only physical health but also mental wellbeing. Barbara O'Neill highlights the strong connection between regular movement and improved mental health, emphasizing how physical activity helps to reduce stress, enhance mood, and combat conditions such as anxiety and depression. This connection is primarily due to the release of endorphins during exercise, which act as natural mood elevators.

One of the most immediate effects of physical activity is its ability to reduce stress. Exercise encourages the body to release endorphins, chemicals in the brain that act as natural painkillers and stress relievers. These endorphins interact with receptors in the brain, reducing the perception of pain and triggering positive feelings. As a result, individuals who engage in regular physical activity often experience lower levels of stress and anxiety.

Exercise is a well-established method for improving mood and combating depression. Physical activity increases the production of neurotransmitters like serotonin and dopamine, which are crucial for regulating mood and emotions. These neurotransmitters are often lower in individuals suffering from depression, making regular exercise a key part of natural mental health management.

The act of moving the body and engaging in rhythmic, repetitive activities such as walking, running, or cycling can also serve as a form of meditation, helping individuals clear their minds and focus on the present moment. This meditative effect, combined with the physical release of stress through movement, offers a powerful tool for managing depression and lifting one's mood.

Studies have shown that people who maintain an active lifestyle are at a lower risk of developing neurodegenerative conditions such as Alzheimer's disease. This protective effect is due to the consistent stimulation of brain cells and the maintenance of healthy blood flow, which keeps the brain functioning optimally as it ages.

Physical activity can also help improve mental clarity by reducing mental fatigue and enhancing energy levels. Exercise increases oxygen intake and improves circulation, which in turn helps the brain function more efficiently. Many people find that after a session of physical activity, they feel more alert, focused, and mentally sharp. This is because the physical exertion helps to eliminate feelings of sluggishness, replacing them with a heightened sense of clarity and vitality.

Chapter 2: Exercises That Promote Healing – Yoga, Walking, and Stretching

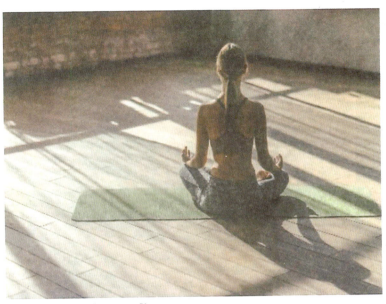

2.1 Yoga: A Gentle Path to Healing

Yoga has long been recognized as a holistic practice that not only enhances physical flexibility, strength, and balance but also promotes relaxation and mindfulness. Its gentle, yet effective, approach makes it an ideal form of exercise for individuals of all ages and fitness levels. Through various poses and controlled breathing, yoga works to improve the body's well-being by addressing both physical and mental health.

Enhancing Flexibility, Strength, and Balance

Yoga's primary benefit lies in its ability to improve flexibility. The stretches involved in many yoga poses target key muscle groups and joints, gradually increasing the body's range of motion. This is particularly beneficial for individuals who experience stiffness or limited mobility. Over time, regular yoga practice helps loosen tight muscles, making movements smoother and less restricted.

In addition to flexibility, yoga is also effective at building strength. Many yoga poses require the use of body weight to engage multiple muscle groups simultaneously, promoting core strength, stability, and endurance. Holding poses like the plank, warrior, or downward-facing dog strengthens the muscles in the arms, legs, and abdomen. The balance component of yoga further reinforces muscular control, helping to prevent falls and injuries, especially in older adults.

Balance training in yoga involves poses such as tree pose or eagle pose, where the individual must maintain their stance while holding a particular position. Proprioception, or the body's awareness of its position in space, is improved by these workouts, which improves stability and coordination. For those recovering from injury or looking to maintain mobility, yoga provides an accessible, gentle means to improve balance.

Supporting Detoxification and Digestion

Beyond the physical benefits, yoga can play a crucial role in detoxification and supporting digestive health. Certain yoga poses stimulate internal organs, promoting the elimination of toxins from the body. Twisting poses, such as revolved chair pose or seated spinal twist, gently massage the abdominal organs, enhancing blood flow and supporting liver and kidney function. These movements help the body's natural detoxification processes by increasing circulation and aiding in the removal of waste products.

Furthermore, yoga supports healthy digestion. Forward bends and twists stimulate the digestive organs, encouraging the movement of food through the digestive tract. Poses such as the seated forward bend or the supine twist apply gentle pressure to the abdomen, helping alleviate issues like constipation or bloating. The deep breathing exercises commonly practiced during yoga sessions also improve oxygen flow to the digestive system, optimizing its function and reducing discomfort.

Alleviating Stress and Promoting Mindfulness

Yoga is widely known for its ability to reduce stress and promote mindfulness. The combination of physical movement and controlled breathing helps calm the nervous system, lowering cortisol levels and reducing feelings of anxiety. Through focused breathing, such as pranayama techniques, individuals learn to center their thoughts and bring their awareness into the present moment, fostering a state of mindfulness.

This mindful awareness is further enhanced by the meditative aspect of yoga. Whether through a dedicated meditation session at the end of a yoga practice or by holding poses with intention and focus, yoga teaches practitioners to tune in to their bodies and quiet the mind. The practice helps individuals develop resilience against stress, improving mental clarity and emotional balance. Regular yoga practice thus becomes a powerful tool for managing the pressures of everyday life while promoting overall mental well-being.

2.2 Walking: The Simplicity of Movement

Walking is one of the simplest and most accessible forms of exercise. Despite its simplicity, it is an incredibly effective way to support physical health, particularly when combined with the restorative benefits of spending time in nature. Walking is suitable for all fitness levels, making it an ideal form of exercise for individuals who may be looking for a low-impact, gentle way to stay active.

Cardiovascular Health and Circulation

Regular walking has been shown to significantly improve cardiovascular health. Walking speeds up the heart rate, strengthening the heart muscle and improving circulation. This improved circulation helps deliver oxygen and nutrients to tissues throughout the body, supporting overall vitality. Regular cardiovascular activity, like walking, reduces the risk of heart disease, hypertension, and stroke by keeping blood pressure within a healthy range.

Walking also helps maintain healthy cholesterol levels. It raises levels of high-density lipoprotein (HDL), the "good" cholesterol, while lowering levels of low-density lipoprotein (LDL), or "bad" cholesterol. Maintaining these healthy levels is crucial for reducing the buildup of plaque in the arteries, which can lead to cardiovascular complications.

Supporting Weight Management and Joint Health

For individuals looking to manage their weight, walking is a highly effective exercise. Walking burns calories, contributing to a healthy energy balance. It is also a weight-bearing exercise, meaning it helps maintain bone density and muscle mass, which are crucial for metabolic health. Engaging in regular walks, particularly at a brisk pace, can help burn fat and prevent unwanted weight gain.

Despite being a weight-bearing activity, walking is gentle on the joints, making it ideal for individuals with joint pain or those at risk of injury. Unlike high-impact exercises such as running or jumping, walking provides a lower-intensity workout that minimizes strain on the knees, hips, and ankles. This makes it a safe and sustainable form of exercise for individuals with conditions like arthritis or those recovering from joint-related injuries.

2.3 The Importance of Stretching for Muscle and Joint Health

Stretching plays a crucial role in maintaining muscle and joint health. It is essential not only for enhancing flexibility but also for preventing injury and promoting overall physical well-being. When muscles and joints are regularly stretched, they remain limber, reducing the likelihood of stiffness, particularly for those with sedentary lifestyles. Regular stretching helps improve circulation, allowing oxygen and nutrients to reach the muscles and joints more efficiently, which in turn supports recovery and reduces discomfort.

Maintaining Flexibility and Mobility

Flexibility is a key component of physical fitness, but it is often overlooked. The body's muscles and joints are designed to move through a full range of motion, and when this range is restricted due to tightness or lack of flexibility, it can lead to discomfort and even injury. Stretching helps maintain the flexibility of muscles and tendons, which is important for smooth, pain-free movement. Whether you are sitting for long periods at a desk or engaging in physical activities, stretching can alleviate tension and improve overall mobility.

For those with sedentary jobs, where sitting for extended periods can lead to tight hips, hamstrings, and lower back pain, regular stretching is especially important. Sitting for long hours can shorten certain muscles, leading to imbalances and reduced mobility over time. Incorporating simple stretching routines that target areas prone to tightness, such as the hip flexors, lower back, and shoulders, can help prevent these issues from developing.

Injury Prevention Through Stretching

In addition to enhancing flexibility, stretching plays a significant role in injury prevention. Muscles that are flexible and well-stretched are less likely to become injured during physical activity. Stretching before and after exercise helps prepare the muscles for movement and aids in the recovery process by reducing muscle stiffness and improving circulation. When muscles are tight and inflexible, they are more prone to strains, tears, and other injuries.

Stretching also improves joint health by promoting the lubrication of joints and reducing the risk of joint stiffness. Regularly stretching the joints, especially those that bear weight like the knees and hips, helps to maintain their integrity and function. By keeping the muscles and joints limber, individuals can reduce their risk of experiencing pain or injury, even as they age.

Stretching Routines for Enhancing Mobility

Barbara O'Neill recommends incorporating simple, effective stretching routines into daily life to maintain mobility and prevent pain. These routines do not need to be time-consuming or complex; even a few minutes of stretching each day can make a significant difference. For those with sedentary jobs, stretching the neck, shoulders, and lower back can help relieve tension that builds up throughout the day. Standing stretches, such as forward folds to stretch the hamstrings and calf muscles, are effective for improving circulation and reducing stiffness in the legs.

Dynamic stretches, which involve movement rather than holding a position, are ideal for warming up before physical activity. Examples include leg swings, arm circles, and gentle lunges to engage the muscles and joints before more intense exercise. After exercise, static stretches, which are held for longer periods, help the muscles cool down and recover, reducing soreness and stiffness.

Chapter 3: Natural Pain Relief for Muscle Recovery – Arnica, Turmeric, and Magnesium

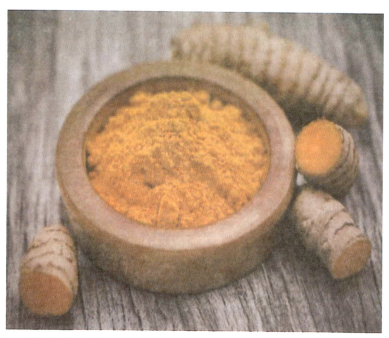

3.1 Natural Solutions for Muscle Recovery

Muscle recovery is an essential part of maintaining overall health, especially after physical activity. Without proper recovery, muscles can become sore, inflamed, and prone to injury. Natural remedies such as arnica, turmeric, and magnesium are highly effective in supporting the body's healing process and reducing inflammation after exercise or physical exertion.

3.2 Arnica: A Time-Tested Remedy for Muscle Pain

Arnica has been widely recognized for its remarkable ability to relieve muscle soreness, bruises, and joint pain due to its powerful anti-inflammatory properties. Arnica comes from the Arnica montana plant and has been used for centuries in traditional medicine to treat various forms of physical trauma. Its anti-inflammatory and analgesic effects make it a go-to remedy for reducing swelling, alleviating pain, and promoting the healing of bruised or injured tissue.

How Arnica Works for Muscle Pain

The key compounds in arnica, including helenalin, are responsible for its potent anti-inflammatory properties. Helenalin acts by inhibiting the production of inflammatory cytokines, which are molecules that contribute to inflammation and pain in the body. When arnica is applied topically, it can penetrate the skin and reduce inflammation in the underlying muscles and tissues, helping to relieve muscle pain and stiffness.

Arnica is particularly effective when applied after physical activity, as it helps soothe sore muscles and prevent stiffness caused by overexertion. It is often used by athletes or individuals recovering from physical strain because of its ability to speed up the healing process. Additionally, it can be useful for reducing the appearance and discomfort of bruising after an injury. Bruises occur when small blood vessels are damaged, and arnica helps to reduce the swelling and discoloration that accompany these minor injuries.

Arnica for Joint Pain

Arnica's anti-inflammatory action also extends to joint pain, making it a valuable remedy for conditions like arthritis. Joint pain often results from inflammation in the joints, leading to stiffness, discomfort, and reduced mobility. By applying arnica gel or oil directly to the affected areas, individuals can experience relief from pain and improved joint flexibility. Arnica helps to reduce inflammation in the synovial membrane, which lines the joints and can become inflamed in cases of arthritis or injury.

Barbara O'Neill recommends using arnica gel or oil for topical application after physical activity to help alleviate muscle soreness and reduce inflammation. Arnica products can be applied several times a day to the affected areas, massaging gently until the product is absorbed into the skin. The convenience of using arnica topically allows for targeted relief without the potential side effects that may come with oral anti-inflammatory medications.

Using Arnica Safely

While arnica is highly effective when used externally, it is important to note that it should not be taken internally unless it is in a homeopathic preparation specifically designed for ingestion. Arnica in its raw form can be toxic if consumed, so it is best used topically as a gel, cream, or oil. For individuals with sensitive skin, it is recommended to do a patch test before using arnica extensively, as some people may experience mild skin irritation.

Arnica offers a natural and time-tested remedy for muscle pain, joint discomfort, and the treatment of bruises, making it a valuable addition to any post-exercise recovery routine.

3.3 Turmeric: A Natural Anti-Inflammatory

Turmeric has earned a reputation as one of the most powerful natural anti-inflammatory agents, largely due to its active compound, curcumin. Curcumin is responsible for the vibrant yellow color of turmeric and has been extensively studied for its ability to combat inflammation and reduce pain. Whether used to relieve muscle soreness after exercise or to manage chronic joint pain, turmeric offers a potent, natural solution for inflammation-related issues.

Turmeric for Joint Health

In addition to its benefits for muscle pain, turmeric is also highly regarded for its ability to support joint health. Inflammatory conditions like arthritis, particularly osteoarthritis and rheumatoid arthritis, cause chronic pain and swelling in the joints. The anti-inflammatory effects of curcumin can help reduce joint pain and improve function, making turmeric an excellent natural alternative to traditional medications.

Turmeric also contains antioxidant properties that protect the body's cells from oxidative stress, which can contribute to inflammation and joint degradation over time. By reducing oxidative stress and inhibiting inflammatory processes, turmeric can slow down the progression of joint damage in individuals suffering from arthritis or other degenerative joint conditions.

Incorporating Turmeric into Your Routine

Barbara O'Neill suggests incorporating turmeric into your daily routine through a variety of methods, such as golden milk, teas, or supplements. Golden milk, a traditional Ayurvedic drink, combines turmeric with milk (or plant-based alternatives), black pepper, and sometimes other warming spices like cinnamon and ginger. The addition of black pepper is particularly important, as it contains piperine, a compound that enhances the absorption of curcumin in the body.

3.4 Magnesium: Essential for Muscle Relaxation

Magnesium is a crucial mineral that plays a vital role in muscle relaxation, preventing cramps, and promoting overall muscle recovery. Its importance is often underestimated, yet it is essential for proper muscle function, nerve transmission, and even energy production. Without adequate magnesium, muscles can become tense and prone to cramping, leading to discomfort and impaired movement.

The Role of Magnesium in Muscle Function

Magnesium is involved in numerous biochemical reactions within the body, many of which are directly linked to muscle function. This mineral helps regulate calcium levels, which is crucial because calcium is responsible for muscle contraction. Magnesium works by balancing calcium's action, ensuring that after a muscle contracts, it can relax properly. Without enough magnesium, muscles can stay in a state of contraction, leading to cramping, stiffness, and tension.

For athletes or individuals who engage in regular physical activity, ensuring an adequate intake of magnesium is especially important. Magnesium supports the recovery process after exercise by reducing muscle soreness and preventing spasms or cramps that can occur due to intense or prolonged activity. Additionally, it aids in reducing the buildup of lactic acid in the muscles, which is a byproduct of exercise and can contribute to post-workout soreness.

Dietary Sources of Magnesium

One of the best ways to maintain proper magnesium levels is through diet. Leafy greens like spinach and kale, legumes like black beans and chickpeas, nuts and seeds like almonds, and whole grains are examples of foods high in magnesium. Additionally, foods like bananas, avocados, and dark chocolate are also good sources of magnesium.

Barbara O'Neill emphasizes that many people do not get enough magnesium from their diet alone, especially if they consume a lot of processed or refined foods, which tend to be low in this important mineral. In such cases, magnesium supplementation may be necessary to support muscle health and overall well-being.

Magnesium supplements come in a variety of forms, such as magnesium oxide, magnesium glycinate, and magnesium citrate. Each has different absorption rates, so it is important to choose a form that is well-tolerated and effectively absorbed by the body. Magnesium glycinate is often recommended for its high bioavailability and gentle effects on the digestive system, making it a good option for individuals who may experience GI issues with other forms of magnesium.

Signs of Magnesium Deficiency

Magnesium deficiency is more common than many people realize and can lead to a variety of symptoms, including muscle cramps, fatigue, and headaches. In more severe cases, magnesium deficiency can cause anxiety, irritability, and even heart palpitations. Because magnesium is involved in nerve transmission, low levels of this mineral can result in nerve-related issues, such as tingling sensations or muscle twitches.

For individuals who frequently experience muscle cramps or tension, increasing magnesium intake through diet or supplementation can provide significant relief. Additionally, magnesium can support better sleep, as it helps relax the muscles and the nervous system, promoting a state of calm that is conducive to rest and recovery.

Chapter 4: Staying Fit at Any Age and Life Stage

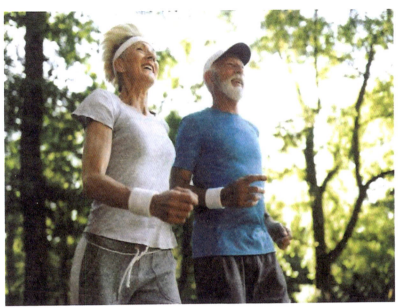

4.1 Maintaining Fitness in Every Stage of Life

Physical activity is essential for maintaining health, strength, and flexibility at every stage of life. While the intensity and type of exercise may vary depending on age, movement remains a critical component of overall well-being, helping to prevent chronic diseases, support mental health, and improve quality of life.

Different life stages have different fitness requirements to be healthy. That's why there are specific recommendations depending on a person's age – that ensures that the exercise don't overexert and cause other problems.

4.2 Fitness Tips for Older Adults

Maintaining physical fitness becomes increasingly important as the body ages, yet it can also become more challenging. For older adults, staying active not only helps preserve physical health but also enhances mental and emotional well-being. Engaging in gentle exercises such as walking, yoga, and swimming offers a safe and effective way for older adults to stay fit without putting undue strain on the body.

Walking: A Simple but Effective Exercise

Walking is one of the simplest forms of exercise and offers a variety of benefits for older adults. It helps improve cardiovascular health, strengthens the muscles, and supports joint mobility. Regular walking can also help maintain a healthy weight, improve balance, and reduce the risk of falls, which is a common concern for older adults.

Yoga to Build Strength and Flexibility

Yoga combines gentle movements with breathwork and mindfulness. The slow, controlled movements in yoga help improve flexibility, balance, and strength, which are critical for maintaining independence as the body ages. Many yoga poses focus on improving balance, a key factor in fall prevention. For older adults, staying steady on their feet is crucial, and regular yoga practice helps to build the necessary core strength and flexibility to maintain stability. Chair yoga, a modified form of yoga, is also available for those with limited mobility, allowing them to enjoy the benefits of yoga while seated.

Swimming: Low-Impact Exercise for Joint Health

Swimming is a highly recommended exercise for older adults, particularly those with joint pain or arthritis. The buoyancy of water supports the body, reducing the impact on the joints while allowing for a full range of motion. Swimming strengthens the muscles, improves cardiovascular health, and enhances flexibility, all without causing the wear and tear associated with high-impact exercises.

In addition to swimming, water aerobics or water walking are also beneficial for joint health. These activities provide resistance without putting stress on the joints, making them ideal for maintaining muscle tone and flexibility in older adults.

Maintaining Bone Density and Joint Health

As the body ages, maintaining bone density and joint health becomes critical to avoid conditions such as osteoporosis and arthritis. Regular movement plays a crucial role in keeping the bones strong and the joints flexible. Weight-bearing exercises, such as walking or light resistance training, help stimulate bone formation and slow down bone loss.

4.3 Integrating Movement into Everyday Life

Incorporating movement into everyday life is essential for maintaining overall health and well-being. Movement doesn't have to be strenuous or time-consuming; small adjustments to daily routines can make a significant difference in staying active. Barbara O'Neill suggests that simple strategies such as taking short walks, standing more frequently, and incorporating regular stretches can be highly effective in keeping the body mobile and promoting circulation.

Short Walks and Standing More Often

One of the easiest ways to integrate movement into a busy schedule is by taking short walks throughout the day. Walking not only helps improve circulation but also boosts energy levels and enhances mental clarity. Even a ten-minute walk can make a difference in combating the sedentary effects of sitting for extended periods. For those with desk jobs, standing up and walking around every hour helps to prevent stiffness and promotes better posture. O'Neill emphasizes that even small movements like standing during phone calls or opting for stairs instead of elevators contribute to overall physical well-being.

Stretching and Regular Movement

Stretching is another simple yet effective way to incorporate movement into a busy life. Frequent stretching promotes injury prevention, decreased muscular tension, and flexibility. It can be easily integrated into daily routines, such as stretching in the morning, during breaks at work, or before bedtime. Simple stretches targeting areas like the neck, shoulders, and lower back can help alleviate the stiffness that often results from sitting or standing for long periods.

Chapter 5: Natural Remedies for Muscle Recovery and Physical Activity Support

Physical activity, whether moderate or intense, places strain on the muscles and body. After exertion, it's essential to support recovery to prevent muscle fatigue, soreness, and injury. Natural remedies have been used for centuries to ease muscle discomfort, reduce inflammation, and accelerate the healing process. In this chapter, we'll explore ten powerful herbal remedies and their application for muscle recovery and physical activity support. Each remedy can be integrated into a holistic recovery routine to enhance the body's natural healing capabilities.

The appendix provides more details for each remedy.

Arnica Gel

Turmeric Golden Milk

Magnesium Oil

Boswellia Capsules

Ginger and Honey Tea

Peppermint Oil (for Muscle Rub)

Comfrey Cream

Rosemary Massage Oil

Chamomile Tea (for Relaxation and Muscle Tension)

Epsom Salt Baths (with Lavender Essential Oil)

St. John's Wort Oil

Ashwagandha Capsules

Lavender Essential Oil (for Massage)

Devil's Claw Capsules

Calendula Oil

Valerian Root (for Relaxation)

Green Tea

Willow Bark Extract

Part 8:
Women's Health and
Hormonal Balance

Chapter 1: Herbal Remedies for Menstrual Health and Menopause

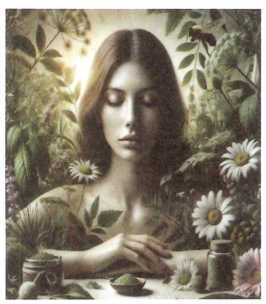

1.1 The Unique Challenges of Women's Health

Women's health is a complex and multifaceted area that requires a specialized approach, especially when considering the unique biological processes that women experience throughout their lives. From puberty through to menopause, hormonal fluctuations play a significant role in determining a woman's physical, emotional, and mental well-being. These hormonal changes, if unbalanced, can lead to a variety of health challenges, including menstrual irregularities, mood swings, fatigue, and other more serious conditions. The key to addressing these challenges lies in understanding the intricate connection between a woman's hormonal system and overall health.

Hormonal Balance Throughout a Woman's Life

Hormones are chemical messengers that regulate many critical functions in the body, including metabolism, reproduction, and mood. In women, hormones such as estrogen, progesterone, and testosterone fluctuate throughout the menstrual cycle and life stages like pregnancy and menopause. These fluctuations are natural, but when hormones become imbalanced, they can cause a range of symptoms that affect both physical and emotional health.

During **puberty**, for instance, the body experiences a surge in hormone production, leading to the development of secondary sexual characteristics and the onset of menstruation. However, for many young women, the transition into menstruation can be accompanied by symptoms such as irregular cycles, severe cramping, or emotional instability due to hormonal imbalances. These symptoms are often signs that the body's delicate hormonal balance is struggling to adjust, which can be exacerbated by factors such as poor diet, stress, or environmental toxins.

The Menstrual Cycle and Its Impact on Health

The menstrual cycle is one of the most visible and impactful expressions of hormonal fluctuations in women's health. Each month, a finely tuned interaction between estrogen and progesterone regulates the cycle, preparing the body for potential pregnancy. When these hormones are in balance, the menstrual cycle tends to be regular, with minimal discomfort. However, when hormonal imbalances occur, women can experience a wide range of symptoms.

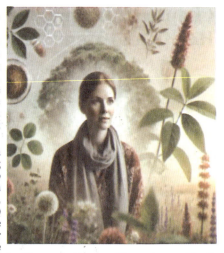

Menstrual irregularities can take many forms, from heavy bleeding and missed periods to painful cramping and emotional disturbances. These issues often point to underlying hormonal imbalances, such as estrogen dominance or low progesterone levels. In some cases, conditions like **polycystic ovary syndrome (PCOS)** or **endometriosis** may be present, both of which are linked to disruptions in normal hormonal activity. For women experiencing these conditions, addressing the root cause of hormonal imbalance is critical to restoring a healthy menstrual cycle and improving overall well-being.

Diet and **lifestyle choices** play a significant role in maintaining hormonal balance throughout the menstrual cycle. A diet rich in whole, nutrient-dense foods supports the body's natural hormone production and helps prevent fluctuations that can lead to menstrual discomfort. For example, foods high in **omega-3 fatty acids**, such as flaxseeds and walnuts, help to regulate inflammation and support balanced hormone levels. Similarly, foods rich in **magnesium** and **vitamin B6** have been shown to alleviate symptoms of premenstrual syndrome (PMS) by promoting better hormone regulation and reducing stress.

Chronic stress can disrupt the delicate balance of hormones by increasing the production of cortisol, a stress hormone that interferes with estrogen and progesterone levels. High cortisol levels over time can lead to issues like irregular periods, exacerbating the emotional and physical symptoms of PMS.

Menopause and Hormonal Decline

Menopause marks a significant transition in a woman's life as hormone production declines and reproductive capacity ceases. This natural process, though inevitable, brings with it unique challenges. The decline in **estrogen** and **progesterone** during menopause can result in symptoms such as **hot flashes**, **night sweats**, and **mood changes**, all of which can impact daily life and well-being.

The hormonal changes that occur during menopause also affect bone health. Estrogen plays a key role in maintaining bone density, and as estrogen levels drop, women become more vulnerable to conditions like **osteoporosis**. Bone health becomes a crucial focus during this stage, with diet and lifestyle interventions playing a major role in preserving bone strength. A diet rich in **calcium** and **vitamin D** is essential to counteract the effects of hormonal decline on the bones. Weight-bearing exercises, such as walking and resistance training, are also recommended to maintain bone density and overall physical health.

In addition to physical symptoms, the emotional impact of menopause should not be overlooked. As hormone levels fluctuate, many women experience **mood swings**, **anxiety**, and even **depression**. These emotional changes are often linked to the body's adjustment to lower estrogen levels, which can influence neurotransmitter activity in the brain. Supporting emotional health during menopause is crucial and can be achieved through a combination of dietary changes, stress management techniques, and, in some cases, **natural hormone therapies**. These therapies, using herbs and supplements that mimic the body's natural hormones, can help ease the transition and reduce the severity of symptoms.

1.2 Menstrual Health: Supporting a Natural Cycle

The menstrual cycle is a vital aspect of a woman's reproductive health, and it is influenced by complex hormonal fluctuations that occur throughout the month. These hormonal changes can sometimes lead to uncomfortable symptoms, such as PMS, cramps, and fatigue. Understanding the underlying causes of these issues and supporting the body with natural remedies can greatly enhance menstrual health and reduce discomfort. In this section, we explore how these fluctuations impact the body and provide practical recommendations for managing menstrual discomfort through the use of herbs and lifestyle changes.

Hormonal Fluctuations and Their Impact on Menstrual Health

Throughout the menstrual cycle, a woman's body undergoes significant hormonal changes, primarily involving the hormones estrogen and progesterone. These fluctuations are necessary for regulating the menstrual cycle, ovulation, and the overall reproductive system. However, when these hormones are out of balance, or when the body is particularly sensitive to these changes, various symptoms can arise.

One common issue is **PMS**, which affects many women in the days leading up to menstruation. Symptoms of PMS can range from mild to severe and include mood swings, irritability, bloating, headaches, and fatigue. These symptoms are often triggered by the rapid drop in estrogen and progesterone levels that occur just before the onset of menstruation. Some women are more sensitive to these changes, which can exacerbate the intensity of PMS symptoms.

Menstrual cramps, or dysmenorrhea, are another prevalent issue that can significantly impact quality of life during menstruation. Prostaglandins, which resemble hormones and induce the uterus to contract and shed its lining, are the cause of these cramps. While some degree of cramping is normal, excessive cramps can indicate an imbalance in hormone levels or inflammation within the body.

Additionally, many women experience **fatigue** during their menstrual cycle, particularly in the luteal phase (the time between ovulation and menstruation). This phase is characterized by higher levels of progesterone, which can lead to feelings of tiredness and lethargy. Combined with the physical toll of menstruation itself, these hormonal shifts can make it challenging to maintain energy levels and focus during this time.

Herbal Remedies for Menstrual Discomfort

To ease the discomfort associated with menstruation, many women turn to natural remedies, particularly herbs that have been used for centuries to support reproductive health. Two of the most highly recommended herbs for menstrual health are **red raspberry leaf** and **vitex** (also known as chasteberry), both of which can help regulate hormonal fluctuations and alleviate symptoms like cramps and PMS.

Red raspberry leaf is a powerful herb known for its ability to tone the uterus and promote overall reproductive health. It contains high levels of vitamins and minerals, including vitamin C, calcium, and magnesium, which are essential for muscle relaxation and reducing cramps. This herb also helps to strengthen the uterine walls, making menstruation less painful and more efficient. Regular consumption of red raspberry leaf tea throughout the menstrual cycle can help to alleviate cramps and reduce the overall discomfort of menstruation.

In addition to its uterine-toning properties, red raspberry leaf is known for balancing hormone levels, which can be particularly beneficial for women who suffer from PMS. By providing the body with essential nutrients, this herb helps to stabilize the hormonal fluctuations that contribute to mood swings, bloating, and other premenstrual symptoms.

Another key herb for menstrual health is **vitex**, or chasteberry, which has a long history of use in supporting women's hormonal balance. Vitex works primarily on the pituitary gland, regulating the production of the hormones estrogen and progesterone. By encouraging the body to produce more progesterone, vitex helps to balance the ratio of estrogen to progesterone, reducing the severity of PMS and promoting a more regular menstrual cycle.

Vitex is particularly effective in addressing symptoms such as **breast tenderness**, **irritability**, and **headaches** that often accompany PMS. Additionally, it can be helpful for women who experience irregular cycles or hormonal imbalances that lead to heavier or more painful periods. Taking vitex regularly can help to promote a more balanced hormonal environment, easing the discomfort associated with menstrual irregularities.

Supporting a Healthy Menstrual Cycle Through Lifestyle Changes

In addition to using herbal remedies, certain lifestyle changes can greatly enhance menstrual health and reduce the severity of symptoms associated with hormonal fluctuations. Diet, exercise, and stress management all play significant roles in supporting a healthy menstrual cycle.

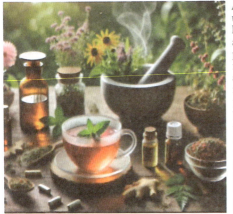

A nutrient-rich diet that focuses on whole, unprocessed foods is essential for maintaining hormonal balance. Foods high in **omega-3 fatty acids**, such as flaxseeds, walnuts, and chia seeds, are particularly beneficial for reducing inflammation and regulating hormone production. These healthy fats also support the production of prostaglandins that reduce menstrual cramps.

Incorporating **leafy greens**, such as spinach and kale, provides the body with magnesium, which helps to relax the muscles of the uterus and alleviate cramps. Additionally, consuming plenty of **fiber-rich foods**, such as fruits, vegetables, and whole grains, can help to regulate estrogen levels by promoting the elimination of excess hormones through the digestive system.

Staying hydrated is also crucial for menstrual health. Drinking plenty of water helps to reduce bloating, a common symptom of PMS, and supports the body's natural detoxification processes, allowing for a smoother menstrual cycle.

Regular physical activity is another key factor in supporting a healthy menstrual cycle. Exercise helps to improve circulation, reduce stress, and regulate hormone levels. Moderate activities like walking, swimming, and yoga are particularly beneficial for reducing menstrual cramps and boosting energy levels. Engaging in these activities throughout the menstrual cycle can also help to reduce the severity of PMS symptoms and support overall hormonal balance.

Stress management is equally important in maintaining a healthy menstrual cycle. Chronic stress can disrupt the delicate balance of hormones in the body, leading to more severe PMS symptoms, irregular periods, and increased menstrual cramps. Incorporating stress-reducing practices like meditation, deep breathing exercises, or spending time in nature can help to calm the nervous system and support hormonal health.

1.3 Herbal Support for Menopause

As women enter menopause, they experience significant hormonal changes that can lead to uncomfortable symptoms such as hot flashes, mood swings, and sleep disturbances. These fluctuations in hormone levels, particularly the decline in estrogen and progesterone, can affect both physical and emotional well-being. In her teachings, Barbara O'Neill emphasizes the importance of using natural remedies to support the body during this transition, suggesting a variety of herbs that help balance hormones and ease menopausal symptoms.

Hormonal Fluctuations and Their Impact

Menopause marks the end of a woman's reproductive years, and with it comes a shift in the body's hormonal balance. The gradual decrease in estrogen and progesterone leads to a wide array of symptoms, which can vary in intensity from woman to woman. Hot flashes, one of the most common symptoms, occur due to changes in the body's thermoregulation. Mood swings are another frequent issue, as the body's fluctuating hormones impact neurotransmitter levels, leading to feelings of irritability, anxiety, or even depression. Additionally, women may experience changes in sleep patterns, weight gain, and a general sense of fatigue.

It is during this time that many seek relief through natural remedies, as they provide a gentler approach to symptom management without the side effects associated with conventional hormone replacement therapies. Herbal remedies can help the body adapt to these changes, restoring balance and offering relief from the discomfort associated with menopause.

Natural Remedies for Menopausal Symptoms

One of the primary herbs recommended to support women through menopause is **black cohosh**. Known for its ability to reduce hot flashes and night sweats, black cohosh works by mimicking the effects of estrogen in the body, thereby alleviating some of the discomforts associated with the hormonal drop during menopause.

It has been traditionally used to address various menopausal symptoms, including mood swings and vaginal dryness, and remains a popular choice among women seeking natural relief.

Wild yam is another powerful herb that plays a role in balancing hormones. Wild yam contains compounds that can be converted into progesterone by the body, helping to address the hormonal imbalances that occur during menopause. By supporting progesterone levels, wild yam helps to alleviate symptoms such as mood swings and irritability, which are commonly linked to declining hormone levels. It is often used in creams and supplements as a natural alternative to synthetic hormones, providing support for women experiencing the emotional and psychological effects of menopause.

Red clover is a third herb that is frequently recommended for menopausal support. Red clover contains phytoestrogens, plant compounds that mimic the activity of estrogen in the body. These phytoestrogens help to reduce the intensity and frequency of hot flashes while also promoting heart and bone health, both of which can be negatively affected by the drop in estrogen during menopause. By gently boosting estrogenic activity, red clover offers a natural way to manage some of the more challenging physical aspects of menopause, such as osteoporosis risk and cardiovascular concerns.

Lifestyle and Diet Considerations

In addition to herbal remedies, supporting the body through menopause also involves making key lifestyle changes. A balanced diet rich in phytoestrogens, found in foods such as flaxseeds, soy, and legumes, can further help to mitigate the symptoms of hormonal fluctuations. Regular exercise is also essential, as it helps to regulate mood, improve sleep, and maintain bone density, all of which are crucial during this stage of life.

Adequate hydration and the avoidance of stimulants like caffeine and alcohol are also important, as they can exacerbate symptoms such as hot flashes and disrupt sleep. Through a combination of herbal remedies and mindful lifestyle changes, women can better navigate the challenges of menopause while maintaining overall health and well-being.

Chapter 2: Natural Approaches to Managing PCOS and Endometriosis

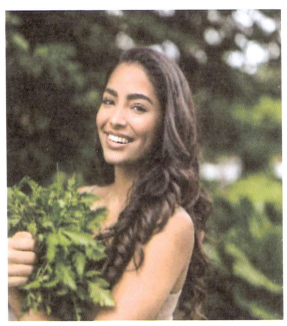

2.1 Understanding PCOS and Its Impact on Hormones

PCOS is a prevalent hormonal disorder affecting many women worldwide, often leading to symptoms such as irregular periods, unexplained weight gain, and fertility challenges. The hormonal imbalance caused by PCOS is primarily linked to excess androgens, which can disrupt the regular functioning of the menstrual cycle. In addressing this complex condition, a holistic approach that focuses on lifestyle and diet is critical for managing the symptoms and improving overall health.

The Impact of PCOS on Hormonal Balance

PCOS disrupts the natural hormonal balance in women by causing an overproduction of androgens, or male hormones, which interferes with the normal development and release of eggs from the ovaries. This hormonal imbalance can result in irregular menstrual cycles, with some women experiencing very few periods per year, while others may have cycles that are unusually long. This disruption can also cause complications such as cysts on the ovaries and anovulation, which can contribute to difficulties in conceiving.

Additionally, the increased androgen levels often lead to physical symptoms such as acne, hair thinning, and excessive hair growth, particularly on the face and body. Many women with PCOS also struggle with insulin resistance, which can exacerbate symptoms by making weight management more challenging. Insulin resistance not only affects metabolism but also contributes to increased androgen production, creating a cycle that worsens the hormonal imbalance.

Dietary Changes for PCOS Management

Barbara O'Neill advocates for dietary modifications as one of the most effective ways to manage PCOS and its related symptoms. A whole-food, plant-based diet that prioritizes nutrient-dense foods can help regulate insulin levels, reduce inflammation, and restore hormonal balance. She emphasizes the importance of avoiding processed foods, sugars, and refined carbohydrates, which can cause spikes in insulin and worsen insulin resistance.

Instead, O'Neill encourages the consumption of low-glycemic foods, such as leafy greens, whole grains, and legumes, which have a stabilizing effect on blood sugar levels. These foods help to prevent the insulin surges that can aggravate PCOS symptoms. Incorporating healthy fats, such as those found in avocados, nuts, and seeds, is also crucial, as they support the production of hormones in a balanced way, helping to regulate the menstrual cycle.

Additionally, eating foods rich in fiber, such as vegetables, berries, and flaxseeds, can aid in improving digestion and eliminating excess estrogen from the body, further contributing to hormonal balance. O'Neill suggests that a diet high in antioxidants from fruits and vegetables can also reduce oxidative stress, which is commonly associated with PCOS and its related metabolic challenges.

2.2 Addressing Endometriosis Naturally

Endometriosis is a chronic and painful condition that occurs when the tissue that normally lines the inside of the uterus, known as the endometrium, grows outside of it. This misplaced tissue can attach itself to various organs in the pelvic region, leading to inflammation, pain, and often fertility issues. Conventional treatments for endometriosis typically involve hormone therapy or surgery, but many women seek natural methods to manage their symptoms. In this section, we explore natural approaches, including lifestyle changes and specific herbal remedies, that can help alleviate the discomfort associated with this condition.

Lifestyle Adjustments for Managing Endometriosis

One of the key factors in managing endometriosis naturally is making adjustments to diet and lifestyle. Inflammation plays a significant role in the pain and discomfort caused by endometriosis, and reducing inflammation through dietary changes can have a profound effect. A diet rich in anti-inflammatory foods, such as leafy green vegetables, fruits, nuts, and seeds, can help to reduce systemic inflammation. Processed foods, refined sugars, and trans fats, which can exacerbate inflammation, should be minimized or eliminated.

In addition to dietary changes, regular exercise can help manage the symptoms of endometriosis. Exercise stimulates the release of endorphins, the body's natural pain relievers, and promotes circulation, which helps reduce the severity of pain. Gentle forms of exercise, such as yoga or walking, are particularly beneficial for women with endometriosis, as they promote relaxation and flexibility without placing excessive strain on the body.

Another important lifestyle change is stress management. Chronic stress can worsen the symptoms of endometriosis by increasing inflammation and hormone imbalances. Techniques such as meditation, deep breathing exercises, and spending time in nature can help reduce stress levels and promote overall well-being.

Herbal Remedies for Endometriosis

Herbal remedies are an integral part of managing endometriosis naturally. Several herbs have been shown to reduce inflammation, ease pain, and balance hormones, providing relief from the symptoms of this condition.

Evening Primrose Oil is one of the most commonly recommended natural treatments for endometriosis. It contains a lot of gamma-linolenic acid (GLA), an omega-6 fatty acid with anti-inflammatory qualities. GLA helps to reduce the inflammation associated with endometriosis, providing relief from pain and discomfort. In addition to its anti-inflammatory effects, evening primrose oil can help regulate hormonal imbalances, which is crucial in managing endometriosis, as the condition is often hormone-driven.

Turmeric is another powerful anti-inflammatory herb that can be highly beneficial for women suffering from endometriosis. The active compound in turmeric, curcumin, has been widely studied for its ability to reduce inflammation and pain. Turmeric's anti-inflammatory properties can help decrease the severity of endometrial tissue growth outside the uterus, easing the pain associated with the condition. Turmeric can be taken as a supplement or added to meals to provide ongoing support for reducing inflammation.

In addition to evening primrose oil and turmeric, **ginger** is another herb that has shown promise in reducing pain and inflammation. Ginger contains compounds called gingerols, which have potent anti-inflammatory effects similar to non-steroidal anti-inflammatory drugs (NSAIDs) but without the harmful side effects. Incorporating ginger tea or supplements into the daily routine can help ease the symptoms of endometriosis.

Other herbs, such as **chaste tree berry** (Vitex agnus-castus), are also helpful in balancing hormones. This herb is known for its ability to regulate the menstrual cycle by influencing the production of progesterone, which can help reduce the severity of endometriosis symptoms.

Chapter 3: Nutrition and Lifestyle Practices for Hormonal Balance

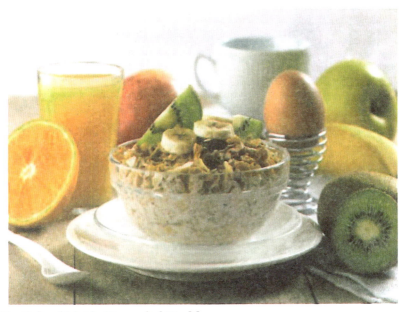

3.1 The Role of Diet in Hormonal Health

Hormonal balance is essential for overall well-being, and diet plays a crucial role in maintaining this delicate balance. A nutrient-dense, plant-based diet is one of the most effective ways to support the body's hormonal system, providing the necessary building blocks for optimal function. Barbara O'Neill emphasizes the importance of eating whole, unprocessed foods rich in essential nutrients, such as healthy fats, fiber, and antioxidants, to ensure that hormones are produced and regulated effectively.

The Importance of Nutrient-Dense Foods for Hormonal Balance

Hormones are chemical messengers that control various functions in the body, from metabolism to mood. They rely on specific nutrients to be synthesized and function properly. A diet that is lacking in these nutrients can lead to hormonal imbalances, which can manifest in a variety of symptoms such as fatigue, mood swings, or irregular menstrual cycles.

One of the key elements for supporting hormonal health is ensuring an adequate intake of **healthy fats**. Hormones like estrogen and progesterone are derived from cholesterol and require fats for their production. Healthy fats, such as those found in **avocados, walnuts**, and **chia seeds**, provide the necessary precursors for hormone synthesis. These fats help stabilize blood sugar levels, which is critical for maintaining hormonal balance, particularly in regulating insulin and cortisol, the stress hormone.

In addition to healthy fats, **fiber** plays an essential role in hormonal regulation. Fiber aids in the elimination of excess hormones, particularly estrogen, through the digestive system. Foods rich in fiber, such as **leafy greens, whole grains**, and **legumes**, help to prevent the reabsorption of excess estrogen in the gut, thus preventing imbalances that could lead to conditions like estrogen dominance. Fiber also supports healthy digestion, which is linked to better overall hormonal health.

Antioxidants are another critical component of a hormone-supportive diet. They protect the body from oxidative stress, which can damage hormone-producing cells and lead to imbalances. Antioxidant-rich foods such as **berries**, **leafy greens**, and **nuts** help to reduce inflammation in the body, further supporting hormone health. In particular, antioxidants found in **vitamin C** and **vitamin E** can directly support the adrenal glands, which produce stress hormones and play a role in overall hormonal balance.

Key Foods That Promote Hormonal Health

Certain foods are particularly beneficial for supporting hormonal balance due to their high nutrient content. **Flaxseeds** are a standout example, as they are rich in **lignans**, a type of phytoestrogen that helps regulate estrogen levels. These lignans can both mimic and balance estrogen in the body, making flaxseeds an excellent addition to the diet for individuals seeking to support reproductive health and mitigate symptoms related to hormonal imbalances.

Leafy greens such as **spinach, kale,** and **Swiss chard** are packed with vitamins, minerals, and antioxidants that support overall health and hormone production. They are high in **magnesium**, which is particularly important for regulating the stress response and maintaining stable blood sugar levels, both of which are crucial for balanced hormones.

In addition to flaxseeds and leafy greens, **omega-3-rich foods** like **walnuts, chia seeds,** and **flaxseeds** play a vital role in hormonal health. Omega-3 fatty acids are anti-inflammatory and help to maintain cell membrane flexibility, which is essential for hormone receptors to function properly. These fatty acids also support the production of hormones like **progesterone**, which helps to balance estrogen and prevent hormonal imbalances.

3.2 Avoiding Hormone Disruptors

Hormone disruptors, found in many aspects of modern life, are chemicals that interfere with the body's natural hormonal balance. These substances can alter the way hormones function, leading to a wide array of health issues, particularly those related to reproductive and endocrine systems. Today, they are present in many everyday items such as processed foods, plastic containers, and chemical-laden personal care products. Understanding how to avoid these disruptors is crucial for maintaining hormonal health.

Environmental Toxins and Hormonal Interference

Many of the toxins we encounter daily act as endocrine disruptors, meaning they mimic or block the action of natural hormones in the body. For example, substances such as **bisphenol A (BPA)**, often found in plastic bottles and food containers, can mimic estrogen, leading to hormonal imbalances. These synthetic chemicals can bind to hormone receptors, altering the body's natural signals. This disruption can cause significant health problems over time, including infertility, weight gain, and increased risk of certain cancers.

In addition to BPA, **phthalates** are another group of chemicals widely used in plastics and personal care products. They, too, interfere with hormonal regulation by affecting how hormones are produced or how cells respond to them. Continuous exposure to these disruptors can have long-term consequences, particularly for individuals who are regularly exposed to plastic food containers, packaged foods, or chemical-laden cosmetics.

Processed foods are another major source of hormone disruptors. Many contain preservatives, artificial flavors, and additives that can interfere with the body's endocrine system. For example, **pesticide residues** on non-organic fruits and vegetables can act as hormone disruptors when ingested over time, impacting the body's ability to maintain a healthy hormonal balance.

Reducing Exposure Through Dietary Choices

To mitigate the effects of hormone disruptors, making conscious dietary choices is essential. One of the key recommendations is to opt for **organic foods** whenever possible. Organic produce is grown without the use of synthetic pesticides, which are often linked to hormonal imbalances. Consuming organic vegetables, fruits, grains, and meats reduces exposure to these harmful chemicals, supporting the body's natural ability to regulate hormones.

Processed foods should also be avoided, as they often contain preservatives and artificial ingredients that can contribute to hormonal disruption. By choosing whole, unprocessed foods, individuals can ensure they are not ingesting additives that could interfere with their endocrine system.

Avoiding Plastics and Choosing Natural Alternatives

Another practical approach to reducing exposure to hormone disruptors is minimizing the use of plastics, especially when it comes to food storage. Plastic containers, particularly those that contain BPA or phthalates, release chemicals into food and beverages, especially when heated. Opting for **glass or stainless steel** containers to store food is a simple and effective way to avoid these toxic compounds.

Similarly, avoiding plastic water bottles in favor of glass or metal alternatives helps reduce daily exposure to these harmful chemicals. Even small, everyday habits like reheating food in plastic containers can lead to the leaching of hormone-disrupting chemicals into the food, compounding their effects over time.

Natural Skincare Products for Hormonal Health

Personal care products are another major source of hormone disruptors. Many conventional skincare and beauty products contain chemicals like **parabens**, which are used as preservatives and can mimic estrogen in the body. Regular use of these products can lead to a build-up of synthetic hormones, which may disrupt the natural hormonal balance.

To avoid this, it is advised to switch to **natural skincare products** that are free from parabens, phthalates, and other synthetic chemicals. Choosing products made from organic or plant-based ingredients ensures that the skin absorbs fewer toxins, reducing the overall hormonal load on the body. Additionally, homemade skincare solutions, such as natural oils and herbal infusions, can provide effective alternatives to chemical-laden commercial products.

3.3 Lifestyle Practices for Hormonal Balance

Maintaining hormonal balance is essential for overall health, as hormones regulate many of the body's key processes, including metabolism, reproduction, and mood. While diet plays a significant role in supporting hormone health, lifestyle factors such as regular exercise, stress management, and adequate sleep are equally important. These elements work together to create a stable internal environment, preventing hormonal fluctuations that can lead to various health issues. In her teachings, Barbara O'Neill emphasizes the need for a holistic approach to hormonal health, incorporating both lifestyle changes and natural practices.

The Role of Exercise in Hormonal Balance

Regular physical activity is one of the most effective ways to support hormonal balance. Exercise stimulates the release of endorphins, which improve mood and help reduce the impact of stress on the body. It also plays a crucial role in regulating insulin levels, which is vital for maintaining balanced blood sugar levels and preventing the development of insulin resistance. Insulin resistance is a key factor in the development of conditions such as PCOS and type 2 diabetes, both of which are closely linked to hormonal imbalances.

Moderate, consistent exercise, such as walking, swimming, or cycling, can also help regulate the production of cortisol, the body's primary stress hormone. By keeping cortisol levels in check, regular exercise prevents the chronic elevation of this hormone, which can lead to weight gain, particularly around the abdomen, and disrupt the body's natural production of other hormones such as estrogen and progesterone.

Stress Management for Hormonal Health

Stress is one of the leading contributors to hormonal imbalance. When the body is under chronic stress, it produces excess cortisol, which can interfere with the production of other key hormones, including thyroid hormones and reproductive hormones. High cortisol levels can also lead to adrenal fatigue, a condition where the adrenal glands become overworked and are no longer able to produce adequate amounts of cortisol. This results in fatigue, weight gain, and mood swings.

The Importance of Sleep for Hormonal Regulation

M of the body's key hormonal processes occur during sleep. For example, the body's production of growth hormone, which is essential for cell repair and regeneration, peaks during deep sleep. Similarly, sleep regulates the production of the hunger hormones ghrelin and leptin, which control appetite and satiety. When sleep is disrupted, ghrelin levels increase, leading to increased hunger and potential weight gain, while leptin levels decrease, making it harder for the body to feel full.

Chapter 4: Supporting Reproductive Health Holistically

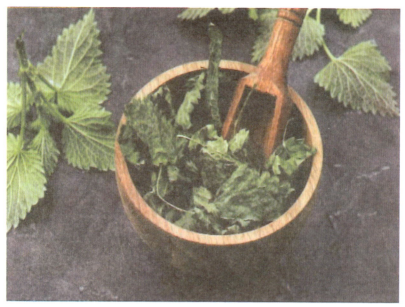

4.1 Fertility Support with Herbs

For women seeking to enhance their fertility, natural herbs offer a powerful way to support reproductive health. Balancing hormones and nourishing the reproductive system are key components of preparing the body for conception. Barbara O'Neill recommends a range of herbs, including maca root, nettle, and red raspberry leaf, each known for its unique properties that promote fertility. These herbs can be used safely in the form of teas, capsules, or infusions, providing a natural and effective means of boosting fertility.

Hormonal Balance and Reproductive Health

Herbs like **maca root** are particularly beneficial for supporting hormonal balance. Maca, a root vegetable native to the Andes, is known as an adaptogen, meaning it helps the body adapt to stress and regulate hormone production. Maca has been traditionally used to improve fertility by stabilizing hormone levels, which is essential for a healthy reproductive system.

Maca is also believed to enhance libido and increase energy levels, both of which are important for women trying to conceive. It works by supporting the endocrine system, helping to regulate the hormones that influence fertility, without directly affecting hormone levels themselves. This makes it a safe and gentle option for women looking to balance their reproductive hormones naturally.

Nettle is another powerful herb for supporting fertility. Nettle is rich in vitamins and minerals, particularly iron, calcium, and magnesium, which are essential for reproductive health. Iron is critical for women looking to conceive, as it helps to build a healthy uterine lining and prevent anemia, which can affect fertility. Nettle also contains vitamin K, which supports proper blood clotting and overall reproductive function.

The mineral-rich nature of nettle makes it an excellent tonic for women's health, strengthening the uterus and preparing the body for pregnancy. When used regularly, nettle helps to nourish the reproductive organs, ensuring they function optimally in preparation for conception.

Strengthening the Reproductive System

For women looking to conceive, **red raspberry leaf** is a key herb for strengthening the reproductive system. Known for its ability to tone the uterine muscles, red raspberry leaf is often used to support reproductive health before and during pregnancy. It helps to prepare the uterus for conception by promoting healthy uterine contractions and increasing blood flow to the pelvic region. This, in turn, creates an optimal environment for implantation.

Red raspberry leaf is also high in vitamins and minerals, particularly vitamin C and magnesium, both of which support reproductive health. Its high content of antioxidants further protects the reproductive organs from oxidative stress, which can negatively affect fertility. By strengthening the uterine muscles, red raspberry leaf helps to ensure a healthy pregnancy once conception occurs.

For those trying to conceive, red raspberry leaf is often taken as a tea, either alone or combined with other fertility-supporting herbs like nettle. Drinking red raspberry leaf tea regularly helps to tone and nourish the reproductive organs, making it a popular choice among women preparing for pregnancy.

Safe Usage of Fertility Herbs

Using these herbs safely is essential for maximizing their benefits while minimizing any potential risks. Fertility-supporting herbs like maca root, nettle, and red raspberry leaf can be consumed in various forms, including teas, capsules, or infusions. For many women, herbal teas are the preferred method, as they allow for easy absorption of nutrients and hydration at the same time.

Maca root can be taken as a powdered supplement or added to smoothies for a more palatable option. The dosage for maca root varies, but most experts recommend starting with 1 to 3 grams per day. It's important to use maca regularly over several months to experience its full benefits, as it works gradually to balance hormones and support fertility.

Nettle is commonly consumed as a tea or infusion. To prepare a nettle infusion, steep a tablespoon of dried nettle leaves in hot water for 10 to 15 minutes. This allows the nutrients to fully extract into the water, providing a mineral-rich drink that can be consumed daily. Alternatively, nettle capsules are available for those who prefer a more convenient option.

Red raspberry leaf is typically taken as a tea, which can be drunk several times a day. Many women find that drinking 2 to 3 cups of red raspberry leaf tea daily helps to strengthen their reproductive system and prepare for pregnancy. For those who prefer capsules, red raspberry leaf supplements are also available, but it's important to follow the dosage instructions to avoid any potential side effects.

While these herbs are generally considered safe, it's always important for women to consult with a healthcare provider, especially if they have any underlying health conditions or are taking other medications. This ensures that the herbs are used safely and effectively as part of a fertility-boosting regimen.

4.2 Natural Birth Control Alternatives

For women seeking alternatives to hormonal birth control, natural methods provide a viable and empowering option. These methods emphasize an understanding of the body's natural rhythms, focusing on fertility awareness and the use of herbal remedies as natural contraceptives. Barbara O'Neill highlights the importance of education and awareness in navigating these methods, allowing women to make informed choices that align with their health and lifestyle.

Fertility Awareness as a Natural Method

Fertility awareness methods (FAM) are grounded in the concept that a woman's fertility is cyclical, with specific phases of higher and lower fertility throughout her menstrual cycle. By tracking these phases accurately, a woman can determine when she is most likely to conceive and either avoid or attempt conception based on her goals. FAM relies on understanding the natural signs of fertility, including basal body temperature, cervical mucus changes, and the position of the cervix.

One of the most widely used fertility tracking methods involves monitoring **basal body temperature (BBT)**. Upon waking each morning, a woman records her body temperature before any physical activity, as even minor movements can alter the reading. During ovulation, there is typically a slight rise in BBT, which indicates that the fertile window is open. This method can be highly effective when used consistently, as it provides clear insight into when ovulation occurs.

Another critical aspect of fertility awareness is tracking **cervical mucus**. Throughout the menstrual cycle, cervical mucus changes in consistency and volume, serving as a natural indicator of fertility. During ovulation, cervical mucus becomes more slippery and clear, resembling egg whites, which facilitates the passage of sperm through the cervix. Recognizing these changes allows women to predict their most fertile days and adjust their behavior accordingly.

For women using fertility awareness as a birth control method, abstaining from intercourse or using barrier methods during the fertile window is essential for preventing pregnancy. FAM can be as effective as some hormonal birth control methods when practiced with diligence and accuracy.

Herbal Remedies for Natural Contraception

In addition to fertility awareness, herbal remedies have long been used as natural contraceptives. One of the most commonly mentioned herbal options is **wild carrot seed**, also known as Queen Anne's Lace. This herb has a historical reputation for its contraceptive properties, and it works by disrupting the implantation of a fertilized egg. Wild carrot seed is typically taken shortly after unprotected intercourse during the fertile period to prevent conception.

Wild carrot seed is consumed in a powdered form or as a tincture, but it must be used with caution and proper understanding, as its effectiveness depends on timing and consistent use. While it is a natural method, it is essential to remember that no contraceptive method, herbal or otherwise, is 100% effective. Therefore, using wild carrot seed requires a thorough understanding of fertility cycles and clear guidance on its application.

Another herbal remedy that may support contraception is **parsley**, which has been traditionally used to stimulate menstruation and potentially disrupt implantation. However, as with all herbal remedies, it is crucial to consult knowledgeable practitioners to ensure the correct use and avoid any unintended side effects.

Practical Guidance for Using Natural Contraceptive Methods

For women interested in natural birth control methods, tracking fertility cycles is the foundation of effectiveness. It begins with careful observation of physical signs, such as those mentioned above, and recording daily findings on a fertility chart. There are also mobile apps designed to help women keep track of their menstrual cycles, offering a convenient and user-friendly way to monitor fertile windows.

However, success with fertility awareness methods requires consistency and discipline. For women new to these techniques, it is recommended to receive education and training from a certified fertility awareness instructor to ensure accurate tracking and interpretation of fertility signals.

Additionally, herbal remedies like wild carrot seed should be used with a deep understanding of their effects and timing. Since herbs can vary in potency and effectiveness, it is important to source high-quality products and follow dosage guidelines carefully. Natural contraceptive methods offer a gentle alternative to hormonal birth control but must be approached with the same level of attention and care.

4.3 Postpartum Health and Recovery

Following childbirth, a woman's body undergoes dramatic changes, both physically and hormonally. The postpartum period is a critical time when the body needs adequate support to restore balance and promote healing. During this phase, it is essential for new mothers to focus on proper nutrition, sufficient rest, and the use of natural remedies to aid recovery and support overall health.

Hormonal Shifts and Nutritional Needs

After giving birth, a woman experiences significant hormonal fluctuations. These changes can affect energy levels, mood, and the body's ability to heal. Hormones such as estrogen and progesterone, which are elevated during pregnancy, drop sharply after delivery. This shift can lead to symptoms like fatigue, mood swings, and difficulty concentrating, often referred to as the "baby blues."

To help balance these hormonal changes, a nutrient-rich diet is crucial. Foods high in vitamins, minerals, and healthy fats provide the essential building blocks for recovery. Omega-3 fatty acids, found in flaxseeds and walnuts, are particularly beneficial for supporting brain health and mood stabilization. Leafy greens, rich in iron and folate, help replenish the body's stores after the blood loss experienced during childbirth. Additionally, a variety of fruits and vegetables provide antioxidants that support cellular repair and overall recovery.

Hydration is another key aspect of postpartum health. Breastfeeding mothers, in particular, need to ensure they are drinking enough water to support milk production. Dehydration can exacerbate fatigue and interfere with the body's natural healing processes. Herbal teas, especially those rich in nutrients, are a gentle way to support hydration and recovery.

Rest and Recovery

Rest is one of the most important factors for postpartum recovery. The body requires time to heal from the physical demands of childbirth, whether it was a vaginal delivery or a cesarean section. Sleep plays a critical role in hormone regulation and tissue repair. However, the responsibilities of taking care of a baby frequently make it difficult for new mothers to get enough sleep. It is important to rest whenever possible, and even short naps can be beneficial in supporting recovery during this time.

In addition to sleep, gentle movement and stretches can aid the recovery process. Walking and light stretching help improve circulation, which is important for healing and reducing postpartum swelling. However, any intense physical activity should be approached cautiously and only after receiving clearance from a healthcare provider.

Herbal Support for Postpartum Health

Herbal remedies have been used for centuries to support women during the postpartum period. These natural solutions can assist with lactation, healing, and overall recovery. One of the key herbs recommended is **fenugreek**, which has been traditionally used to support milk production. Fenugreek stimulates the milk ducts, making it an excellent choice for mothers who may be struggling with breastfeeding. Its natural properties help boost lactation while also providing important nutrients that can support the mother's overall health.

Comfrey is another important herb in the postpartum recovery toolkit. Known for its ability to support wound healing, comfrey can be used externally to soothe and heal tissues affected by childbirth. For mothers recovering from perineal tears or episiotomies, comfrey compresses or salves can help speed up the healing process and reduce discomfort. It has natural anti-inflammatory properties that make it ideal for soothing soreness and promoting tissue regeneration.

Other supportive herbs include **raspberry leaf**, which is often used to tone the uterus and aid in postpartum recovery. Raspberry leaf helps the uterus return to its normal size more quickly and can ease postpartum cramping. Its astringent properties also support the body's overall recovery by promoting tissue healing.

In addition to these specific herbs, adaptogenic herbs such as **ashwagandha** can help balance the stress response and support emotional well-being during the postpartum period. Adaptogens help the body cope with stress and restore hormonal balance, which can be beneficial for new mothers adjusting to the demands of caring for a newborn.

Chapter 5: 10 Herbal Remedies for Women's Health and Hormonal Balance

Herbal remedies have long been used to support women's health, particularly in addressing issues related to hormonal balance. Each herb has specific properties that can help alleviate symptoms of hormonal imbalance, menstrual discomfort, and other reproductive health concerns. Below are 10 powerful herbal remedies that can be used to support women's health and promote hormonal balance. Following the guidance on when, how, and how much to use these herbs can help optimize their effectiveness.

1. Red Raspberry Leaf Tea

Red raspberry leaf tea is a well-known remedy for supporting reproductive health, especially for women during pregnancy. It is rich in vitamins and minerals, such as calcium, magnesium, and iron, which are essential for a healthy reproductive system. Red raspberry leaf is also known for its ability to tone the uterus, making it beneficial for women experiencing menstrual cramps or preparing for childbirth.

How to Use: To make red raspberry leaf tea, steep one teaspoon of dried leaves in hot water for 10-15 minutes. This tea can be consumed up to three times a day. For women who are pregnant, it is typically recommended to begin drinking the tea during the second or third trimester to help tone the uterus in preparation for labor.

2. Black Cohosh Capsules

Black cohosh is frequently used to support women experiencing menopausal symptoms such as hot flashes, night sweats, and mood swings. This herb has been shown to have estrogen-like effects, making it particularly useful for women going through perimenopause or menopause. Black cohosh is also known to help with menstrual pain and irregular cycles.

How to Use: Black cohosh is most commonly available in capsule form. It is generally recommended to take 40-80 milligrams of black cohosh daily, but doses may vary based on individual needs. For best results, black cohosh should be taken consistently for at least a few weeks to see improvements in menopausal symptoms.

3. Vitex (Chasteberry) Tincture

Vitex, also known as chasteberry, is one of the most effective herbs for balancing hormones in women. It works by influencing the pituitary gland, which helps regulate the production of hormones such as progesterone and estrogen. Vitex is particularly useful for women with irregular menstrual cycles, PMS, or conditions like PCOS. It is also helpful for women looking to support fertility.

How to Use: Vitex is commonly used in tincture form. A typical dose is 20-40 drops of the tincture, taken once a day, usually in the morning. For hormonal balance, it is best to use vitex consistently over several months, as its effects build gradually over time.

4. Evening Primrose Oil

Evening primrose oil is rich in gamma-linolenic acid (GLA), an essential fatty acid that has anti-inflammatory properties and supports hormone regulation. This oil is particularly useful for alleviating PMS symptoms such as breast tenderness, bloating, and irritability. It is also used to support skin health, making it a popular choice for women experiencing hormonal acne.

How to Use: Evening primrose oil is available in both capsule and liquid forms. For PMS relief, a daily dose of 1,000-2,000 milligrams is generally recommended, starting a week or two before the onset of menstruation. It can be taken throughout the month for overall hormonal support.

5. Maca Root Powder

Maca root is an adaptogen that helps the body adapt to stress, making it a popular choice for women dealing with hormonal imbalances caused by stress or adrenal fatigue. Maca root is also known for boosting energy, improving mood, and enhancing libido. It is beneficial for women going through menopause, as it helps balance hormone levels without directly affecting estrogen production.

How to Use: Maca root powder can be added to smoothies, teas, or other beverages. A typical dose ranges from one to three teaspoons per day. It is important to start with a lower dose and gradually increase as needed to assess how the body responds.

6. Turmeric Tea

Turmeric is renowned for its anti-inflammatory properties and is particularly beneficial for women experiencing painful menstrual cramps or conditions like endometriosis. Turmeric helps reduce inflammation in the body, making it useful for supporting overall hormonal health and reducing pain associated with menstruation.

How to Use: To make turmeric tea, mix one teaspoon of turmeric powder with hot water, a dash of black pepper, and a bit of honey for sweetness. This tea can be consumed once or twice daily to help reduce inflammation and support hormonal balance.

7. Wild Yam Cream

Wild yam is often used as a natural source of progesterone. While it doesn't contain progesterone itself, it contains compounds that can help the body produce and regulate this important hormone. Wild yam cream is commonly used by women experiencing menopause or those looking to balance estrogen dominance.

How to Use: Wild yam cream is typically applied topically to areas of the body where the skin is thin, such as the wrists or inner arms. A small amount of cream is massaged into the skin once or twice daily. It's important to use wild yam cream consistently to see its full effects over time.

8. Spearmint Tea (for PCOS)

Spearmint tea is particularly beneficial for women with PCOS, as it helps reduce androgen levels, which are often elevated in women with this condition. By lowering androgens, spearmint tea can help alleviate symptoms such as excess hair growth (hirsutism) and acne, both of which are common in PCOS.

How to Use: To make spearmint tea, steep one to two teaspoons of dried spearmint leaves in hot water for 10 minutes. It is recommended to drink this tea twice a day for best results in managing PCOS symptoms.

9. Red Clover Infusion

Red clover is a powerful herb for supporting hormonal balance, especially in women going through menopause. It contains phytoestrogens, which are plant-based compounds that mimic estrogen in the body. This makes red clover particularly useful for alleviating menopausal symptoms such as hot flashes and night sweats.

How to Use: Red clover is often consumed as an infusion. To make it, steep one tablespoon of dried red clover flowers in hot water for 15-20 minutes. This infusion can be consumed once or twice daily to support hormonal balance and reduce menopausal symptoms.

10. Nettle Tea

Nettle is a nutrient-dense herb that supports women's health by providing essential vitamins and minerals, including iron, calcium, and magnesium. Nettle tea is particularly beneficial for women who experience heavy menstrual bleeding, as it helps replenish lost iron and supports the health of the reproductive system.

How to Use: To make nettle tea, steep one teaspoon of dried nettle leaves in hot water for 10-15 minutes. This tea can be consumed once or twice a day, particularly during the menstrual cycle to support overall reproductive health.

Part 9:
Men's Health and Vitality

Chapter 1: Common Health Concerns for Men – Prostate Health, Vitality, and Stress

1.1 Prostate Health: An Essential Aspect of Men's Wellbeing

Prostate health is a significant concern for men, especially as they age. The prostate gland, a small organ located below the bladder, plays a crucial role in male reproductive health by producing fluids that nourish and transport sperm. However, as men grow older, the prostate becomes susceptible to several conditions, such as benign prostatic hyperplasia (BPH) and prostate cancer. Barbara O'Neill highlights the importance of maintaining prostate health through proactive measures, which include regular checkups, dietary adjustments, and the use of herbal remedies. Understanding these factors is key to preserving overall wellbeing and reducing the risk of prostate-related issues.

The Role of the Prostate in Men's Health

The prostate gland is integral to male reproductive function, contributing to the production of seminal fluid. This fluid not only helps transport sperm during ejaculation but also provides essential nutrients to sustain sperm cells. Despite its small size, the prostate has a significant influence on a man's sexual and reproductive health. However, as men age, the prostate often enlarges, leading to conditions such as BPH, which affects urinary function and can cause discomfort. BPH is a non-cancerous enlargement of the prostate that can lead to symptoms like frequent urination, difficulty in starting urination, and a weak urine flow.

While BPH is not life-threatening, it can impact the quality of life for many men. In addition, prostate cancer is another serious concern that affects older men. It is one of the most common types of cancer in men, and regular screening is critical for early detection. Prostate-specific antigen (PSA) tests and digital rectal exams (DRE) are common methods used to monitor prostate health and detect potential problems early. Barbara emphasizes the importance of these checkups, especially for men over the age of 50, as part of a proactive approach to maintaining prostate health.

Nutrition and Its Impact on Prostate Health

Diet plays a vital role in supporting prostate health and reducing the risk of conditions such as BPH and prostate cancer. O'Neill advocates for a whole-food, plant-based diet that is rich in nutrients and low in processed foods. She suggests that reducing the consumption of saturated fats and red meat can help lower the risk of prostate issues, as diets high in animal fats have been linked to an increased risk of prostate cancer.

Instead, she recommends incorporating foods that are rich in antioxidants, vitamins, and minerals, which can protect the prostate and support overall health. Foods such as tomatoes, which are high in lycopene, a powerful antioxidant, have been shown to support prostate health by reducing oxidative stress and inflammation. Cruciferous vegetables like broccoli, cauliflower, and kale are also recommended, as they contain compounds that have been associated with a reduced risk of cancer. These vegetables help in detoxifying the body and supporting the natural functions of the liver, which plays an indirect role in hormone regulation and cancer prevention.

Additionally, maintaining proper hydration and consuming a high-fiber diet is crucial for reducing the buildup of toxins in the body, which can negatively impact the prostate. Fiber-rich foods such as whole grains, legumes, and fruits promote better digestion and aid in the elimination of harmful substances from the body.

1.2 Supporting Vitality and Energy Levels Naturally

As men age, it is common to experience a gradual decline in energy and vitality. Fatigue, low libido, and reduced stamina can be distressing, but they are often linked to factors that can be addressed naturally. These issues, according to holistic health principles, are frequently tied to stress, poor nutrition, and hormonal imbalances. The goal is to restore balance through a combination of proper nutrition, sleep, and physical activity, all of which can naturally enhance vitality and energy levels.

Nutrition: The Foundation of Energy

Nutrition plays a pivotal role in supporting vitality and energy. As Barbara O'Neill often emphasizes, the body requires a steady supply of nutrients to maintain energy and stamina. Diets that are high in processed foods, sugars, and unhealthy fats can lead to energy crashes and exacerbate feelings of fatigue. These foods cause blood sugar levels to spike and then crash, leaving the body without the consistent fuel it needs to function optimally.

Instead, a diet rich in whole foods—especially fruits, vegetables, lean proteins, and healthy fats—provides sustained energy throughout the day. Foods that are particularly beneficial for boosting energy include those rich in B vitamins, such as whole grains, legumes, and leafy greens. B vitamins are essential for energy production as they help convert food into fuel the body can use. Omega-3 fatty acids, found in foods like flaxseeds, walnuts, and oily fish, also play an important role in maintaining brain health and energy levels by reducing inflammation and supporting cellular function.

Additionally, it is important to avoid nutrient deficiencies that can lead to fatigue. For example, low levels of iron or magnesium can contribute to tiredness and reduced stamina. Ensuring that the diet is rich in iron from sources such as leafy greens, legumes, and lean meats can help prevent fatigue. Similarly, magnesium, found in nuts, seeds, and whole grains, supports energy production and muscle function, helping to reduce feelings of tiredness.

Hormonal Imbalances and Energy Levels

As men age, hormonal imbalances, particularly a decline in testosterone levels, can significantly affect energy and vitality. Testosterone plays a key role in maintaining muscle mass, strength, libido, and overall energy. When testosterone levels drop, men may experience a range of symptoms, including fatigue, reduced motivation, and a decline in sexual desire.

Balancing hormones naturally can help alleviate these symptoms and restore vitality. One way to support hormone balance is through proper nutrition. Consuming foods that are rich in zinc, such as pumpkin seeds, and healthy fats like those found in avocados, can promote healthy testosterone levels. In addition, minimizing exposure to environmental toxins, such as those found in plastics and pesticides, can help maintain hormonal health by reducing the body's toxic load, which can disrupt hormone function.

Herbs such as **ashwagandha** and **tribulus terrestris** are known to support hormonal balance and enhance vitality. These adaptogenic herbs help regulate stress hormones while promoting overall hormonal health, which can lead to increased energy and improved stamina.

The Importance of Sleep for Energy Restoration

Adequate sleep is one of the most important factors in restoring energy and vitality. During sleep, the body undergoes crucial repair processes, including cellular regeneration and the balancing of hormones. Without sufficient rest, these processes are disrupted, leaving the body in a state of depletion. Sleep deprivation also negatively affects cognitive function and mood, further diminishing one's sense of well-being.

Physical Activity: Boosting Energy and Stamina

Regular physical activity is another key factor in maintaining energy and vitality. Exercise helps increase circulation, bringing oxygen and nutrients to cells and tissues throughout the body. It also stimulates the production of endorphins, hormones that improve mood and reduce stress. Engaging in physical activity on a regular basis helps prevent fatigue by enhancing cardiovascular health and muscle strength.

Chapter 2: Natural Herbs to Support Testosterone and Energy Levels

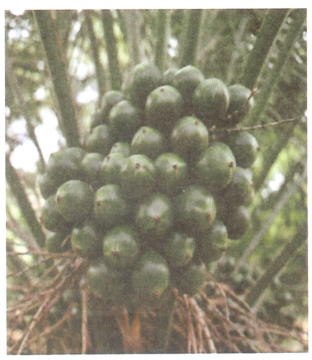

2.1 Saw Palmetto: A Traditional Remedy for Prostate Health

Saw palmetto is a powerful herb traditionally used for supporting prostate health, especially in men experiencing BPH. As the prostate enlarges, it can put pressure on the urinary tract, leading to symptoms such as difficulty urinating, increased frequency, and nocturia (the need to urinate at night). By using saw palmetto, men can alleviate these symptoms and support overall urinary health in a natural, non-invasive way.

Saw Palmetto and BPH Symptom Relief

One of the primary uses of saw palmetto is to reduce the symptoms associated with BPH. The enlargement of the prostate is a common issue among men, especially as they age, and can lead to significant discomfort. Saw palmetto functions by preventing testosterone from being converted into dihydrotestosterone (DHT), a hormone that promotes the growth of the prostate. By blocking this conversion, saw palmetto helps to reduce the size of the prostate and alleviate the symptoms that come with its enlargement. This is particularly important for men looking for natural alternatives to pharmaceutical treatments, which often come with undesirable side effects.

The anti-inflammatory properties of saw palmetto also play a significant role in reducing swelling and irritation in the prostate area. Inflammation is a key contributor to the discomfort and urinary problems associated with BPH, and by lowering inflammation, saw palmetto not only helps ease symptoms but also promotes overall prostate health.

Balancing Hormones and Supporting Prostate Function

Another significant benefit of saw palmetto is its ability to help balance hormones, particularly in men as they age. Hormonal imbalances, especially related to testosterone and estrogen levels, can contribute to prostate issues. Saw palmetto helps to regulate these hormones, ensuring that the body maintains a healthy balance. By inhibiting the production of DHT, the herb helps to prevent excessive prostate growth while still supporting the natural levels of testosterone in the body. This is crucial not only for prostate health but also for maintaining overall male vitality.

In addition to supporting hormonal balance, saw palmetto promotes the health of the urinary tract. Men experiencing BPH often deal with symptoms like frequent urination, incomplete bladder emptying, and discomfort. By addressing the underlying hormonal and inflammatory issues, saw palmetto helps to improve urinary function, making it easier for men to maintain a healthy and active lifestyle without the constant discomfort of BPH symptoms.

Saw Palmetto in Men's Health Formulas

Because of its wide range of benefits for prostate health and hormone regulation, saw palmetto is commonly included in men's health supplements and formulas. These products often combine saw palmetto with other herbs known for their benefits to male reproductive health, such as nettle root or pygeum. Together, these herbs work synergistically to support not only prostate function but also overall male hormonal health, helping to combat the effects of aging on the male body.

2.2 Nettle Root: Supporting Hormonal Balance

Nettle root is a powerful herb known for its ability to support hormonal balance, particularly in men. It has been traditionally used to promote prostate health and maintain healthy testosterone levels. As an anti-inflammatory agent, nettle root helps reduce swelling and discomfort in the prostate, making it a valuable remedy for men experiencing hormonal imbalances or issues related to prostate health. The herb's wide range of benefits is rooted in its unique ability to influence hormone regulation naturally.

Nettle Root and Prostate Health

Prostate health is a significant concern for men, especially as they age. Enlarged prostate, also known as BPH, is a common issue that can cause urinary discomfort and other complications. Nettle root has long been recognized for its role in addressing these symptoms by reducing inflammation and supporting the prostate. The process by which the enzyme 5-alpha-reductase transforms testosterone into dihydrotestosterone (DHT) is inhibited by the root. High levels of DHT are associated with prostate enlargement, so by blocking this conversion, nettle root can help to prevent and reduce the severity of BPH symptoms.

In addition to its effects on DHT, nettle root also has the ability to bind to sex hormone-binding globulin (SHBG), a protein that regulates the availability of testosterone in the body. By lowering the amount of SHBG, nettle root increases the amount of free testosterone, which is crucial for maintaining vitality and overall hormonal health in men. This makes nettle root a highly effective herb for men who are looking to support their prostate and hormonal balance naturally.

Nettle Root and Testosterone Balance

Testosterone is an essential hormone for male health, influencing energy levels, muscle mass, and overall vitality. As men age, testosterone levels naturally decline, which can lead to fatigue, reduced libido, and muscle loss. Nettle root has been shown to help support healthy testosterone levels by preventing its conversion into DHT, as well as increasing the amount of free testosterone available in the body. This makes it an important herb for men who want to maintain their energy and hormonal balance as they age.

In addition to supporting testosterone, nettle root also contains anti-inflammatory compounds that reduce inflammation in the body, particularly in areas like the prostate where inflammation can affect hormonal health. By reducing inflammation, nettle root helps to alleviate the discomfort and imbalance caused by hormonal issues.

How to Use Nettle Root for Hormonal Health

Nettle root can be consumed in several forms, making it a versatile herb for daily use. One of the most popular ways to take nettle root is as a tea. Preparing nettle root tea involves steeping dried nettle root in hot water for several minutes, allowing the active compounds to infuse the water. Drinking this tea regularly can help to promote hormonal balance, reduce inflammation, and support prostate health.

For those who prefer a more concentrated form, nettle root supplements are also available. These supplements provide a standardized dose of the herb and are often used to maintain consistent hormonal support. Whether consumed as a tea or in supplement form, nettle root is a valuable addition to any regimen aimed at supporting hormonal health and vitality.

2.3 Zinc: Essential for Testosterone Production

Testosterone is a critical hormone for men's health, playing a pivotal role in energy levels, muscle mass, and overall reproductive health. One of the key elements that supports the production of testosterone is zinc. Barbara O'Neill emphasizes the importance of zinc in maintaining healthy testosterone levels, noting that a deficiency in this essential mineral can lead to reduced energy, decreased libido, and impaired reproductive function.

The Role of Zinc in Testosterone Production

Zinc is involved in various biological processes, but one of its most crucial roles is in the production of testosterone. This hormone is essential not only for reproductive health but also for maintaining strength, vitality, and overall well-being in men. Zinc acts as a cofactor for several enzymes that regulate testosterone production in the testes. When zinc levels are sufficient, the body can effectively produce and maintain optimal hormone levels, ensuring proper reproductive function and energy balance.

A deficiency in zinc can disrupt this process. Low zinc levels are directly correlated with decreased testosterone, which can lead to symptoms such as fatigue, reduced muscle mass, and a lowered sex drive. Furthermore, low testosterone can contribute to more severe health problems over time, including osteoporosis, mood disorders, and infertility. Therefore, ensuring adequate zinc intake is essential for preserving not only testosterone levels but also overall health and vitality.

Zinc-Rich Foods for Hormonal Balance

The body does not store zinc, meaning that regular consumption of zinc-rich foods is essential to maintaining its levels. Certain foods are particularly beneficial for providing the body with the necessary amount of this mineral to support testosterone production.

One of the most well-known sources of zinc is **oysters**, which are extremely rich in this mineral. Consuming oysters regularly can significantly boost zinc levels and contribute to healthy testosterone production. Other seafood, such as crab and lobster, are also excellent sources of zinc.

For those who prefer plant-based options, **pumpkin seeds** are a fantastic source of zinc. They are easy to incorporate into the diet and can be added to salads, smoothies, or eaten as a snack. Pumpkin seeds provide a convenient way to boost zinc intake without relying on animal products. Other seeds and nuts, such as sesame seeds and cashews, also contain good amounts of zinc.

Whole grains, such as quinoa and oats, and **legumes**, like chickpeas and lentils, provide additional sources of zinc, especially for individuals following a vegetarian or vegan diet. These foods not only support testosterone production but also contribute to overall health by providing fiber, vitamins, and minerals that are important for daily well-being.

Zinc Supplements for Maintaining Optimal Levels

In addition to dietary sources, zinc supplements can be beneficial for men who struggle to meet their daily zinc requirements through food alone. Supplementing with zinc is particularly useful for those who have conditions that may interfere with zinc absorption or who follow a diet that is naturally low in zinc-rich foods. Zinc supplements come in various forms, such as zinc gluconate or zinc picolinate, and can be taken daily to help maintain optimal testosterone levels and support reproductive health.

However, it is important to note that excessive supplementation can lead to adverse effects, such as GI discomfort or interference with the absorption of other minerals like copper. Therefore, it is recommended to monitor zinc intake carefully and to consult with a healthcare provider if necessary to determine the appropriate dosage.

2.4 Adaptogenic Herbs for Stress and Vitality

Adaptogenic herbs are known for their ability to help the body cope with stress and maintain balance, supporting overall vitality and energy levels. These herbs work by regulating the body's stress response, making them valuable tools for promoting resilience in the face of mental, physical, and emotional strain.

Ashwagandha and Rhodiola Rosea are two of the most well-known adaptogens, frequently recommended for their ability to reduce the effects of stress and boost energy. By supporting adrenal health, these herbs help regulate hormone production, which is crucial for maintaining both vitality and optimal testosterone levels.

The Role of Ashwagandha in Stress Reduction

Ashwagandha, a powerful adaptogen, has been used for centuries in Ayurvedic medicine to promote physical strength and mental clarity. It is highly valued for its ability to regulate the body's cortisol levels, the hormone responsible for the "fight or flight" response. When stress is chronic, cortisol remains elevated for prolonged periods, leading to fatigue, impaired cognitive function, and a weakened immune system. Ashwagandha works by helping to lower cortisol levels, allowing the body to return to a state of balance.

Furthermore, ashwagandha has a reputation for promoting adrenal health, which is critical for stress management over the long run. The adrenal glands are responsible for producing hormones like cortisol and adrenaline, which play a critical role in the body's stress response. Over time, chronic stress can deplete the adrenal glands, leading to what is commonly referred to as "adrenal fatigue." Ashwagandha helps to restore adrenal function, enabling the body to better manage stress without becoming overwhelmed.

This adaptogen is also noted for its role in boosting testosterone levels and supporting vitality, particularly in men. By reducing stress and improving adrenal health, Ashwagandha helps to maintain healthy levels of testosterone, which is essential for energy, mood, and overall well-being.

Rhodiola Rosea: Enhancing Energy and Resilience

Rhodiola Rosea is another adaptogenic herb highly regarded for its ability to enhance energy and improve mental resilience. This herb grows in cold regions and has been traditionally used to combat fatigue and improve physical endurance. Like Ashwagandha, Rhodiola helps regulate the body's stress response, but it is particularly effective in boosting energy levels and reducing mental fatigue.

One of Rhodiola's primary actions is its effect on the adrenal glands. By supporting adrenal health, Rhodiola helps the body produce and regulate the hormones needed to maintain energy and focus throughout the day. This adaptogen has been shown to improve cognitive function, particularly under conditions of stress, making it an excellent choice for those who experience mental exhaustion or burnout.

Rhodiola also supports testosterone production by balancing the stress response. Stress, particularly chronic stress, can suppress the production of testosterone, leading to reduced energy levels, decreased motivation, and even mood disturbances. By promoting adrenal balance, Rhodiola helps to ensure that testosterone levels remain stable, supporting both physical and mental vitality.

Supporting Adrenal Health with Adaptogens

Adrenal health is key to maintaining overall vitality, particularly when it comes to managing stress. The adrenal glands are responsible for producing several hormones, including cortisol, adrenaline, and testosterone. When these glands are overworked due to chronic stress, they can become depleted, leading to symptoms of adrenal fatigue, such as low energy, difficulty concentrating, and reduced physical endurance.

Adaptogens like Ashwagandha and Rhodiola work by supporting the adrenal glands, allowing them to function more efficiently even under stressful conditions. By reducing the burden on the adrenals, these herbs help to balance hormone production, ensuring that cortisol levels do not remain elevated for too long. This, in turn, supports the body's ability to produce sufficient amounts of testosterone, which is critical for maintaining energy, strength, and overall vitality.

Chapter 3: Holistic Practices for Improving Male Stamina and Stress Management

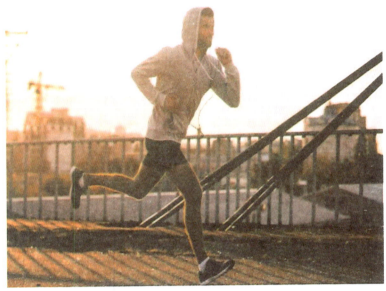

3.1 The Role of Regular Physical Activity in Male Health

Physical activity is a critical component of maintaining overall health, especially for men. It not only helps in maintaining muscle mass and cardiovascular fitness but also plays a key role in regulating hormones and managing stress. Barbara O'Neill emphasizes that regular exercise is an essential part of a holistic approach to male health, impacting everything from energy levels to emotional well-being.

As men age, the natural decline in testosterone levels can result in a gradual loss of muscle mass, a condition known as sarcopenia. This loss of muscle can lead to decreased strength and vitality, making everyday tasks more difficult and reducing overall quality of life. Regular physical activity, particularly weight-bearing exercises, is essential for maintaining muscle mass and strength. Weight training stimulates the muscles, promoting growth and preventing the age-related decline that many men experience. It also helps in increasing bone density, reducing the risk of osteoporosis, which can affect men later in life.

Cardiovascular health is another critical area where exercise has a profound impact. Activities such as running, swimming, cycling, or even brisk walking increase heart rate and improve blood circulation, helping to strengthen the heart muscle. Regular cardiovascular exercise lowers blood pressure, improves cholesterol levels, and reduces the risk of heart disease, one of the leading causes of death among men. Consistent aerobic activity also boosts lung capacity, allowing the body to use oxygen more efficiently, which in turn improves stamina and endurance.

3.2 Stress Management Techniques for Long-Term Vitality

Chronic stress is one of the most pervasive factors contributing to a decline in overall health, particularly when it comes to hormone regulation. Elevated stress levels lead to the overproduction of cortisol, a hormone released by the adrenal glands in response to stress. While cortisol is necessary for managing acute stress, prolonged exposure to elevated cortisol levels can interfere with various physiological functions, including testosterone production. Testosterone is crucial for maintaining energy levels, muscle mass, and overall vitality, especially in men. Therefore, reducing chronic stress is essential for preserving long-term health and well-being.

3.3 The Importance of Sleep for Hormonal Balance

Sleep plays a critical role in maintaining the body's natural rhythms and supporting hormonal balance. Disruptions in sleep can have a significant impact on the body's production of hormones, particularly testosterone, which is essential for energy, vitality, and overall well-being. Barbara O'Neill highlights the importance of getting quality sleep to sustain optimal hormonal function and offers practical strategies to improve sleep hygiene, along with natural remedies to promote restful sleep.

Hormones are regulated by the body's circadian rhythms, which are closely tied to sleep patterns. When these rhythms are disrupted—due to inadequate or poor-quality sleep—the body's ability to produce and regulate hormones is compromised. Testosterone, in particular, is highly sensitive to changes in sleep. This hormone, crucial for both men and women, plays a key role in maintaining muscle mass, energy levels, and overall vitality. It is primarily produced during the deeper stages of sleep, especially REM (rapid eye movement) cycles. Therefore, insufficient sleep can lead to a reduction in testosterone production, which in turn affects energy, mood, and physical performance.

Lack of sleep also influences other hormones, including cortisol, which is often referred to as the "stress hormone." Elevated cortisol levels due to insufficient rest can further disrupt hormonal balance by interfering with the production of testosterone and other vital hormones. This hormonal imbalance can lead to feelings of fatigue, irritability, and a decline in overall health. Barbara explains that by prioritizing good sleep, individuals can help reset their natural rhythms, which in turn supports healthy hormone levels.

Chapter 4: Nutrition for Men's Health and Vitality

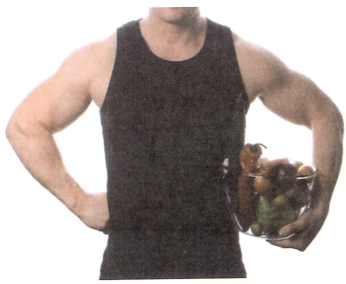

4.1 A Nutrient-Dense Diet for Male Hormonal Health

The importance of nutrition in maintaining optimal male hormonal health cannot be overstated. A diet rich in whole, plant-based foods is essential for supporting the body's natural balance of hormones, particularly testosterone, which is crucial for maintaining energy, stamina, and overall vitality. While there are various factors that influence hormonal health, the role of nutrition is one of the most impactful and controllable. Barbara O'Neill highlights how adopting a nutrient-dense diet can help men achieve and sustain healthy hormone levels naturally.

The Role of Antioxidants, Vitamins, and Minerals in Hormonal Health

Hormonal function is closely tied to the availability of specific nutrients, many of which can be obtained through a diet rich in whole, plant-based foods. Antioxidants, such as vitamins C and E, play a crucial role in protecting cells from oxidative stress, which can otherwise lead to hormonal imbalances. Oxidative stress is known to damage cells, including those responsible for hormone production, thus making antioxidants a key component in maintaining healthy hormone levels.

Vitamins and minerals are equally important for hormonal health. Zinc, in particular, is one of the most critical minerals for testosterone production. A deficiency in zinc can result in reduced testosterone levels, leading to symptoms such as fatigue, low libido, and decreased muscle mass. Foods rich in zinc, such as nuts, seeds, and whole grains, should be a staple in any diet aimed at supporting male hormonal health. Magnesium is another essential mineral that helps regulate testosterone levels and supports muscle function, energy metabolism, and overall vitality.

In addition to these nutrients, maintaining a balanced intake of B vitamins is vital for energy production and hormone regulation. B vitamins, found abundantly in leafy greens, nuts, and seeds, assist in the conversion of food into energy and play a role in the synthesis of hormones, ensuring that the body can produce adequate levels of testosterone and other critical hormones.

Key Foods for Boosting Testosterone and Maintaining Stamina

Several specific foods have been identified as particularly beneficial for supporting male hormonal health. Nuts and seeds, such as walnuts, flaxseeds, and chia seeds, are excellent sources of essential fatty acids, including omega-3s. These healthy fats are necessary for hormone production, particularly testosterone, and help to reduce inflammation, which can otherwise disrupt hormonal balance.

Leafy greens, such as spinach, kale, and Swiss chard, are rich in antioxidants and minerals like magnesium, which contribute to testosterone regulation. These greens also provide fiber, which supports overall digestion and helps the body to eliminate excess hormones, preventing imbalances. By including a variety of leafy greens in the diet, men can ensure they are providing their bodies with the essential nutrients needed for optimal hormonal function.

Healthy fats, such as those found in avocados, olive oil, and coconut oil, are another important component of a diet aimed at supporting testosterone levels. These fats provide the building blocks for hormone production and help the body absorb fat-soluble vitamins like A, D, E, and K, which are also crucial for maintaining healthy testosterone levels. Incorporating healthy fats into the diet not only supports hormonal balance but also provides sustained energy and improves overall stamina.

Whole grains and legumes also play a role in supporting male hormonal health. These foods provide a steady release of energy, preventing spikes and crashes in blood sugar levels that can negatively affect hormone production. Additionally, they are rich in fiber, which helps to maintain a healthy digestive system and ensures that the body can effectively eliminate toxins and excess hormones.

4.2 The Role of Omega-3 Fatty Acids in Men's Health

Omega-3 fatty acids play a crucial role in maintaining men's health, especially in reducing inflammation and supporting brain function. These essential fats, found abundantly in flaxseeds, chia seeds, and fatty fish like salmon, provide multiple health benefits that go beyond just physical wellness. They are vital for preserving mental clarity, maintaining steady energy levels, and promoting long-term cognitive function. In her teachings, Barbara O'Neill discusses how incorporating these healthy fats into daily meals can contribute to a man's overall vitality and well-being.

Omega-3s and Inflammation Reduction

One of the key benefits of omega-3 fatty acids is their powerful anti-inflammatory properties. Although the body naturally responds to injury or infection with inflammation, chronic inflammation can cause a number of health problems, such as heart disease, joint discomfort, and even mental health difficulties. Omega-3s help reduce this chronic inflammation by decreasing the production of inflammatory molecules such as cytokines and eicosanoids.

In men, inflammation is often linked to conditions like cardiovascular disease and arthritis. By reducing inflammation, omega-3 fatty acids not only protect the heart and joints but also support overall metabolic function. These healthy fats play a vital role in regulating blood pressure, reducing triglycerides, and improving circulation, all of which are essential for maintaining cardiovascular health. In this way, omega-3s contribute to a healthier, more resilient body, protecting against the long-term risks associated with chronic inflammation.

Omega-3s and Brain Health

In addition to their anti-inflammatory benefits, omega-3 fatty acids are critical for brain health. They support the structure and function of brain cells, particularly in the membranes of neurons, where they help ensure optimal communication between cells. This is particularly important for maintaining mental clarity and cognitive function as men age. Omega-3s, especially docosahexaenoic acid (DHA), are integral to supporting memory, focus, and overall brain performance.

Low levels of omega-3s have been associated with cognitive decline, mental fatigue, and even mood disorders. By ensuring adequate intake of these fats, men can support their brain's ability to process information efficiently and maintain energy levels throughout the day. Omega-3s help to protect against the oxidative stress that can impair brain function, making them essential for long-term mental well-being.

Incorporating Omega-3-Rich Foods into Daily Meals

One of the simplest ways to ensure a sufficient intake of omega-3s is by incorporating omega-3-rich foods into daily meals. Flaxseeds, chia seeds, and walnuts are excellent plant-based sources of alpha-linolenic acid (ALA), a type of omega-3 that can be converted into the more potent forms, eicosapentaenoic acid (EPA) and DHA, within the body. For those following a plant-based diet, these seeds can easily be added to smoothies, salads, or yogurt to increase omega-3 intake.

For those who consume fish, fatty fish like salmon, mackerel, and sardines are some of the best dietary sources of EPA and DHA. Including these types of fish in meals at least twice a week provides a reliable and direct source of omega-3s. Cooking fish with healthy oils, such as olive oil, can enhance its flavor while preserving its nutritional value. Additionally, fish oil supplements are available for individuals who may struggle to incorporate enough omega-3s into their diet through food alone.

In daily meal planning, simple strategies like sprinkling flaxseeds or chia seeds on oatmeal or adding them to baked goods can boost omega-3 consumption without much effort. Chia seeds, in particular, absorb liquid and can be used to make chia pudding, a nutritious and delicious way to include more omega-3s in breakfast or snacks.

4.3 Avoiding Hormonal Disruptors

Hormonal balance is essential for maintaining overall health, but it is increasingly challenged by exposure to harmful substances in everyday life. Many of these substances, found in processed foods, plastics, and household products, can disrupt the body's natural hormonal function, leading to a range of health issues. In her teachings, Barbara O'Neill highlights the importance of avoiding these hormonal disruptors and emphasizes the role of clean eating and reducing environmental toxin exposure to support hormonal health.

The Impact of Processed Foods and Refined Sugars on Hormones

Processed foods and refined sugars are significant contributors to hormonal imbalances. These products are often stripped of nutrients and contain additives that can interfere with the body's natural hormone regulation. High sugar consumption, for instance, leads to spikes in insulin levels, a hormone that plays a key role in regulating blood sugar. When consumed in excess, refined sugars can cause insulin resistance, which not only affects metabolic health but also has a ripple effect on other hormones, such as estrogen and cortisol.

Barbara warns that many processed foods contain artificial preservatives and additives, which can further stress the endocrine system. These chemicals can mimic or block hormone receptors, disrupting the body's delicate hormonal balance. In particular, artificial sweeteners, flavor enhancers, and food dyes have been linked to disruptions in thyroid function and reproductive hormones.

To protect hormonal health, it is crucial to avoid processed foods and instead focus on whole, nutrient-dense options. Incorporating fresh fruits, vegetables, whole grains, and lean proteins into the diet helps to stabilize blood sugar levels and support the natural production of hormones. Additionally, choosing organic produce minimizes exposure to pesticides and chemicals that can act as endocrine disruptors.

Dangers of Hormone-Disrupting Chemicals in Plastics and Packaged Goods

Another major source of hormonal disruption comes from chemicals commonly found in plastics and packaged goods. Substances like **bisphenol A (BPA)** and **phthalates**, which are used in the production of plastics, can leach into food and beverages, particularly when exposed to heat. These chemicals are known endocrine disruptors, meaning they can interfere with the body's hormone systems by mimicking estrogen or blocking hormonal signals.

Exposure to these substances has been related to a number of health concerns, including trouble with reproduction, child development, and even some types of cancer. Barbara stresses the importance of avoiding plastic containers, particularly for storing food or liquids. Instead, she recommends using glass or stainless steel containers, which do not contain harmful chemicals that can leach into food.

Packaged goods also pose a risk, as they often contain preservatives and chemicals designed to prolong shelf life. These substances can accumulate in the body over time, disrupting hormone production and function. Reducing the use of plastics and opting for fresh, unpackaged foods is a crucial step in minimizing exposure to these toxins.

Clean, Organic Eating for Hormonal Health

To further protect hormonal health, it is essential to prioritize clean, organic eating. Organic foods are grown without the use of synthetic pesticides, herbicides, or fertilizers, all of which can contain hormone-disrupting chemicals. By choosing organic produce, individuals reduce their exposure to these harmful substances, which can interfere with the body's natural hormonal rhythms.

In addition to organic produce, it is important to be mindful of meat and dairy products. Conventional animal farming often relies on hormones to promote growth and increase production. Consuming meat and dairy from animals treated with synthetic hormones can introduce these substances into the human body, leading to hormonal imbalances. Choosing organic, hormone-free options helps to avoid these risks and supports the body's natural hormonal function.

Moreover, Barbara advocates for a diet rich in **phytoestrogens**, which are naturally occurring plant compounds that can help balance estrogen levels in the body. Foods such as flaxseeds, soy, and legumes contain phytoestrogens that can support hormonal health without the negative effects associated with synthetic chemicals.

Chapter 5: 10 Natural Remedies for Men's Health and Vitality

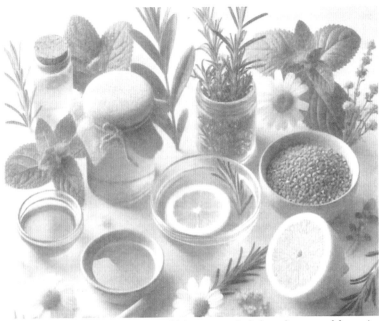

Maintaining optimal health and vitality is essential for men, particularly as they age and face unique health challenges. From supporting hormonal balance to boosting energy levels, natural remedies can play a significant role in enhancing men's well-being. Below are ten natural remedies, along with recommendations for how, when, and why to use them, that can support various aspects of men's health.

1. Saw Palmetto Capsules

Saw palmetto is widely known for its benefits in supporting prostate health. It functions by preventing testosterone from being converted into the hormone dihydrotestosterone (DHT), which is connected to prostate hypertrophy. For men experiencing symptoms of BPH, such as frequent urination, saw palmetto can provide relief.

How to use: Take saw palmetto in capsule form, typically 160 mg twice daily.

When to use: It is best taken with meals to aid absorption.

Why to use: Saw palmetto is ideal for men over 40 or those experiencing prostate issues. Regular use can help reduce inflammation in the prostate and support overall urinary health.

2. Nettle Root Tea

Nettle root has been used traditionally to promote urinary tract health and support prostate function. It contains compounds that help reduce symptoms of BPH and may enhance testosterone levels, making it a great addition to a health regimen focused on men's vitality.

How to use: Brew nettle root tea by steeping 1-2 teaspoons of dried nettle root in hot water for 10-15 minutes.

When to use: Drink 1-2 cups daily, ideally in the morning and evening.

Why to use: Regular consumption of nettle root tea can help alleviate urinary issues and support hormonal balance, particularly for men over 50.

3. Zinc Supplement

Zinc is an essential mineral that plays a crucial role in testosterone production and immune function. It is also important for prostate health and overall reproductive wellness. Deficiencies in zinc can lead to decreased testosterone levels and an increased risk of prostate issues.

How to use: Take a zinc supplement containing 15-30 mg per day.

When to use: It is best taken with a meal to prevent stomach upset.

Why to use: Zinc supplementation is important for men who are looking to maintain healthy testosterone levels and support reproductive health, especially if dietary intake is insufficient.

4. Ashwagandha Powder

Ashwagandha is an adaptogenic herb that helps the body manage stress while enhancing physical performance and stamina. It also has a positive effect on testosterone levels, making it particularly beneficial for men seeking to improve both physical and mental vitality.

How to use: Mix 1 teaspoon of ashwagandha powder into water, smoothies, or herbal teas.

When to use: Take once or twice daily, preferably in the morning and before bed.

Why to use: Ashwagandha helps combat fatigue, stress, and low energy levels, supporting overall vitality and well-being.

5. Rhodiola Rosea Tincture

Rhodiola Rosea is another adaptogen known for its ability to reduce fatigue and enhance mental clarity and endurance. It works by improving the body's resistance to stress and promoting better energy levels, making it ideal for men dealing with the demands of a busy lifestyle.

How to use: Take 30-40 drops of Rhodiola Rosea tincture in water.

When to use: Once or twice daily, preferably in the morning or early afternoon. Avoid taking it in the evening as it may interfere with sleep.

Why to use: Rhodiola is particularly beneficial for men who experience mental and physical fatigue, helping to restore energy and focus.

6. Pumpkin Seeds (Zinc-Rich Snack)

Pumpkin seeds are a natural source of zinc and magnesium, two minerals that are essential for testosterone production and prostate health. These seeds are also rich in antioxidants, which help reduce inflammation.

How to use: Eat a small handful (about 1 ounce) of raw or roasted pumpkin seeds daily.

When to use: They can be eaten as a snack anytime during the day.

Why to use: Regular consumption of pumpkin seeds supports prostate health, hormonal balance, and overall vitality due to their high zinc content.

7. Maca Root Powder

Maca root is traditionally used to boost energy, stamina, and libido. It is particularly valued for its ability to balance hormones and improve sexual function in men, making it a popular choice for enhancing vitality and reproductive health.

How to use: Mix 1-2 teaspoons of maca root powder into smoothies, oatmeal, or yogurt.

When to use: Take daily, preferably in the morning for an energy boost.

Why to use: Maca root supports physical performance and sexual health, making it an excellent choice for men seeking to enhance both energy and reproductive function.

8. Tribulus Terrestris Extract

Tribulus Terrestris is a natural herb known for its ability to increase testosterone levels and enhance libido. It is often used by athletes to improve strength and stamina, and it has been traditionally employed to address male fertility and sexual performance issues.

How to use: Take 250-500 mg of Tribulus Terrestris extract daily.

When to use: It can be taken once or twice a day with meals.

Why to use: This herb is particularly beneficial for men looking to boost testosterone naturally, improve physical performance, and enhance sexual health.

9. Valerian Root for Sleep

Valerian root is a calming herb that has been used for centuries to promote better sleep and reduce anxiety. Adequate sleep is crucial for maintaining hormonal balance, mental clarity, and overall vitality, making valerian root an important remedy for men who struggle with insomnia or poor sleep quality.

How to use: Take valerian root in capsule form (400-900 mg) or as a tea before bed.

When to use: 30 minutes to an hour before bedtime.

Why to use: Valerian root helps men achieve deep, restful sleep, which is essential for energy recovery, stress management, and maintaining healthy testosterone levels.

10. Omega-3 Fish Oil

Omega-3 fatty acids are essential for heart health, cognitive function, and reducing inflammation throughout the body. They also play a role in maintaining healthy testosterone levels and supporting overall vitality. Omega-3 fish oil supplements are a convenient way to ensure adequate intake of these crucial fats.

How to use: Take 1-2 grams of omega-3 fish oil daily.

When to use: It can be taken with meals, either in the morning or at night.

Why to use: Omega-3 supplements help reduce inflammation, support heart health, and maintain cognitive function, all of which are important for long-term vitality in men.

Each of these natural remedies can support different aspects of men's health and vitality, from boosting energy and testosterone levels to promoting restful sleep and reducing inflammation. Integrating these remedies into daily routines can lead to significant improvements in overall well-being, particularly when paired with a healthy lifestyle.

Part 10:
Aging Gracefully – Supporting Longevity and Vitality

Chapter 1: Slowing the Aging Process with Nutrition and Natural Supplements

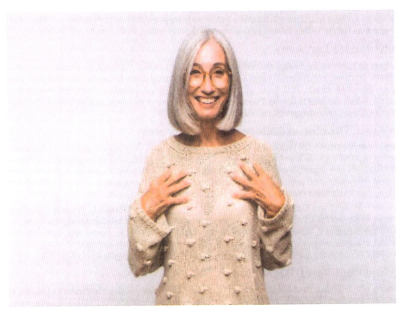

1.1 The Aging Process: A Holistic Perspective

The aging process is an inevitable part of life, but its pace and effects can be greatly influenced by the choices we make, particularly in terms of diet, lifestyle, and stress management. The holistic perspective views aging not as a decline in health, but as a natural progression that can be embraced gracefully when the body is nourished and supported properly. By understanding how factors such as chronic inflammation, poor nutrition, and stress accelerate aging, and by adopting practices that include nutrient-dense foods and natural remedies, it is possible to promote longevity and vitality well into the later years of life.

The Role of Chronic Inflammation in Accelerating Aging

One of the key factors that contribute to premature aging is chronic inflammation. Inflammation is the body's natural response to injury or infection, but when it becomes chronic, it can damage tissues and organs over time. Chronic inflammation is often triggered by poor dietary choices, environmental toxins, and prolonged stress. This ongoing inflammatory state accelerates the breakdown of cells and leads to the development of age-related conditions such as arthritis, cardiovascular disease, and cognitive decline.

Poor Diet and Its Impact on Aging

A poor diet is another major contributor to the acceleration of aging. Diets high in processed foods, sugars, unhealthy fats, and artificial additives can lead to nutritional deficiencies that prevent the body from functioning optimally. When the body lacks essential nutrients, it cannot adequately repair cells, manage inflammation, or detoxify harmful substances. Over time, this results in the deterioration of vital systems, leading to premature aging and an increased risk of chronic diseases.

Nutrient-poor foods also contribute to oxidative stress, a condition where harmful molecules known as free radicals accumulate in the body, damaging cells and tissues. This oxidative damage is a key factor in the aging process, as it leads to the breakdown of DNA, proteins, and lipids, which are essential for maintaining healthy cellular function. To combat this, it is important to consume a diet rich in antioxidants, which neutralize free radicals and protect the body from oxidative stress.

The Importance of Nutrient-Dense Foods in Slowing Aging

To slow the effects of aging and support the body's natural repair processes, it is essential to consume a diet that is rich in nutrient-dense foods. These foods provide the vitamins, minerals, and antioxidants needed to keep the body's systems functioning efficiently. Nutrient-dense foods such as leafy greens, berries, nuts, seeds, and whole grains help to reduce inflammation, support detoxification, and promote cellular repair.

1.2 Nutrition for Longevity

A key aspect of maintaining health and vitality as we age lies in the nutrients we consume. A diet rich in antioxidants, vitamins, and minerals plays a crucial role in slowing down the aging process by protecting the body from oxidative stress. This form of stress is caused by an imbalance between free radicals and antioxidants, which can lead to the deterioration of cells over time. A well-balanced diet, therefore, is essential to supporting longevity by preserving cellular health and function.

Antioxidants, Vitamins, and Minerals to Combat Aging

Oxidative stress is a significant factor in the aging process. Free radicals—unstable molecules produced by the body during metabolic processes—can damage cells, proteins, and DNA, leading to aging and various chronic diseases. The body uses antioxidants as a defense against this harm. By neutralizing free radicals, antioxidants protect cells from harm and support the body's ability to repair and regenerate tissues. A diet abundant in antioxidant-rich foods helps reduce the impact of oxidative stress and promotes healthy aging.

Vitamins such as A, C, and E are particularly important in this regard. Vitamin C, found in citrus fruits and leafy greens, is known for its ability to boost collagen production, which helps maintain the integrity of the skin as we age. Vitamin E, which can be found in nuts and seeds, works to protect skin cells from oxidative damage and maintain overall skin health. These vitamins, along with other essential minerals like selenium and zinc, help maintain the body's ability to repair itself and function optimally throughout the aging process.

The Role of Plant-Based, Whole Foods in Longevity

Plant-based, whole foods are central to promoting longevity due to their high concentration of phytonutrients, fiber, and healthy fats. Phytonutrients are naturally occurring compounds in plants that provide health benefits beyond basic nutrition. Foods such as leafy greens, berries, nuts, seeds, and legumes are particularly rich in these nutrients, which have been shown to reduce inflammation, improve heart health, and support overall well-being.

Leafy greens like spinach, kale, and Swiss chard are especially beneficial for their high content of vitamins and minerals, including calcium and magnesium, which support bone health as we age. Berries, such as blueberries and strawberries, are packed with antioxidants like anthocyanins, which protect against cognitive decline and help maintain brain health. Nuts and seeds provide healthy fats, including omega-3 fatty acids, which are known to reduce inflammation and support heart health—an important factor in longevity.

Beans, lentils, and chickpeas are examples of legumes that are a great source of fiber and plant-based protein. These foods help regulate blood sugar levels, lower cholesterol, and improve digestive health, all of which contribute to a longer, healthier life. In addition, the fiber in plant-based foods supports gut health by promoting the growth of beneficial bacteria in the digestive system.

1.3 Natural Supplements to Support Longevity

As the body ages, maintaining optimal health becomes increasingly dependent on proper nutrition and supplementation. Some key supplements play a vital role in supporting bone strength, cognitive function, and cardiovascular health, helping to slow the aging process. In her teachings, Barbara O'Neill emphasizes the importance of specific nutrients, such as Vitamin D, magnesium, omega-3 fatty acids, and antioxidants, for promoting longevity and protecting the body from the damage associated with aging.

The Role of Antioxidants in Slowing the Aging Process

In addition to vitamins and minerals, antioxidants are critical for protecting the body from the oxidative damage that accelerates the aging process. One of the most potent antioxidants is **CoQ10** (Coenzyme Q10), a compound naturally produced by the body that plays a key role in energy production at the cellular level.

CoQ10 levels decrease with age, and supplementation can help restore these levels, supporting heart health and reducing the risk of age-related diseases. CoQ10 also functions as an antioxidant, neutralizing free radicals that can damage cells and contribute to aging.

Resveratrol, another powerful antioxidant, is found in grapes, berries, and red wine. Resveratrol has gained attention for its potential to extend lifespan by activating certain genes associated with longevity and cellular repair. It also supports cardiovascular health by improving circulation and reducing inflammation, both of which are critical for preventing heart disease and maintaining overall vitality as the body ages.

Turmeric, a spice commonly used in traditional medicine, contains **curcumin**, its active compound known for its potent anti-inflammatory and antioxidant effects. Curcumin helps to reduce oxidative stress in the body, which is a key contributor to cellular aging. By neutralizing free radicals and reducing inflammation, turmeric supports the body's natural repair processes and can help slow the visible and internal signs of aging.

Chapter 2: Herbal Remedies for Cognitive Function and Memory Retention

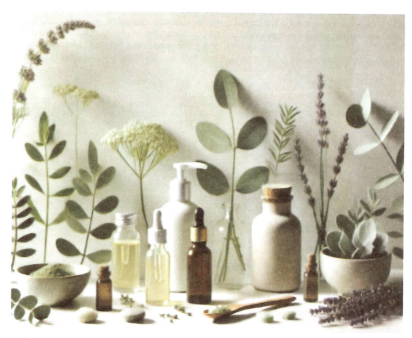

2.1 Understanding Cognitive Decline with Age

As the body naturally ages, cognitive function often begins to show signs of decline. Memory loss, brain fog, and difficulty concentrating are common complaints among older adults. These issues are not just the result of aging itself but are frequently caused by underlying factors such as inflammation, poor circulation, and oxidative stress in the brain. Addressing these root causes can help slow the progression of cognitive decline and support brain health.

There are several systems and natural effects on the body that contribute to cognitive functionality and its decline:

- Inflammation and Cognitive Decline
- Poor Circulation and Cognitive Function
- Oxidative Stress and Brain Health

Part 18 provides more details, but the following are some of the primary herbal remedies to keep your brain sharp as you age.

2.2 Ginkgo Biloba: A Natural Brain Booster

Ginkgo Biloba has long been recognized for its powerful effects on memory and cognitive function. As one of the oldest living tree species, its leaves have been used in traditional medicine for centuries to treat a variety of ailments, particularly those affecting the brain. In her teachings, Barbara O'Neill advocates the use of Ginkgo Biloba to enhance mental clarity and support healthy brain function as we age. This potent herb works by improving circulation to the brain and reducing oxidative stress, making it an excellent natural remedy for maintaining cognitive sharpness.

2.3 Turmeric: Reducing Inflammation for Cognitive Health

Turmeric is a powerful natural remedy known for its potent anti-inflammatory properties, largely attributed to its active ingredient, curcumin. Curcumin plays a vital role in protecting the brain from age-related cognitive decline by reducing chronic inflammation that can impair brain function. This natural compound is well-regarded for its ability to support overall brain health, and its inclusion in daily nutrition can serve as a preventive measure against cognitive impairments. In her teachings, Barbara O'Neill emphasizes the importance of turmeric as a key component in maintaining brain health and reducing inflammation.

2.4 Bacopa: Enhancing Memory and Learning

Bacopa is an herb widely recognized for its ability to support memory retention and improve cognitive function. Traditionally used in Ayurvedic medicine, Bacopa has gained attention for its potential to enhance learning abilities, reduce stress, and prevent cognitive decline. The herb works by influencing neurotransmitters in the brain, helping to promote mental clarity and focus while also offering a calming effect that can reduce anxiety-related memory issues.

Chapter 3: Supporting Physical Strength and Energy as We Age

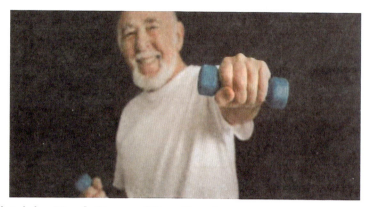

3.1 Maintaining Muscle Mass and Bone Density

As we age, the preservation of muscle mass and bone density becomes increasingly critical for maintaining overall health and mobility. Muscle mass naturally decreases with age, a condition known as sarcopenia, while bones become more fragile due to a decline in density, leading to osteoporosis. Both conditions significantly increase the risk of falls, fractures, and a reduced quality of life. In her teachings, Barbara O'Neill emphasizes the importance of a proactive approach to maintaining muscle mass and bone density through regular exercise, proper nutrition, and, when necessary, supplementation.

The Role of Strength Training and Resistance Exercises

Weight-bearing and resistance exercises are among the most effective methods for maintaining both muscle mass and bone density. Strength training, which includes exercises such as lifting weights, using resistance bands, or engaging in bodyweight exercises like squats and lunges, plays a crucial role in stimulating muscle growth and preserving bone strength. When muscles contract against resistance, they pull on the bones, promoting the rebuilding of bone tissue and helping to prevent bone loss over time.

These types of exercises are particularly important for older adults because they target the very issues that lead to sarcopenia and osteoporosis. By regularly engaging in resistance training, individuals can slow the natural decline of muscle mass, thereby improving strength, balance, and overall functional mobility. For bones, the stress caused by weight-bearing movements signals the body to increase bone density, effectively reducing the risk of osteoporosis-related fractures. Strength training is not only a preventative measure but can also help reverse some of the muscle and bone loss that has already occurred.

Incorporating a mix of different resistance exercises is key to targeting various muscle groups and promoting even bone density throughout the body. Movements like squats and lunges engage large muscle groups in the legs, helping to strengthen the bones in the hips and thighs, which are especially prone to fractures in older adults. Meanwhile, upper body exercises such as push-ups or dumbbell presses work to maintain strength and density in the arms and shoulders, areas that also tend to weaken with age.

Nutrition and Supplementation for Bone and Muscle Health

Exercise alone, however, is not enough to fully protect against muscle and bone loss. Proper nutrition is essential to provide the body with the necessary building blocks for maintaining and rebuilding these tissues. Protein, for instance, is a key nutrient for muscle growth and repair. As muscle mass decreases with age, it becomes even more important to ensure adequate protein intake to support muscle maintenance.

In addition to protein, calcium and vitamin D are essential for bone health. Calcium is the primary mineral found in bones, while vitamin D is necessary for the proper absorption of calcium from the diet. Ensuring that the body receives adequate amounts of these nutrients can help slow the progression of bone density loss. Foods such as leafy green vegetables, almonds, and fortified plant-based milks are excellent sources of calcium, while sunlight exposure and foods like mushrooms provide vitamin D.

For those who are unable to meet their nutritional needs through diet alone, supplementation may be necessary. Calcium and vitamin D supplements can be particularly helpful for individuals at risk of osteoporosis. Magnesium, another mineral important for bone health, can also be taken as a supplement to support bone strength and density. Additionally, supplements such as collagen and protein powders may be useful for older adults struggling to maintain adequate muscle mass through diet alone.

3.2 Herbs to Boost Physical Energy

Physical energy and stamina are essential for maintaining an active and healthy lifestyle, particularly as we age. There are a variety of natural herbs that can help boost energy levels and support vitality, allowing the body to adapt to stress and maintain resilience. These herbs, known as adaptogens, are highly regarded for their ability to enhance endurance and balance the body's stress response. Among the most commonly recommended adaptogenic herbs are ginseng, ashwagandha, and maca root. These powerful herbs can be easily incorporated into daily routines to support energy and overall well-being.

Ginseng: The Energizing Adaptogen

Ginseng, a well-known adaptogen, is celebrated for its ability to boost both physical and mental energy. It has been traditionally used in Chinese medicine for centuries to enhance stamina, improve immune function, and increase endurance. Ginseng works by supporting the body's stress response and helping it adapt to physical and mental challenges. By improving energy metabolism at the cellular level, it can help reduce feelings of fatigue and promote sustained energy throughout the day.

Incorporating ginseng into daily routines is simple. It can be consumed as a tea or taken in powdered form mixed into smoothies or beverages. For those who prefer supplements, ginseng capsules are also widely available. Regular use of ginseng can help the body maintain a steady supply of energy, improve focus, and support long-term vitality.

Ashwagandha: Balancing Energy and Reducing Stress

Ashwagandha is another potent adaptogen known for its ability to support physical energy while also balancing stress. It is particularly effective in reducing cortisol levels, the stress hormone that can drain energy and weaken the body over time. By helping to balance cortisol and other stress-related hormones, ashwagandha promotes a sense of calm and well-being while simultaneously boosting physical stamina.

Ashwagandha is often recommended for individuals who experience chronic fatigue or stress-related exhaustion. It can be easily incorporated into daily life by adding it to smoothies, teas, or even in powdered form mixed with warm milk. As a supplement, ashwagandha is available in capsule form and can be taken consistently to support long-term energy and resilience.

Maca Root: Natural Energy Booster

Maca root, native to the Andes mountains of Peru, is another powerful herb for boosting energy and stamina. It is especially valued for its ability to improve endurance and support hormone balance, which is crucial for maintaining energy levels as we age. Maca root is rich in vitamins, minerals, and amino acids, all of which contribute to its energizing properties. It is also known for enhancing physical performance, making it a popular choice among athletes and those looking to increase their overall vitality.

Maca root can be easily integrated into daily routines by adding the powdered form to smoothies, juices, or baked goods. It has a slightly nutty flavor that blends well with other foods, making it a versatile addition to a healthy diet. Maca supplements are also available for those who prefer a more concentrated form of the herb.

Incorporating Adaptogenic Herbs into Daily Routines

Barbara O'Neill emphasizes the importance of consistency when using adaptogenic herbs to boost energy. These herbs are most effective when incorporated into daily routines over time, allowing the body to gradually adapt and respond to their benefits. Whether through teas, powders, or supplements, regular use of ginseng, ashwagandha, and maca root can significantly improve energy levels and overall vitality.

For those new to these herbs, starting with small amounts and gradually increasing the dosage is often recommended to allow the body to adjust. Many of these herbs can be combined in teas or smoothies, making it easy to create energy-boosting blends that can be consumed throughout the day. By incorporating these powerful adaptogens into a daily routine, individuals can experience a natural and sustained increase in physical energy, supporting both daily activities and long-term health.

3.3 Natural Support for Joint Health

As the body ages, maintaining healthy joints becomes increasingly important. Joint pain and stiffness, often the result of inflammation and wear on cartilage, can severely impact mobility and quality of life. One of the key principles in managing joint health naturally is to focus on reducing inflammation, which is often at the root of joint issues such as arthritis. Barbara O'Neill advocates for the use of anti-inflammatory herbs as a natural remedy to support joint health and ease pain, particularly focusing on **Boswellia**, **ginger**, and **turmeric**. These herbs can be incorporated into both the diet and used in topical applications, providing holistic support for aching joints.

Anti-Inflammatory Herbs for Joint Health

Boswellia, also known as frankincense, is one of the most potent natural anti-inflammatories. It works by inhibiting the production of pro-inflammatory enzymes, which are often elevated in cases of arthritis and other joint disorders. The active compounds in Boswellia, known as boswellic acids, help to reduce pain and swelling in the joints, making movement more comfortable. Unlike conventional anti-inflammatory drugs, Boswellia is gentler on the stomach, which makes it a suitable option for long-term use.

Ginger is another powerful anti-inflammatory herb recommended for joint health. Known for its warming properties, ginger can improve circulation and reduce inflammation in the affected joints. It contains compounds called gingerols, which have been shown to reduce pain and stiffness in conditions like osteoarthritis. Ginger can be consumed in various forms, such as fresh, powdered, or in teas, and can also be added to meals to enhance its benefits. Its anti-inflammatory properties make it a versatile remedy that supports overall health as well as joint function.

Turmeric, rich in curcumin, is perhaps one of the most well-known natural remedies for joint inflammation. Curcumin has strong antioxidant and anti-inflammatory effects, making it highly effective in reducing joint pain and improving mobility. Turmeric works by blocking certain molecules involved in the inflammatory process, thereby reducing joint stiffness and swelling. It is often recommended for individuals suffering from chronic joint pain due to conditions like rheumatoid arthritis.

Practical Advice on Using Herbs for Joint Support

These anti-inflammatory herbs can be used in several ways to support joint health. Incorporating them into the diet is one of the simplest methods. **Boswellia** is commonly available in supplement form, which can be taken daily to manage inflammation. However, it is important to ensure that the supplement contains a standardized amount of boswellic acids to achieve the desired effects.

Ginger can be easily added to meals as a spice or consumed as a tea. Fresh ginger root can be sliced and steeped in hot water to create a soothing tea that helps to reduce inflammation from the inside. Ginger can also be added to smoothies or soups for an extra anti-inflammatory boost. Additionally, ginger oil can be used topically, massaged into sore joints to provide relief from stiffness and pain.

Turmeric is highly versatile and can be used in cooking or taken as a supplement. When using turmeric for joint health, it is important to combine it with black pepper or a source of healthy fat, such as coconut oil, to improve the absorption of curcumin in the body. Turmeric powder can be added to curries, soups, or smoothies, making it an easy addition to a daily diet. For those who prefer topical application, turmeric-infused oils or balms can be applied to the joints to relieve localized pain and stiffness.

Topical Applications for Joint Pain Relief

In addition to dietary use, these herbs can be applied topically to further alleviate joint pain. **Boswellia**, **ginger**, and **turmeric** can be infused into oils or balms and massaged directly onto the affected joints. Topical applications allow the active compounds in these herbs to penetrate the skin and provide targeted relief to the inflamed area.

For instance, a **ginger oil** massage can stimulate blood flow to the affected joints, reducing stiffness and pain. Similarly, **turmeric** balms can be applied to inflamed joints to reduce swelling and enhance mobility. These balms are especially useful when the pain is localized, allowing the herbs to work directly where they are needed most.

Chapter 4: Lifestyle Tips for Supporting Longevity

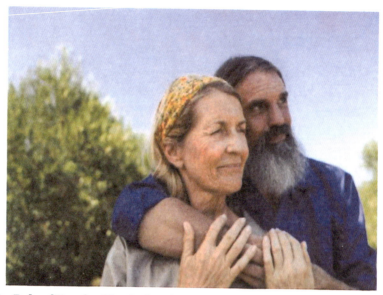

4.1 The Role of Regular Physical Activity

Maintaining regular physical activity is a cornerstone of good health. Barbara O'Neill emphasizes that staying active throughout life is essential not only for maintaining physical health but also for supporting mental and emotional well-being. Regular movement helps keep the cardiovascular system strong, supports mental clarity, and is a key factor in promoting longevity. The importance of consistent physical activity cannot be overstated, as it plays a central role in ensuring that the body remains resilient and capable of self-healing throughout the aging process.

Recommended Low-Impact Activities

For individuals looking to maintain physical activity without placing undue strain on the body, low-impact exercises are particularly beneficial. These activities are gentle on the joints but highly effective in promoting mobility, strength, and endurance. Walking is one of the simplest and most accessible forms of exercise that offers significant health benefits. It helps to improve circulation, maintain muscle tone, and boost energy levels without overtaxing the body.

Swimming is another excellent low-impact activity. The buoyancy of water supports the body, reducing stress on the joints while providing resistance that helps build muscle strength and endurance. Swimming is particularly beneficial for individuals with joint pain or arthritis, as it allows for full-body movement without discomfort.

Yoga and tai chi are also recommended for their ability to promote flexibility, balance, and mental calmness. These practices focus on slow, controlled movements that improve posture, core strength, and joint mobility. In addition to their physical benefits, yoga and tai chi encourage mindfulness and relaxation, helping to reduce stress and promote mental clarity.

4.2 Managing Stress and Promoting Emotional Wellbeing

Chronic stress is a leading factor in the acceleration of the aging process. Part 7 covers the different methods of managing stress.

Supporting Emotional Health with Mindfulness and Gratitude

In addition to managing stress, practices that support emotional resilience and mental clarity are essential for promoting overall wellbeing, particularly as individuals age. Mindfulness, the practice of staying present in the moment, is one of the most effective ways to cultivate emotional balance. By focusing on the present rather than worrying about the future or dwelling on the past, mindfulness helps to reduce anxiety and promote mental calm. Practicing mindfulness regularly can help individuals navigate the challenges of aging with a clearer mind and a more peaceful heart.

Gratitude journaling is another valuable tool for emotional wellbeing. By taking time each day to reflect on things to be grateful for, individuals can shift their focus away from stressors and toward positive aspects of their lives. This practice helps to foster a more optimistic outlook, which is crucial for emotional resilience. It encourages individuals to appreciate the present, enhancing feelings of contentment and reducing the impact of stress on mental health.

4.3 The Importance of Sleep and Restorative Health

As we age, the importance of sleep becomes increasingly critical for maintaining overall health and well-being. Sleep is not merely a time for rest; it plays a vital role in the body's natural processes of cellular repair, brain function, and energy restoration. Without sufficient and high-quality sleep, the body begins to age prematurely, and cognitive functions such as memory, concentration, and problem-solving skills start to decline. Sleep, therefore, is a cornerstone of restorative health, ensuring that the body and mind can function at their optimal levels.

Part 27 details how to create a better environment and mindset to get the best sleep.

Chapter 5: 12 Natural Remedies for Aging Gracefully

Aging is a natural part of life, but many seek ways to do so gracefully, maintaining vitality and health well into their later years. Through her holistic approach, Barbara O'Neill highlights the use of natural remedies to support the aging process, ensuring that the body remains resilient, energized, and balanced. Below are 12 remedies that have been traditionally used to support cognitive function, energy levels, joint health, and overall well-being during the aging process. Each remedy offers specific benefits, and when taken in the correct amounts, they can make a significant difference in promoting graceful aging.

1. Ginkgo Biloba Extract

Ginkgo biloba is well-known for its ability to enhance cognitive function, making it an excellent remedy for those looking to maintain mental sharpness as they age. Ginkgo biloba improves circulation to the brain, which enhances memory, focus, and mental clarity.

Dosage: Ginkgo biloba extract is typically taken in doses of 120-240 mg per day, divided into two or three doses.

How to take it: It can be consumed in capsule or liquid form, with or without food. Regular use over several weeks is often needed to see noticeable improvements in cognitive function.

2. Turmeric Capsules

Turmeric is rich in curcumin, a potent anti-inflammatory compound that supports joint health and reduces inflammation in the body. Inflammation is one of the key contributors to many age-related conditions, including arthritis and cardiovascular disease.

Dosage: 500-1,000 mg of turmeric extract (with at least 95% curcuminoids) per day is recommended.

How to take it: For best results, take turmeric capsules with meals. Combining turmeric with black pepper enhances curcumin absorption in the body.

3. Bacopa Monnieri Tincture

Bacopa monnieri is another herb that has long been used to enhance memory and cognitive function. It helps reduce anxiety and stress, which are often heightened with age, while also promoting clearer thinking and better memory retention.

Dosage: 300 mg of bacopa extract (standardized to contain 50% bacosides) per day is the standard dosage.

How to take it: Bacopa is best taken with food, as the absorption of its active compounds is improved when combined with fats. Bacopa tinctures can also be added to water or juice.

4. Ashwagandha Powder

Ashwagandha is an adaptogenic herb that helps the body manage stress, a crucial factor in maintaining health as we age. It also supports energy levels, improves endurance, and boosts mental clarity.

Dosage: 300-500 mg of ashwagandha root extract, taken once or twice daily.

How to take it: Ashwagandha can be taken in capsule or powder form. The powder can be added to smoothies or warm drinks. Consistency in daily intake is key for long-term benefits.

5. Maca Root Supplement

Maca root is a powerful adaptogen known to enhance energy levels and stamina. It can also help regulate hormonal balance, making it especially beneficial for those experiencing the hormonal fluctuations associated with aging.

Dosage: 1,500-3,000 mg of maca root powder per day.

How to take it: Maca is commonly taken in powder form, which can be added to smoothies or oatmeal. It is also available in capsules for ease of use.

6. CoQ10 Supplement

Coenzyme Q10 (CoQ10) is a naturally occurring antioxidant that supports heart health and cellular energy production. As we age, our levels of CoQ10 decline, which can contribute to fatigue and reduced vitality.

Dosage: 100-200 mg of CoQ10 per day.

How to take it: CoQ10 is best taken with a meal containing fats, as it is fat-soluble and is absorbed more effectively in the presence of dietary fat.

7. Resveratrol Capsules

Resveratrol, a polyphenol found in red grapes and berries, is widely recognized for its anti-aging properties. It supports cardiovascular health and has been shown to protect against oxidative damage, which is a major contributor to the aging process.

Dosage: 150-500 mg of resveratrol per day.

How to take it: Resveratrol can be taken in capsule form with or without food. For best results, a consistent daily dose is recommended.

8. Boswellia Extract

Boswellia, also known as frankincense, is a natural anti-inflammatory remedy that is particularly beneficial for joint health. It helps reduce the symptoms of osteoarthritis and other inflammatory conditions that commonly arise with aging.

Dosage: 300-500 mg of boswellia extract (standardized to contain 30-65% boswellic acids) per day.

How to take it: Boswellia can be taken in capsule or tablet form, preferably with meals. Regular use is necessary to experience its full anti-inflammatory benefits.

9. Ginseng Tea

Ginseng is a well-known tonic herb that boosts energy levels, supports immune function, and enhances overall vitality. It is particularly helpful for combating age-related fatigue and improving stamina.

Dosage: 200-400 mg of ginseng extract per day or 1-2 cups of ginseng tea.

How to take it: Ginseng can be consumed as a tea or in capsule form. For the tea, steep ginseng root or tea bags in hot water for 5-10 minutes. Ginseng is best taken in the morning to avoid interfering with sleep.

10. Magnesium Supplement

Magnesium is an essential mineral that supports muscle function, bone health, and relaxation. Many people are deficient in magnesium, particularly as they age, which can lead to muscle cramps, poor sleep, and elevated stress levels.

Dosage: 200-400 mg of magnesium per day.

How to take it: Magnesium can be taken in tablet or powder form, preferably in the evening to promote relaxation and better sleep. Magnesium citrate or magnesium glycinate are well-absorbed forms of the mineral.

11. Valerian Root Tea

Valerian root is a natural remedy for sleep disturbances, which often become more prevalent with age. It helps promote relaxation and deeper sleep, which is essential for the body's repair and regeneration processes.

Dosage: 300-600 mg of valerian root extract or 1 cup of valerian tea before bed.

How to take it: Valerian can be consumed in capsule form or as a tea. For the tea, steep valerian root or a tea bag in hot water for 5-10 minutes before consuming.

12. Omega-3 Fish Oil

Omega-3 fatty acids are crucial for maintaining cardiovascular health, cognitive function, and joint flexibility. As we age, the anti-inflammatory properties of omega-3s help protect against conditions like heart disease and arthritis.

Dosage: 1,000-2,000 mg of EPA and DHA (the active components of omega-3) per day.

How to take it: Omega-3 supplements are typically taken in soft gel form, with meals. It is important to choose high-quality fish oil supplements to ensure purity and effectiveness.

Part 11: Detoxification and Cleansing the Body Naturally

Chapter 1: Barbara O'Neill's Approach to Detox – Liver, Kidney, and Colon Health

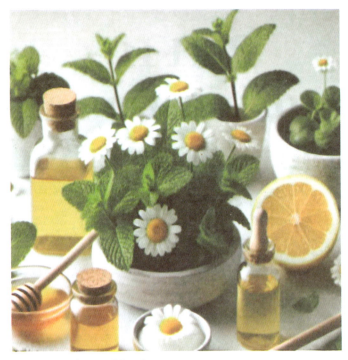

1.1 The Importance of Detoxification

Detoxification is one of the most crucial processes for maintaining optimal health. The body has several natural detox pathways, including the liver, kidneys, colon, skin, and lungs. These organs work in tandem to filter and eliminate toxins, chemicals, and waste products that accumulate from both internal metabolic processes and external sources such as the environment and diet. Over time, the body's detox systems can become overwhelmed, especially when poor diet, environmental pollutants, and chronic stress are present. In this section, the importance of detoxification and how to support the body's natural cleansing processes will be explored in depth.

Hydration is a critical component for all types of detoxification as it helps flush the toxins out of the body.

The Body's Natural Detoxification Pathways

The liver plays a central role in detoxification by filtering blood and metabolizing toxins into safer compounds that can be eliminated from the body. This complex organ processes everything from medications and alcohol to natural waste products generated from normal bodily functions. Additionally, it converts fat-soluble toxins into water-soluble substances, which can then be excreted through the kidneys or the intestines. When the liver is functioning optimally, it supports the entire body by preventing the buildup of harmful substances. However, when burdened by excessive toxins, the liver's efficiency can diminish, leading to various health complications.

The kidneys also serve as vital organs in the detoxification process. They filter out waste products and excess substances from the blood, regulating fluid and electrolyte balance in the body. By removing harmful compounds through urine, the kidneys help prevent the buildup of toxins. Adequate hydration is key to keeping the kidneys functioning properly, as water is essential for flushing out waste products.

The colon is responsible for eliminating solid waste from the body. When the colon is functioning well, it aids in the regular removal of toxins that pass through the digestive system. A sluggish or overloaded colon can result in constipation and reabsorption of toxins, which can further burden the liver and other organs. Keeping the colon healthy requires regular fiber intake, proper hydration, and avoiding processed foods that can slow down its function.

The skin, as the body's largest organ, also plays an important role in detoxification through perspiration. Sweat helps to release toxins, particularly heavy metals and other waste products. By maintaining a healthy balance of sweating, either through exercise or saunas, the skin can support the body's overall detox efforts.

Finally, the lungs are essential for detoxification, as they remove carbon dioxide and other volatile compounds through breathing. Breathing deeply and engaging in regular physical activity ensures that the lungs can effectively eliminate these waste products and deliver oxygen to the body's cells.

Toxin Buildup and Overloaded Systems

Over time, the body's natural detoxification systems can become overwhelmed by the sheer volume of toxins present in modern life. Barbara O'Neill emphasizes that a combination of poor dietary choices, environmental pollutants, and chronic stress can overload the detox pathways, leading to toxin buildup. Processed foods, for example, contain artificial additives, preservatives, and other chemicals that the liver must work harder to process. Additionally, environmental toxins such as heavy metals, pesticides, and pollutants from air and water further strain the body's detox systems.

Chronic stress compounds the problem by diverting the body's resources toward survival, thus diminishing the energy available for detoxification. When the body is in a constant state of "fight or flight," it prioritizes short-term survival over long-term health, which can result in reduced liver function, sluggish digestion, and impaired kidney filtration. This creates a vicious cycle where toxins accumulate faster than the body can eliminate them.

The consequences of toxin buildup are far-reaching. In addition to fatigue and digestive issues, a burdened detox system can manifest in skin problems, hormone imbalances, and weakened immunity. Many chronic diseases, including cardiovascular issues, autoimmune disorders, and even some cancers, have been linked to prolonged exposure to toxins and a failure to detoxify effectively. Thus, regular detoxification is not just a reactive measure but a proactive approach to health.

Detox Practices to Avoid Overloading the System

In addition to diet and exercise, certain detox practices can further enhance the body's ability to eliminate toxins. Barbara O'Neill advocates for regular detox programs that target the liver, kidneys, and colon. These programs often involve periods of cleansing, where the diet is simplified to reduce the burden on the digestive system and provide the liver with the nutrients it needs to regenerate. Juice fasting, for instance, allows the body to rest from the energy-intensive process of digestion while flooding it with vitamins, minerals, and antioxidants that support detoxification.

Another practice she recommends is intermittent fasting, which gives the digestive system a break and allows the liver and kidneys to focus on clearing out waste. This approach can be particularly beneficial for individuals who experience bloating, sluggish digestion, or difficulty concentrating due to toxin overload. During fasting, the body shifts its energy toward repair and detoxification, allowing it to process and eliminate toxins more efficiently.

1.2 Understanding the Liver's Role in Detox

The liver plays an essential role in maintaining the body's overall health by acting as its primary detoxification organ. It is responsible for filtering toxins from the bloodstream and converting harmful substances into forms that can be safely eliminated. Every day, the liver processes various chemicals, drugs, and metabolic waste products, ensuring that the body remains free from harmful accumulations that can lead to disease. The detoxification function of the liver is vital, and understanding how it works is a key step in supporting overall health and well-being.

The Liver's Function in Detoxification

The liver's detoxification process is both complex and efficient. As the body's largest internal organ, it performs several essential functions, the most critical of which is detoxification. It filters blood coming from the digestive tract before passing it to the rest of the body. During this filtration, the liver neutralizes toxins, chemicals, and drugs, converting them into water-soluble forms that can be eliminated through urine or bile.

In particular, the liver plays a central role in breaking down and removing harmful substances such as alcohol, medications, and environmental pollutants. One of the key processes in the liver's detoxification mechanism involves enzymes that convert fat-soluble toxins into water-soluble compounds. These enzymes facilitate the transformation of potentially dangerous substances, allowing them to be safely excreted by the kidneys or intestines. Without the liver's ability to filter and eliminate these toxins, harmful chemicals would accumulate in the bloodstream, leading to potentially severe health problems over time.

The liver also metabolizes hormones and other natural substances produced by the body. Excess hormones, such as estrogen, are broken down and removed by the liver to maintain hormonal balance. This process is crucial for preventing conditions related to hormonal imbalances, such as estrogen dominance, which can contribute to various health issues, including reproductive problems and even certain types of cancer.

Detoxifying Chemicals, Drugs, and Metabolic Waste

One of the liver's primary tasks is to detoxify chemicals that enter the body through food, water, and the environment. In modern life, individuals are exposed to a variety of toxins on a daily basis, including pesticides, food additives, and industrial pollutants. The liver works tirelessly to neutralize these substances, protecting the body from their harmful effects. Additionally, the liver is responsible for metabolizing drugs and medications, including over-the-counter pain relievers and prescription drugs. While these substances are often necessary for treating various health conditions, their repeated use can place a significant burden on the liver.

Apart from external toxins, the liver must also deal with metabolic waste products generated by the body's normal functions. For example, ammonia is a toxic by-product of protein metabolism. The liver converts ammonia into urea, which is then excreted through the urine. This conversion is essential for preventing the buildup of toxic substances in the bloodstream, which could lead to conditions such as hepatic encephalopathy, a disorder that affects brain function due to liver failure.

1.3 Supporting Kidney Health

The kidneys play a crucial role in maintaining overall health, especially during detoxification processes. They are responsible for filtering the blood, removing waste products, and balancing essential minerals and fluids in the body. Maintaining optimal kidney function is particularly important when undergoing detox, as the kidneys work hard to cleanse the body of toxins and regulate its internal environment. Without proper support, the detox process can become less effective, leading to an accumulation of waste that may negatively impact health.

The Role of the Kidneys in Detoxification

The kidneys are integral to the body's filtration system, processing approximately 200 liters of blood daily. Their primary function is to filter out waste products, excess minerals, and toxins, converting them into urine for elimination. In addition, the kidneys help to maintain a balance of electrolytes, such as sodium, potassium, and calcium, which are vital for various bodily functions including nerve signaling and muscle contractions. Without the efficient functioning of the kidneys, these waste products and excess minerals can build up in the bloodstream, contributing to health issues such as high blood pressure and kidney stones.

One of the key responsibilities of the kidneys during detoxification is to manage the body's fluid balance. During detox, it is common for the body to release stored toxins from tissues, which are then carried to the kidneys for elimination. The kidneys must be functioning optimally to handle this increased load of waste material. If the kidneys are not properly supported, the detox process can strain the organs, leading to dehydration, mineral imbalances, and potentially impaired kidney function.

1.4 The Colon: Cleansing for Digestive Health

The colon plays a crucial role in maintaining overall health, particularly in the realm of digestion and detoxification. When the colon is not functioning properly, waste can accumulate and lead to a variety of health issues, including inflammation and toxic overload. Regular cleansing of the colon is essential to prevent this buildup and ensure that the body's waste is eliminated efficiently, avoiding the reabsorption of toxins into the bloodstream. Barbara O'Neill emphasizes the importance of colon health as part of a broader approach to maintaining a clean and functional digestive system, which is foundational for overall well-being.

The Impact of Waste Buildup in the Colon

One of the key concerns with an unhealthy colon is the buildup of waste material. When food is not properly digested or waste is not effectively eliminated, it can stagnate in the colon, leading to a host of digestive problems. The accumulation of this waste can create an environment ripe for harmful bacteria, yeasts, and parasites to thrive. These pathogens can contribute to inflammation in the digestive tract, resulting in discomfort, bloating, and conditions like IBS. Moreover, prolonged waste retention can lead to constipation, which further exacerbates these issues by preventing the timely removal of toxins from the body.

When the colon becomes inflamed due to waste buildup, this inflammation can extend beyond the digestive system, affecting the overall health of the body. Inflammation is often considered a precursor to chronic diseases, as it weakens the immune system and creates an environment where disease can flourish. Keeping the colon free from waste buildup is, therefore, an essential step in reducing inflammation and preventing broader health issues.

The Role of Colon Health in Detoxification

The colon is one of the body's primary organs for detoxification. Alongside the liver and kidneys, the colon ensures that waste products and toxins are removed from the body. If the colon is not functioning properly, however, toxins can be reabsorbed into the bloodstream, leading to a condition known as "autointoxication." This occurs when harmful substances, which should have been eliminated, instead re-enter the body and circulate through the bloodstream, causing symptoms such as fatigue, headaches, skin problems, and even mood disorders.

Maintaining colon health through regular cleansing supports the body's natural detoxification processes. By ensuring that waste is promptly and efficiently eliminated, the colon helps prevent the buildup of toxins that could otherwise overwhelm the body's systems. Proper colon function allows the liver and kidneys to focus on their detoxification roles without being burdened by a backup of waste in the digestive tract.

Methods for Colon Cleansing

In line with the philosophy of natural healing, one of the most effective ways to maintain a clean colon is through diet. Eating a high-fiber diet is critical, as fiber helps move waste through the digestive system more efficiently. Fiber acts like a broom, sweeping through the intestines and preventing waste from lingering too long in the colon. Foods like fruits, vegetables, whole grains, and legumes are rich in fiber and are integral to keeping the colon clean and functional.

In addition to dietary changes, hydration plays a vital role in supporting colon health. Drinking sufficient water helps to soften stool and ensures that waste can pass smoothly through the intestines. Without adequate hydration, the colon may struggle to eliminate waste, leading to constipation and a higher risk of toxic buildup.

Herbal remedies are another natural method for colon cleansing. Herbs like **psyllium husk**, which is high in soluble fiber, help to bulk up stool and promote healthy bowel movements. **Aloe vera** is known for its soothing properties and can help reduce inflammation in the digestive tract, making it a useful addition to a colon cleansing routine. **Slippery elm** is another herb that can be beneficial, as it forms a gel-like substance that coats and soothes the digestive lining, promoting healing in the colon.

Finally, regular physical activity is essential for maintaining colon health. Exercise stimulates the muscles in the intestines, encouraging regular bowel movements and helping to prevent constipation. Incorporating movement into daily routines can aid the body's natural detoxification process and keep the colon functioning properly.

Chapter 2: Detoxifying Herbs for Liver, Kidney, and Colon Health

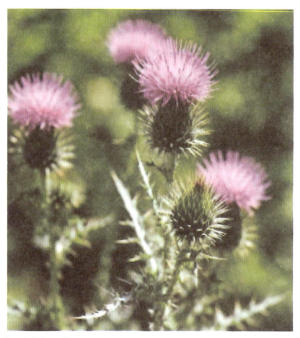

2.1 Milk Thistle: A Liver Protector

Milk thistle has long been regarded as one of the most powerful herbs for liver support, and its active compound, silymarin, plays a crucial role in protecting the liver from damage. The liver is responsible for detoxifying the body, processing nutrients, and breaking down toxins. However, modern lifestyles, which often include exposure to environmental pollutants, processed foods, and medications, place an immense burden on the liver. When overwhelmed, the liver's ability to function optimally can be compromised, leading to a range of health issues. Milk thistle works by strengthening liver function and aiding in the repair of damaged liver cells, making it an essential tool in maintaining overall health.

Silymarin: Repairing and Protecting the Liver

The primary component of milk thistle is silymarin, a potent antioxidant known for its ability to regenerate liver cells and protect them from further harm. This compound acts as a shield, helping the liver detoxify harmful substances more efficiently. Silymarin is particularly effective at neutralizing free radicals, which are unstable molecules that can damage cells and accelerate aging. By preventing oxidative damage, milk thistle not only aids in liver repair but also helps protect it from future harm.

The liver's regenerative ability is one of its most remarkable features, and milk thistle helps to enhance this natural process. Whether the liver has been damaged by toxins, alcohol, or poor dietary choices, silymarin supports the production of new, healthy cells to replace the damaged ones. This process allows the liver to recover from chronic stress and continue performing its vital detoxification functions.

Forms of Milk Thistle for Liver Detoxification

Milk thistle is most commonly used in the form of tea or tinctures. Both forms provide a concentrated dose of silymarin, allowing the liver to benefit from its protective and regenerative properties. Tea is an easily accessible way to incorporate milk thistle into a daily routine. Prepared by steeping the herb in hot water, the tea delivers a gentle but effective dose of silymarin, making it suitable for regular use.

Tinctures, on the other hand, offer a more potent form of milk thistle. These concentrated liquid extracts provide a stronger dose of the herb's active compounds, and only a small amount is needed to achieve therapeutic benefits. Tinctures are often recommended for those who require more intensive liver support, particularly after prolonged exposure to toxins or alcohol.

2.2 Dandelion Root: Enhancing Liver and Kidney Detox

Dandelion root has long been valued for its potent detoxifying properties, particularly in supporting the liver and kidneys, two of the body's primary detoxification organs. In her teachings, Barbara O'Neill emphasizes the importance of keeping these organs functioning optimally, as they play a critical role in filtering and eliminating toxins from the body. Dandelion root is one of the key natural remedies she suggests for this purpose, as it acts both as a diuretic and a stimulant for bile production, making it an essential herb in promoting detoxification processes.

Dandelion Root as a Diuretic

One of the main actions of dandelion root is its ability to function as a natural diuretic. Diuretics increase the amount of urine produced by the kidneys, which helps the body to expel excess fluid and waste products more efficiently. This is particularly beneficial for individuals who experience water retention or have difficulty eliminating toxins due to sluggish kidney function. By encouraging the kidneys to flush out excess water, dandelion root helps to reduce the strain on the body's detoxification pathways, making it easier for the kidneys to filter out waste and maintain fluid balance.

In addition to its diuretic properties, dandelion root contains high levels of potassium, an essential mineral that is often depleted when using synthetic diuretics. This natural source of potassium helps to maintain electrolyte balance, ensuring that the body does not lose vital nutrients during the detoxification process. This makes dandelion root a more gentle and sustainable option compared to other diuretics, which can sometimes cause nutrient imbalances.

Stimulating Bile Production for Liver Health

Dandelion root also plays a crucial role in supporting liver detoxification by stimulating the production of bile. Bile is essential for breaking down fats in the digestive system and for aiding in the elimination of toxins. When the liver produces more bile, it enhances the body's ability to metabolize fats and remove fat-soluble toxins, which can otherwise accumulate and contribute to health problems. This makes dandelion root especially useful for individuals who may have a congested or sluggish liver.

2.3 Burdock Root: Blood Purification and Detox

Burdock root has been widely recognized for its powerful ability to purify the blood and support detoxification processes in the body. Its primary action lies in its capacity to help the body eliminate accumulated toxins from the bloodstream, making it a valuable herb for maintaining overall health. The root has been used traditionally for centuries and is especially noted for its role in enhancing the body's natural detoxification pathways.

Blood Purification and Toxin Elimination

One of the main benefits of burdock root is its ability to cleanse the blood by facilitating the removal of toxins that build up over time. This accumulation of toxins can stem from environmental pollutants, processed foods, and various chemicals encountered in daily life. By supporting the body's natural detoxification mechanisms, burdock root helps to reduce the toxic load on the system, which in turn promotes healthier organ function and overall vitality.

Burdock root is known to stimulate lymphatic drainage, which helps in clearing waste products from the tissues and reducing the burden on the body's detoxification organs. It also promotes circulation, allowing for better distribution of nutrients and the removal of waste materials from cells. These combined effects make burdock root an ideal herb for long-term detox support.

Kidney Health and Heavy Metal Detoxification

In her teachings, Barbara O'Neill highlights the importance of kidney health in maintaining the body's detoxification capabilities. The kidneys play a vital role in filtering out toxins from the blood and excreting them through urine. Burdock root is especially beneficial for promoting kidney function, as it aids in the efficient elimination of waste and helps prevent the accumulation of harmful substances within the body.

One of the most significant advantages of burdock root is its ability to assist in the detoxification of heavy metals. Heavy metals such as lead, mercury, and cadmium can accumulate in the body over time, leading to various health issues. Burdock root helps the kidneys expel these toxic metals, preventing their buildup and supporting the body's long-term health.

Consumption for Detox Support

Burdock root can be consumed in various forms to support detoxification, with tea and supplements being the most common methods. Drinking burdock root tea is an easy and gentle way to introduce its detoxifying properties into the daily routine. When used as a tea, it provides a mild diuretic effect, promoting the elimination of waste through urine.

For more concentrated detox support, burdock root can be taken in supplement form, which is often recommended for those looking to use the herb for extended periods. The use of supplements allows for a consistent dosage, ensuring the body receives ongoing benefits from this powerful blood purifier.

Chapter 3: Detox and Cleansing

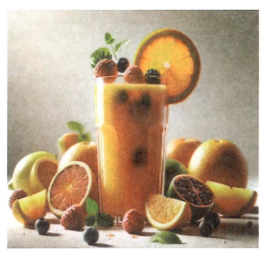

3.1 The 3-Day Liver Detox

The liver is one of the most vital organs in the body, responsible for filtering toxins, metabolizing nutrients, and supporting overall health. To ensure optimal liver function, regular detoxification can be an essential part of maintaining health and vitality. A 3-day liver detox, as outlined in Barbara O'Neill's teachings, focuses on cleansing and rejuvenating the liver through a carefully designed dietary and lifestyle regimen. This detox plan emphasizes the consumption of nutrient-rich foods and herbs known for their liver-supporting properties, along with key daily practices that enhance the detoxification process.

Foods to Support Liver Health

A key component of the 3-day liver detox program is the incorporation of specific foods known to support liver function. Leafy greens, such as spinach, kale, and arugula, are central to the detox process due to their high content of chlorophyll. Chlorophyll helps to eliminate toxins from the bloodstream and supports the liver's natural detoxification processes. Cruciferous vegetables, including broccoli, cauliflower, and Brussels sprouts, are also emphasized in the detox plan. These vegetables contain compounds that enhance the liver's ability to produce detoxifying enzymes, aiding in the breakdown and elimination of harmful substances.

Herbs like milk thistle and dandelion root are integral to the liver detox. Milk thistle is known for its ability to protect liver cells and regenerate damaged tissue, making it a powerful ally in liver health. Dandelion root supports the liver by promoting bile production, which helps to break down fats and facilitates the elimination of toxins. Both of these herbs can be consumed in the form of teas or supplements during the detox to provide additional liver support.

Healthy fats, such as those found in avocados, flaxseeds, and olive oil, are included in the detox program to provide the liver with the necessary building blocks for cell repair. These fats support the liver's ability to metabolize and store energy while also assisting in the detoxification of fat-soluble toxins.

What to Avoid During the Detox

During the 3-day liver detox, it is essential to avoid foods and substances that place additional strain on the liver. Processed foods, which are often high in trans fats, refined sugars, and artificial additives, can overwhelm the liver and slow down the detoxification process. Eliminating these foods from the diet allows the liver to focus on repairing itself and clearing out accumulated toxins.

Caffeine is another substance to avoid during the detox. While moderate amounts of caffeine can have some health benefits, it can also place a burden on the liver, particularly if consumed in large quantities. During the detox, it is best to substitute caffeine with herbal teas, which can provide similar energy-boosting effects without adding stress to the liver.

Alcohol is particularly harmful to liver health and should be completely avoided during the detox program. Alcohol is processed directly by the liver, and its consumption can lead to inflammation and damage to liver cells. By eliminating alcohol, the liver is given the opportunity to repair any damage and restore its natural function.

Two Additional Methods for Liver Detoxification

In addition to the 3-day liver detox program, there are other natural methods that can support and enhance liver health. These detox methods emphasize nourishing the liver, promoting its detoxification pathways, and protecting it from potential harm. Below are two more approaches that can be used to help cleanse and rejuvenate the liver, ensuring it functions optimally.

1. Juice Fasting for Liver Detox

Juice fasting is a powerful way to support liver detoxification by flooding the body with vitamins, minerals, and antioxidants while giving the digestive system a break. This method typically lasts for 1 to 3 days, during which solid foods are avoided, and only freshly pressed juices from fruits and vegetables are consumed. By providing the liver with an abundance of nutrients and hydration, juice fasting helps to flush out toxins and promote cellular regeneration.

Step-by-Step Guide to Juice Fasting:

Prepare Your Juices

The juices consumed during this detox should be made from fresh, organic fruits and vegetables. Key ingredients that support liver detoxification include:

Beets: Known for their high content of betaine, which aids in liver cell repair.

Carrots: Rich in beta-carotene, which helps the liver break down toxins.

Apples: Provide malic acid, which helps cleanse the liver and promote bile production.

Leafy Greens: Kale, spinach, and chard are packed with chlorophyll, which supports the liver's detoxification pathways.

Aim to drink a variety of juices throughout the day to ensure a wide range of nutrients. A good formula includes a combination of vegetables and a smaller portion of fruit to keep the sugar content low.

Drink Regularly Throughout the Day

During the fast, drink one glass of juice every 2 to 3 hours. In between juice servings, it is important to stay hydrated by drinking plenty of water or herbal teas. This will assist in flushing toxins from the liver and kidneys.

Include Lemon Water

As with the 3-day liver detox, starting your day with a glass of warm lemon water helps to stimulate bile production and kickstart the liver's detox processes. Adding lemon to your juices throughout the day can further enhance liver detoxification due to its high vitamin C content.

Rest and Gentle Movement

Since juice fasting provides fewer calories than a regular diet, it's important to avoid intense physical activity during the detox. Instead, focus on gentle movements like walking or yoga to stimulate circulation and support the body's detoxification processes.

Gradual Reintroduction of Solid Foods

Once the juice fast is complete, it's important to ease back into eating solid foods. Start with light, nutrient-dense meals such as vegetable broths, salads, and steamed vegetables. Avoid processed foods, sugars, and alcohol to allow the liver to continue the detox process post-fast.

2. Castor Oil Pack Liver Detox

A castor oil pack is an external method of detoxifying the liver that has been used for centuries to support liver health and promote detoxification. Castor oil, when applied topically over the liver, penetrates the skin and helps to improve circulation, reduce inflammation, and promote the movement of lymphatic fluid. This method is gentle and can be used regularly to maintain liver health.

Step-by-Step Guide to Castor Oil Pack Detox:

Prepare Your Materials

For this detox, you will need:

Organic, cold-pressed castor oil.

A piece of soft flannel cloth large enough to cover your liver area.

Plastic wrap or a towel.

A heating pad or hot water bottle.

Apply the Castor Oil

Soak the flannel cloth in castor oil until it is saturated but not dripping. Lie down on your back in a comfortable position, and place the cloth over your liver, located on the right side of your abdomen, just below the ribcage.

Cover with Plastic Wrap or Towel

To prevent the oil from staining your clothes or sheets, place a layer of plastic wrap or an old towel over the flannel. This will also help to seal in the warmth during the detox session.

Apply Heat

Place a heating pad or hot water bottle over the covered castor oil pack. The heat helps to increase circulation and allows the castor oil to penetrate more deeply into the tissues. Relax for 30 to 60 minutes while the pack is in place. This is an ideal time for meditation or deep breathing exercises to enhance the detoxification process.

Remove and Cleanse the Area

After the session, remove the pack and gently clean the area with warm water or a mild soap to remove any remaining oil. The castor oil pack can be stored in a plastic bag and reused for several detox sessions.

Repeat Regularly

For best results, use the castor oil pack 2 to 3 times a week for a few weeks. This method can be particularly beneficial for those looking to reduce liver inflammation and support detoxification over time.

3.2 Kidney Cleanse Protocol

The kidneys play a vital role in detoxifying the body by filtering waste products and excess fluids from the bloodstream. Over time, however, factors such as poor diet, dehydration, and exposure to toxins can impair kidney function, leading to a buildup of waste and a decreased ability to maintain overall health. A kidney cleanse protocol is designed to support the kidneys in their role of waste elimination, allowing them to function optimally and preventing the development of more serious health conditions. In this section, we will outline a natural kidney cleanse protocol that focuses on diet, hydration, and the use of specific herbs known to enhance kidney function.

Hydration: The Foundation of a Kidney Cleanse

The first and most important step in any kidney cleanse protocol is hydration. Proper hydration is essential for kidney function, as water helps the kidneys filter waste and flush it out through urine. Without adequate water intake, the kidneys cannot function efficiently, leading to the buildup of waste products and the potential formation of kidney stones.

To begin the kidney cleanse, it is recommended to increase water consumption to at least eight to ten glasses of purified water per day. This helps ensure that the kidneys are consistently receiving the water they need to carry out their filtering process. Water not only aids in flushing toxins but also helps dissolve minerals that could form kidney stones, keeping the urinary system free from blockages.

In addition to pure water, herbal teas can be a beneficial part of the hydration process. Herbal infusions made from plants known to support kidney function, such as nettle leaf or dandelion root, help boost the body's ability to detoxify through urine. Nettle, in particular, is known for its diuretic properties, which encourage the kidneys to expel waste more efficiently.

Diet and Nutrient Support for Kidney Health

Incorporating a nutrient-rich diet is essential for supporting kidney health during a cleanse. A focus on whole, unprocessed foods, including fruits, vegetables, and healthy fats, provides the body with the vitamins and minerals necessary to promote optimal kidney function. Fruits and vegetables with high water content, such as cucumbers, watermelon, and celery, are particularly beneficial, as they help hydrate the body and support the cleansing process.

Leafy greens, berries, and cruciferous vegetables are also rich in antioxidants, which protect the kidneys from oxidative stress caused by free radicals. Foods such as parsley and cilantro are often included in a kidney cleanse protocol for their natural detoxifying properties, as they help flush out heavy metals and other toxins that can burden the kidneys.

Limiting the intake of sodium, processed sugars, and animal proteins is also important during a kidney cleanse. High levels of sodium can lead to fluid retention and place additional stress on the kidneys, while processed sugars can contribute to inflammation and interfere with the body's natural detoxification processes. Animal proteins, particularly those from red meat, produce more metabolic waste products that the kidneys must filter out, so it is advised to reduce protein consumption or opt for plant-based sources like legumes and seeds during the cleanse.

Herbs for Kidney Cleansing

Herbs play a central role in natural kidney cleanses, as many have diuretic properties that help increase urine output and assist the kidneys in flushing toxins more efficiently. Several herbs are particularly effective in supporting kidney health:

Dandelion root: Known for its strong diuretic properties, dandelion root helps the kidneys excrete more urine, thereby removing waste products more efficiently. It also contains vitamins A, C, and K, which support overall kidney function and detoxification.

Nettle leaf: Nettle is another potent diuretic that helps reduce fluid retention and promote the elimination of waste. It also has anti-inflammatory properties that can help protect the kidneys from damage caused by toxins or inflammation.

Marshmallow root: This herb is known for its soothing and anti-inflammatory properties. It helps protect the delicate tissues of the urinary tract and supports the kidneys by increasing urine production, which aids in flushing out waste.

Horsetail: Horsetail is a traditional herbal remedy used to support kidney function. It has diuretic properties that increase urine flow, helping to cleanse the kidneys and prevent the formation of kidney stones. Additionally, it is rich in antioxidants that help protect kidney cells from damage.

Corn silk: Corn silk is a natural diuretic that has been used for centuries to promote kidney health. It helps reduce inflammation in the urinary system and supports the kidneys by promoting the excretion of excess fluid and toxins.

These herbs can be consumed as teas, tinctures, or supplements during the kidney cleanse to enhance the detoxification process and improve overall kidney health. It is recommended to incorporate them into the diet for the duration of the cleanse to maximize their benefits.

Supporting the Cleanse with Gentle Exercise and Rest

In addition to hydration, diet, and herbal support, incorporating gentle exercise and adequate rest is essential during a kidney cleanse. Exercise helps improve circulation, which supports the kidneys in their filtering process by delivering more oxygen and nutrients to the tissues. Activities such as walking, yoga, or swimming are gentle on the body but still effective in promoting detoxification.

Rest is equally important, as the kidneys work best when the body is in a relaxed state. Ensuring adequate sleep and allowing the body time to recover during the cleanse will help optimize kidney function and ensure that the detoxification process is as effective as possible.

3.3 Colon Cleansing for Digestive Health

The health of the digestive system plays a crucial role in maintaining overall well-being. When the colon becomes sluggish or impacted due to poor dietary choices or lack of proper elimination, it can lead to various health issues, from bloating and constipation to more serious conditions such as inflammation and toxin buildup. A colon cleanse aims to restore the health and efficiency of the digestive tract, allowing for better nutrient absorption and the elimination of waste. One such program involves the use of fiber-rich foods, herbal laxatives, and probiotics, which work together to thoroughly cleanse the colon.

Fiber-Rich Foods for Colon Cleansing

A central aspect of colon cleansing is the inclusion of fiber-rich foods in the diet. Fiber is essential for promoting regular bowel movements and preventing the buildup of waste material in the digestive tract. Foods such as flaxseeds and chia seeds are highly recommended because of their high fiber content and their ability to absorb water, forming a gel-like substance that helps move waste through the intestines. These seeds act as natural bulking agents, increasing stool mass and encouraging the body to eliminate toxins more effectively.

Flaxseeds are particularly rich in both soluble and insoluble fibers. Soluble fiber dissolves in water and forms a gel that aids in the slow digestion of food, while insoluble fiber adds bulk to stool, making it easier to pass. Chia seeds, on the other hand, are known for their ability to expand in the stomach, promoting satiety while assisting in the smooth movement of waste through the digestive system.

Another crucial component of a fiber-rich colon cleanse is the inclusion of fermented vegetables. Foods like sauerkraut, kimchi, and pickles introduce beneficial bacteria into the gut, helping to break down food and maintain a healthy balance of microorganisms. Fermented foods act as natural probiotics, supporting gut health by ensuring that harmful bacteria do not overgrow in the colon.

Herbal Laxatives for Cleansing

Alongside fiber-rich foods, herbal laxatives are an important element in promoting thorough cleansing of the colon. Unlike chemical laxatives that can be harsh on the digestive system, herbal alternatives work gently to stimulate bowel movements and alleviate constipation. Some common herbs used for this purpose include senna, cascara sagrada, and aloe vera, all of which have a mild laxative effect and help stimulate the colon muscles to encourage the elimination of waste.

Senna, in particular, is known for its active compounds called sennosides, which irritate the lining of the bowel, causing a laxative effect. Similarly, cascara sagrada works by encouraging peristalsis—the wave-like contractions of the intestinal muscles that move waste toward the rectum. Aloe vera, widely known for its soothing properties, also acts as a natural laxative by stimulating the bowel and aiding in detoxification. These herbal remedies are recommended as short-term solutions to cleanse the colon effectively and should not be used for prolonged periods to avoid dependence.

Probiotics for Gut Health

Probiotics are a vital part of any colon cleanse program, as they help restore the balance of bacteria in the gut after cleansing. When the colon is cleansed, both harmful and beneficial bacteria can be flushed out, making it essential to replenish the good bacteria that support digestion and nutrient absorption. Fermented vegetables, as previously mentioned, are a natural source of probiotics, but they can also be supplemented with probiotic capsules or powders for a more concentrated dose.

Probiotics not only aid digestion but also play a role in maintaining the integrity of the gut lining, preventing the development of conditions like leaky gut, where toxins and undigested food particles pass through the intestinal walls into the bloodstream. By introducing beneficial bacteria into the digestive system, probiotics help enhance immune function, promote healthy bowel movements, and reduce inflammation.

Step-by-Step Colon Cleanse Methods

In addition to the fiber-rich foods, herbal laxatives, and probiotics, there are other colon cleanse methods that can be incorporated into a regular routine to promote digestive health. Here are two step-by-step methods for cleansing the colon:

Method 1: Water-Based Colon Cleanse

Start the day with lemon water: Upon waking, drink a glass of warm water with freshly squeezed lemon juice. Lemon helps alkalize the body and stimulates the liver, promoting detoxification.

Hydrate with plenty of water throughout the day: Drink at least 2-3 liters of water daily. Water is essential for keeping the colon hydrated and aiding in the smooth passage of stool. Staying hydrated ensures that the fiber consumed has enough liquid to form soft, bulky stools.

Incorporate fiber-rich meals: For breakfast, have a smoothie made with chia seeds, flaxseeds, and greens like spinach or kale. Fiber will bind to toxins and push them through the digestive system.

Use herbal teas: In the evening, drink a cup of herbal tea made with senna or cascara sagrada to gently stimulate the bowels. These herbs work overnight to encourage bowel movements the following morning.

End the cleanse with probiotics: The next day, replenish the gut by consuming fermented foods or a high-quality probiotic supplement to restore healthy gut bacteria.

Method 2: Juice-Based Colon Cleanse

Begin with a green juice: In the morning, consume a green juice made from celery, cucumber, spinach, and ginger. These ingredients are not only rich in nutrients but also help reduce inflammation and stimulate digestion.

Drink an herbal laxative tea: Mid-morning, have an herbal tea that includes aloe vera or senna to promote detoxification. These herbs work to stimulate bowel movements naturally without the harsh effects of chemical laxatives.

Incorporate psyllium husk: Before lunch, mix a tablespoon of psyllium husk into a glass of water and drink it quickly. Psyllium acts as a natural fiber supplement that bulks up stool and aids in the removal of waste.

Continue hydrating with water or coconut water: Drink water consistently throughout the day to support hydration and prevent constipation. Coconut water is an excellent alternative for replenishing electrolytes lost during detoxification.

Conclude the cleanse with a probiotic-rich meal: End the day with a light dinner consisting of fermented vegetables, such as kimchi or sauerkraut, and a simple soup made from nutrient-dense vegetables like carrots, zucchini, and spinach. This ensures that the body receives probiotics while being gently nourished.

Chapter 4: Detoxing Gently for Long-Term Health

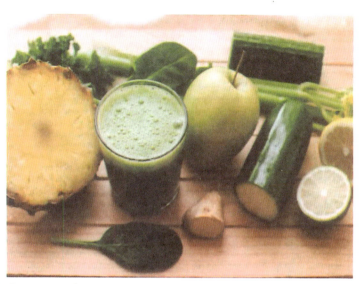

4.1 Daily Detox Practices

Daily detoxification is a natural process that the body engages in to eliminate toxins and maintain optimal health. Incorporating simple habits into everyday life can support the body's detox pathways and keep it functioning at its best without resorting to intensive or extreme cleansing protocols. Barbara O'Neill advises adopting a range of practices that can help the body gently cleanse itself on a regular basis, ensuring that toxins are efficiently removed and overall well-being is maintained.

Herbal Teas for Gentle Detoxification

One of the key practices recommended is the inclusion of herbal teas in a daily routine. Certain herbs have detoxifying properties that can support the liver, kidneys, and lymphatic system in their natural detox processes. **Dandelion tea**, for example, is known for its ability to promote liver function and enhance bile production, aiding in the digestion and elimination of toxins. Similarly, **nettle tea** is often used for its ability to cleanse the blood and support kidney health by promoting the elimination of waste through urine.

Herbal teas not only support detoxification but also provide antioxidants that help neutralize free radicals, protecting the body from oxidative stress. Drinking these teas regularly is a simple, non-invasive way to encourage detox without overwhelming the body's systems. O'Neill emphasizes the importance of choosing organic, high-quality herbs to ensure that the detox benefits are maximized and that no additional toxins, such as pesticides, are introduced into the body.

Clean Eating for Ongoing Detox Support

Another cornerstone of daily detox practices is maintaining a clean, nutrient-dense diet. A clean diet consists primarily of whole, unprocessed foods, such as fruits, vegetables, whole grains, nuts, and seeds, which provide the essential vitamins, minerals, and fiber necessary to support the body's natural detox functions. Fiber, in particular, plays a crucial role in eliminating toxins by promoting healthy bowel movements, ensuring that waste is efficiently removed from the digestive system.

Cruciferous vegetables like **broccoli, kale, and Brussels sprouts** are especially beneficial for detoxification, as they contain compounds that support liver function and help in breaking down and eliminating harmful substances from the body. Additionally, including foods rich in **antioxidants**, such as berries and leafy greens, protects the cells from damage caused by toxins and supports overall cellular health. This type of diet reduces the burden on the liver and kidneys, allowing them to function more efficiently in their detox roles.

Dry Brushing for Lymphatic Health

Dry brushing is a simple yet effective daily detox practice that promotes lymphatic circulation. The lymphatic system is responsible for removing waste products from the body's tissues and plays a key role in detoxification. By stimulating the lymph nodes through dry brushing, individuals can encourage the flow of lymph fluid, helping to clear out toxins and improve overall skin health.

This practice involves using a natural bristle brush to gently brush the skin in circular motions, starting from the extremities and moving toward the heart. Dry brushing not only supports detoxification but also exfoliates the skin, removing dead skin cells and promoting healthy skin regeneration. Regular dry brushing can improve skin texture, increase circulation, and enhance the body's ability to remove waste through the skin, which is one of the largest detox organs.

The Importance of Regular Exercise and Sweating

Exercise is a fundamental part of daily detox practices because it encourages sweating, one of the body's primary methods of eliminating toxins. Through perspiration, the body expels heavy metals, chemicals, and other harmful substances, reducing the overall toxic load. Physical activity also increases circulation, ensuring that blood and lymph flow efficiently throughout the body, delivering oxygen and nutrients to cells and tissues while removing waste products.

Engaging in moderate exercise, such as walking, cycling, or yoga, on a daily basis can help keep the detox pathways active and effective. Sweating during exercise not only aids in detoxification but also supports cardiovascular health, improves mood, and enhances energy levels. Additionally, regular movement helps prevent the stagnation of lymph fluid, reducing the risk of toxin buildup and supporting the immune system in fighting off infections.

4.2 Avoiding Common Detox Mistakes

Detoxification is a natural process that the body carries out daily, but in the quest for better health, many people turn to extreme detox programs that can sometimes do more harm than good. It is crucial to approach detoxification carefully, ensuring that the body receives the nourishment it needs while eliminating toxins. Barbara O'Neill highlights the potential dangers of extreme detox methods, such as prolonged fasting or restrictive juice cleanses, which may deprive the body of essential nutrients, ultimately weakening its natural healing capacity.

The Risks of Extreme Detox Programs

Detox programs have gained popularity, often promising quick results and radical transformations. However, many of these programs involve drastic measures like extended fasting or consuming only juices for several days. While the intent behind these programs is often to "cleanse" the body, they can actually lead to nutrient deficiencies and a weakened immune system. O'Neill cautions against such approaches because they fail to provide the body with the necessary nutrients, particularly proteins, fats, and key vitamins that are essential for repair and detoxification processes.

Prolonged fasting, for example, can deplete the body's stores of glycogen, leaving individuals feeling fatigued and mentally foggy. Moreover, this kind of fasting may force the body to break down muscle tissue for energy, which can further reduce strength and endurance. Similarly, juice cleanses, though rich in vitamins and antioxidants, lack the proteins and fats needed to sustain energy levels and maintain cellular repair. Without these key nutrients, the detoxification process becomes less efficient, as the liver and other detox organs rely on a balanced intake of macronutrients to function optimally.

A Balanced Approach to Detoxification

Rather than resorting to extreme detox methods, O'Neill advocates for a balanced and sustainable approach to detoxification. The body has built-in mechanisms to detoxify itself through the liver, kidneys, lungs, skin, and digestive system. Supporting these organs with the right nutrients and lifestyle habits allows for gentle, ongoing detoxification without putting the body under undue stress.

A balanced detox plan should include a nutrient-dense diet, rich in whole foods such as vegetables, fruits, whole grains, and lean proteins. Foods like leafy greens, which are high in chlorophyll, support the liver in its detoxifying role, while fiber from whole grains and vegetables helps to remove waste products from the digestive tract. Adequate protein intake is crucial, as amino acids are essential for phase two of liver detoxification, where toxins are converted into water-soluble compounds for elimination.

Hydration is also a key component of effective detoxification. Drinking plenty of water helps to flush out toxins through the kidneys, while herbal teas such as dandelion and milk thistle can further support liver function. These gentle, natural methods allow the body to detoxify at its own pace, ensuring that it remains nourished and balanced throughout the process.

Avoiding Detox Symptoms

Extreme detox programs often result in unpleasant symptoms like headaches, fatigue, and irritability, which are commonly referred to as "detox symptoms." These occur when the body is overwhelmed by the release of toxins that it cannot efficiently process and eliminate. O'Neill warns that these symptoms are often a sign that the detoxification process is too aggressive and that the body is not being adequately supported.

To avoid these symptoms, it is important to take a gradual approach to detoxification, ensuring that the body is well-nourished and not deprived of essential nutrients. Incorporating a variety of whole foods into the diet helps to buffer the detox process, allowing the liver and kidneys to function more effectively. Additionally, incorporating rest and gentle movement, such as walking or yoga, can help to promote lymphatic drainage and circulation, further aiding the detox process.

4.3 Detoxifying the Environment

Detoxification goes beyond cleansing the body from within. It also involves removing harmful chemicals from the spaces we inhabit daily. Many household items and personal care products contribute to the toxic load on the body, as they contain substances that can accumulate over time and interfere with the body's natural detox processes. Barbara O'Neill encourages a holistic approach to health, which includes detoxifying the environment to reduce exposure to these external toxins. By creating a toxin-free living space, individuals can support their body's overall health and reduce the risk of long-term health issues.

Reducing Exposure to Toxins in Household Cleaners

One of the primary sources of environmental toxins is household cleaners. Many commercial cleaning products contain harsh chemicals that can linger in the air or on surfaces, contributing to respiratory issues, skin irritation, and even hormonal disruption. These substances, including synthetic fragrances, bleach, and ammonia, are often absorbed through the skin or inhaled, placing additional strain on the body's detoxification organs, particularly the liver and lungs.

Switching to natural, non-toxic cleaning alternatives is an effective way to reduce exposure to these harmful substances. Simple ingredients such as vinegar, baking soda, and lemon juice can be used to clean various surfaces around the home without introducing harmful chemicals. These natural options not only disinfect but also neutralize odors, providing a safe and effective alternative to traditional chemical-laden products. Additionally, using essential oils such as tea tree, lavender, or eucalyptus can add antimicrobial properties while leaving a pleasant, natural scent in the home.

Detoxifying Personal Care Products

Personal care products, including shampoos, lotions, and cosmetics, often contain chemicals that can disrupt the endocrine system and burden the body's detox pathways. Ingredients such as parabens, sulfates, and synthetic fragrances are common culprits that can cause skin irritation and hormonal imbalances. Reducing exposure to these chemicals by choosing natural alternatives is essential for maintaining long-term health.

Barbara O'Neill recommends carefully reading labels and selecting products made with plant-based ingredients and free from synthetic additives. For example, switching to natural deodorants made from coconut oil or baking soda can help avoid aluminum-based compounds, which have been linked to various health concerns. Similarly, opting for shampoos and conditioners that use natural oils and botanicals can help avoid sulfates and parabens that are harsh on both the scalp and the body. Many natural brands offer alternatives that nourish the skin and hair without introducing harmful chemicals into the system.

Cookware and Food Storage Choices

The kitchen is another area where toxins can accumulate, often through the use of non-stick cookware or plastic food containers. Non-stick pans, while convenient, often release harmful chemicals when heated, particularly if the surface becomes scratched. These chemicals, such as perfluorinated compounds (PFCs), can leach into food and accumulate in the body over time, potentially causing adverse health effects.

To reduce exposure to these toxins, switching to stainless steel, cast iron, or ceramic cookware is highly recommended. These materials are free from harmful chemicals and provide safe alternatives for cooking. Additionally, replacing plastic food containers with glass or stainless steel helps prevent chemicals like BPA (bisphenol A) from leaching into food, especially when containers are heated or exposed to acidic contents.

Practical Tips for Creating a Toxin-Free Living Space

Detoxifying the environment doesn't have to be overwhelming. Small, gradual changes can have a significant impact on reducing the toxic load on the body. Start by identifying the products used most frequently in the home, such as cleaners, personal care products, and cookware, and find natural alternatives that align with health goals. Whenever possible, choose products labeled as organic, non-toxic, and free from synthetic additives.

In addition to these practical changes, improving ventilation in the home is another simple way to detoxify the environment. Regularly opening windows to allow fresh air circulation can help remove airborne toxins that may accumulate from indoor products or materials. Incorporating air-purifying plants, such as aloe vera or spider plants, can also enhance indoor air quality by filtering out toxins naturally.

Chapter 5: 12 Natural Remedies for Detoxification

Detoxification is a vital process for maintaining health, as it allows the body to eliminate accumulated toxins and waste products that can impair its natural functions. By supporting the liver, kidneys, digestive system, and lymphatic system, detoxification can help restore balance and promote optimal health. The following are twelve natural remedies that can assist in detoxifying the body, each with specific instructions for how and when to use them.

1. Milk Thistle Tincture

Milk thistle is renowned for its powerful liver-protective properties. It contains **silymarin**, a compound that supports liver detoxification and regeneration. Milk thistle tincture can be taken to cleanse and protect the liver, especially after exposure to environmental toxins or poor dietary habits.

How to use: Take 15–20 drops of milk thistle tincture in a small glass of water, 2–3 times daily.

When to use: Best taken before meals to support liver function and improve digestion.

Duration: Milk thistle can be used for a few weeks during a detox program or longer for ongoing liver support.

2. Dandelion Root Tea

Dandelion root is another excellent herb for detoxification, particularly for liver and kidney health. It acts as a gentle diuretic, helping to increase urine output and remove toxins through the kidneys. It also stimulates bile production, assisting in digestion and the elimination of waste.

How to use: Brew 1–2 teaspoons of dried dandelion root in boiling water and steep for 10–15 minutes. Drink 1–2 cups daily.

When to use: Morning or afternoon, ideally on an empty stomach.

Duration: Dandelion root tea can be consumed daily during detoxification or as needed for kidney and liver health.

3. Burdock Root Capsules

Burdock root is well-known for its blood-purifying properties. It helps to cleanse the bloodstream and support the liver's detoxification processes. Burdock root also has anti-inflammatory effects, which can aid in reducing the burden of toxins on the body.

How to use: Take 1–2 capsules of burdock root extract, 2–3 times daily.

When to use: Best taken with meals to enhance absorption.

Duration: Burdock root can be used for several weeks during a detox regimen or periodically for blood purification.

4. Nettle Leaf Tea

Nettle leaf is a potent diuretic that helps the body eliminate excess fluid and toxins through the kidneys. It is also rich in vitamins and minerals, supporting overall health while detoxifying. Nettle leaf tea is gentle enough to be used regularly.

How to use: Steep 1–2 teaspoons of dried nettle leaves in boiling water for 10 minutes. Drink 1–3 cups per day.

When to use: Throughout the day, ideally between meals.

Duration: Nettle tea can be consumed daily during detoxification or as a regular part of a health regimen.

5. Parsley Juice

Parsley is a powerful detoxifying herb, especially for the kidneys. Its diuretic properties help flush out toxins while providing essential nutrients like vitamin C, iron, and chlorophyll, which support the body's natural cleansing processes.

How to use: Blend a handful of fresh parsley with water or other vegetables to make a juice. Drink 1 small glass daily.

When to use: Early in the day to kickstart detoxification.

Duration: Parsley juice can be used daily for a week or two during an intensive detox, or a few times a week for ongoing support.

6. Warm Lemon Water

Lemon is an excellent natural detoxifier that stimulates liver function and aids in digestion. Drinking warm lemon water in the morning helps cleanse the digestive system, alkalize the body, and promote hydration.

How to use: Squeeze the juice of half a lemon into a glass of warm water. Drink once daily.

When to use: First thing in the morning, on an empty stomach.

Duration: Warm lemon water can be consumed daily as part of a healthy morning routine.

7. Turmeric Golden Milk

Turmeric contains **curcumin**, a powerful antioxidant and anti-inflammatory compound that supports liver detoxification and protects against oxidative damage. Golden milk is a soothing, anti-inflammatory drink that can be easily incorporated into a detox program.

How to use: Mix 1 teaspoon of turmeric powder into warm plant-based milk, and add a pinch of black pepper (to enhance absorption). Drink 1 cup daily.

When to use: In the evening as a calming and detoxifying beverage.

Duration: Golden milk can be enjoyed daily during detox or whenever inflammation needs to be reduced.

8. Psyllium Husk (Fiber)

Psyllium husk is a natural fiber that helps to cleanse the digestive tract by promoting regular bowel movements. It acts as a gentle bulk-forming laxative, helping to remove waste and toxins from the colon.

How to use: Mix 1 tablespoon of psyllium husk with a glass of water. Drink immediately, followed by another glass of water.

When to use: Once daily, preferably before bed or first thing in the morning.

Duration: Psyllium husk can be used for short-term cleansing (1–2 weeks) or periodically for digestive health.

9. Ginger Detox Tea

Ginger is a warming herb that promotes digestion, increases circulation, and supports detoxification. It helps to break down toxins in the liver and can ease digestive discomfort during detoxification.

How to use: Grate 1 inch of fresh ginger and steep in hot water for 10 minutes. Drink 1–2 cups per day.

When to use: After meals to aid digestion or between meals for detox support.

Duration: Ginger tea can be consumed daily during a detox or as needed to support digestion.

10. Aloe Vera Juice

Aloe vera is known for its soothing and healing properties, particularly for the digestive system. It acts as a gentle laxative, helping to cleanse the colon and improve bowel movements while also providing hydration and nutrients.

How to use: Drink 1–2 tablespoons of pure aloe vera juice mixed with water, once daily.

When to use: Early in the morning or before meals.

Duration: Aloe vera juice can be used for short-term detoxification (1–2 weeks) or periodically to support digestive health.

11. Activated Charcoal (for Toxin Binding)

Activated charcoal is highly effective at binding toxins and chemicals in the digestive tract, helping to remove them from the body. It can be used for acute detoxification, particularly after exposure to toxins or during periods of cleansing.

How to use: Take 1–2 capsules of activated charcoal with a large glass of water, as needed.

When to use: Only during specific detoxification periods or after exposure to toxins.

Duration: Activated charcoal should be used short-term, for a few days at a time, to avoid nutrient depletion.

12. Apple Cider Vinegar Tonic

Apple cider vinegar is a well-known detoxifier that helps to balance pH levels, support digestion, and cleanse the liver. It can also aid in detoxifying the lymphatic system and improving skin health.

How to use: Mix 1 tablespoon of raw, unfiltered apple cider vinegar in a glass of water. Drink once daily.

When to use: Before meals to support digestion and detoxification.

Duration: Apple cider vinegar can be consumed daily for a few weeks as part of a detox regimen or regularly for ongoing health benefits.

Part 12:
Heart Health – Circulatory and Cardiovascular Wellness

Chapter 1: The Heart's Vital Role in Overall Health

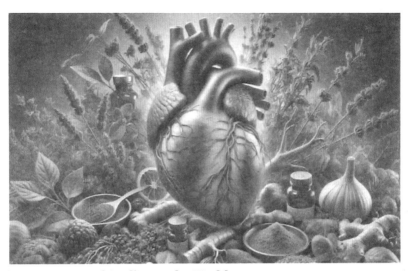

1.1 The Importance of Cardiovascular Health

The cardiovascular system plays a crucial role in maintaining overall health, with the heart at its core, acting as the body's central engine. Every beat of the heart pumps oxygen-rich blood to the organs, muscles, and tissues, providing them with the nutrients they need to function effectively. The health of this system directly impacts longevity, vitality, and quality of life. However, in today's world, many factors such as poor diet, lack of exercise, and chronic stress contribute to the decline of cardiovascular health. In her teachings, Barbara O'Neill highlights the importance of protecting and strengthening the heart through a combination of lifestyle changes, a balanced diet, and natural remedies.

The Role of the Heart as the Body's Central Engine

The heart is a powerful muscle responsible for circulating blood throughout the body. Its continuous pumping action ensures that oxygen and vital nutrients reach every cell, while also removing waste products like carbon dioxide. O'Neill emphasizes the heart's critical role in sustaining life, explaining that when the heart weakens or becomes compromised, every other system in the body is affected. A well-functioning heart is essential not only for physical endurance but also for cognitive function, energy levels, and emotional well-being.

Given the heart's importance, it is crucial to understand the factors that can lead to its decline. Conditions like atherosclerosis, where plaque builds up in the arteries, or hypertension, which causes increased pressure in the blood vessels, are just two examples of how cardiovascular health can deteriorate. These conditions can reduce the heart's efficiency, leading to further complications such as heart attacks or strokes. Recognizing these risks, O'Neill stresses the importance of taking proactive steps to maintain a healthy heart.

Impact of Poor Cardiovascular Health

When cardiovascular health is compromised, the consequences are far-reaching. Poor heart health can lead to a range of conditions that drastically reduce the quality of life. Hypertension, often referred to as high blood pressure, is a common issue that puts extra strain on the heart and arteries. Left unchecked, it can damage the blood vessels and increase the risk of heart attacks, strokes, and kidney disease. High cholesterol levels also contribute to heart disease by promoting the accumulation of fatty deposits in the arteries, leading to blockages that restrict blood flow.

Heart disease itself is a leading cause of death worldwide, and its symptoms are often subtle or go unnoticed until significant damage has already occurred. Shortness of breath, fatigue, and chest pain are common indicators, but many people do not experience symptoms until the condition has progressed. This makes prevention and early intervention crucial in protecting cardiovascular health.

Lifestyle Changes for Cardiovascular Health

One of the most effective ways to protect and strengthen the heart is through lifestyle changes. O'Neill emphasizes that even small, consistent changes in daily habits can have a profound impact on heart health. One of the key recommendations is regular physical activity. Exercise helps to strengthen the heart muscle, improve circulation, and regulate blood pressure. Activities such as walking, swimming, or cycling are particularly beneficial for maintaining cardiovascular fitness. Additionally, exercise promotes weight management, which is critical since obesity is a significant risk factor for heart disease.

In addition to exercise, reducing stress is vital for cardiovascular health. Chronic stress elevates cortisol levels, which can lead to increased blood pressure and inflammation in the body. These factors contribute to the wear and tear of the heart and blood vessels over time. Incorporating stress-reducing practices like deep breathing, meditation, or spending time in nature can help lower cortisol levels and create a more heart-friendly environment.

Sleep is another essential component of cardiovascular health. O'Neill highlights the importance of restorative sleep in maintaining a healthy heart. Poor sleep quality has been linked to hypertension, heart disease, and metabolic disorders. Establishing a regular sleep routine and creating a restful environment can help ensure the body and heart receive the rest they need to function optimally.

1.2 Circulation and the Role of the Cardiovascular System

Proper circulation is fundamental to maintaining overall health, as it ensures that essential nutrients and oxygen are delivered throughout the body, supporting healing, energy production, and detoxification. The cardiovascular system plays a critical role in this process, moving blood through a network of arteries, veins, and capillaries. This system not only transports oxygen and nutrients to the cells but also helps to remove waste products and toxins from the body, maintaining the body's internal balance.

Importance of Healthy Circulation

One of the key messages Barbara O'Neill conveys is that optimal circulation is vital for ensuring the body functions as it should. When blood flows efficiently, tissues and organs receive the nutrients and oxygen they need to perform essential tasks like cellular repair and detoxification. Poor circulation, on the other hand, can lead to a range of health issues, from fatigue and poor concentration to more serious conditions like high blood pressure, atherosclerosis, and cardiovascular disease.

A healthy circulatory system also supports the body's natural healing processes. For instance, when a part of the body is injured, the blood delivers immune cells, oxygen, and nutrients to the damaged area, promoting faster healing. Proper blood flow ensures that the body's self-repair mechanisms work efficiently, which is critical for maintaining health and preventing illness.

Flexibility of Blood Vessels and Cardiovascular Health

One of the most crucial aspects of maintaining healthy circulation is ensuring that the blood vessels remain flexible and free from blockages. Blood vessels, particularly arteries, need to be able to expand and contract as blood flows through them. When blood vessels become stiff or constricted, it becomes harder for blood to circulate, leading to increased pressure on the cardiovascular system.

The flexibility of blood vessels can be compromised by several factors, including poor diet, lack of exercise, and exposure to toxins. Diets high in unhealthy fats, sugars, and processed foods contribute to the buildup of plaque in the arteries, a condition known as atherosclerosis. Plaque formation restricts blood flow and makes the arteries less flexible, which can lead to high blood pressure and increase the risk of heart attacks or strokes. The body's detoxification processes also become less efficient when circulation is impaired, as the blood cannot effectively remove waste products from the body.

In her teachings, Barbara highlights the importance of consuming a nutrient-dense diet to support cardiovascular health. Foods rich in antioxidants, healthy fats, and fiber help to reduce inflammation in the blood vessels and prevent plaque buildup. For example, incorporating foods high in omega-3 fatty acids, such as flaxseeds and walnuts, can improve the flexibility of the arteries and support overall cardiovascular function. Antioxidant-rich fruits and vegetables, like berries and leafy greens, are also vital for protecting blood vessels from oxidative damage, which can lead to stiffness and blockages.

Preventing Atherosclerosis

Atherosclerosis, or the hardening of the arteries due to plaque buildup, is a leading cause of cardiovascular diseases. It occurs when cholesterol, fats, and other substances accumulate on the artery walls, forming plaques that can restrict blood flow. Over time, these plaques can rupture, leading to blood clots that may cause heart attacks or strokes. Preventing atherosclerosis is, therefore, essential for maintaining healthy circulation and protecting cardiovascular health.

Barbara emphasizes that one of the most effective ways to prevent atherosclerosis is through dietary changes. Reducing the intake of processed foods, trans fats, and sugars is crucial for minimizing the risk of plaque formation. Instead, she advocates for a diet rich in whole, plant-based foods that provide the body with the nutrients

Chapter 2: Natural Remedies for Supporting Heart Health

2.1 Hawthorn: Nature's Heart Tonic

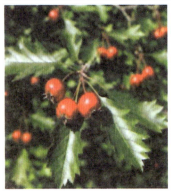

Hawthorn is widely recognized as a powerful herb for heart health, often referred to as "the herb for the heart" due to its well-documented ability to strengthen the cardiovascular system. It has been traditionally used to support heart function and has gained prominence in modern natural health circles for its effectiveness in enhancing circulation, reducing blood pressure, and strengthening the heart muscle. One of the primary ways hawthorn works is by improving the flow of blood to and from the heart, ensuring that the heart receives adequate oxygen and nutrients to function optimally.

Strengthening the Heart Muscle

Hawthorn's ability to strengthen the heart muscle is one of its most important functions. It contains flavonoids, which are compounds that promote better blood flow in the coronary arteries, improving the heart's strength and endurance. This is particularly beneficial for individuals dealing with conditions such as heart failure or chronic fatigue, where the heart's capacity to pump blood efficiently may be compromised. By supporting the heart muscle, hawthorn helps to improve overall cardiovascular endurance and energy levels, allowing the heart to work more effectively without becoming overly strained.

In addition to enhancing the heart muscle's strength, hawthorn helps to balance the heart's rhythm, making it useful for those who experience irregular heartbeats or palpitations. Its gentle action on the heart allows it to be used long-term, providing ongoing support to cardiovascular health.

Improving Circulation and Reducing Blood Pressure

Hawthorn is also effective in improving circulation throughout the body. By relaxing the blood vessels, it helps to reduce resistance in the arteries, allowing blood to flow more freely. This not only improves oxygen delivery to vital organs but also helps to reduce high blood pressure, one of the key risk factors for heart disease. Regular use of hawthorn has been shown to dilate blood vessels, particularly in the coronary arteries, which supply the heart with blood.

Furthermore, hawthorn's action as a vasodilator means that it helps reduce the workload on the heart by allowing blood to circulate more easily, making it especially useful for those with hypertension. The gentle lowering of blood pressure over time can help reduce the risk of more severe cardiovascular events, such as heart attacks or strokes.

2.2 Flaxseed: Reducing Inflammation with Omega-e Fatty Acids

Flaxseeds, known for their rich content of omega-3 fatty acids, play a vital role in supporting heart health by reducing both inflammation and cholesterol levels. Incorporating flaxseeds into the diet is a powerful way to address two key factors that contribute to cardiovascular disease. Omega-3 fatty acids are essential for maintaining the balance of healthy fats in the body, and flaxseeds provide a plant-based source that is particularly beneficial for those seeking to reduce their intake of animal products.

One of the key reasons flaxseeds are so effective in promoting heart health is their high concentration of alpha-linolenic acid (ALA), a type of omega-3 fatty acid. ALA is converted in the body into other forms of omega-3s, which help to reduce inflammation throughout the body. Inflammation is a common contributor to a wide range of chronic diseases, including heart disease, arthritis, and autoimmune conditions. By reducing inflammation, flaxseeds help to protect the cardiovascular system and prevent the progression of conditions related to chronic inflammation.

Chronic inflammation can cause damage to the arteries, contributing to the buildup of plaque and the eventual narrowing of blood vessels. This can lead to an increased risk of heart attacks and strokes. Consuming flaxseeds regularly helps reduce the levels of inflammatory markers in the body, lowering the risk of these dangerous health events.

2.3 Garlic: A Natural Cholesterol and Blood Pressure Reducer

Garlic has long been celebrated for its medicinal properties, particularly in supporting heart health. As a key component of Barbara O'Neill's holistic approach to wellness, garlic plays a vital role in maintaining a healthy cardiovascular system. This powerful herb is widely recognized for its ability to lower cholesterol levels and reduce blood pressure, two critical factors that contribute to overall heart health. Additionally, garlic acts as a natural blood thinner, reducing the risk of dangerous blood clots and promoting better circulation throughout the body.

Garlic for Lowering Cholesterol

One of the most well-documented benefits of garlic is its ability to lower cholesterol levels. High cholesterol, especially LDL cholesterol, can lead to the buildup of plaque in the arteries, increasing the risk of heart disease and stroke. Garlic contains compounds, particularly **allicin**, that help reduce the production of cholesterol in the liver. When consumed regularly, garlic has been shown to decrease overall cholesterol levels, including LDL (the "bad" cholesterol), while potentially raising HDL (the "good" cholesterol). This balancing effect helps to maintain healthy arteries and supports long-term cardiovascular health.

In her teachings, the emphasis on whole foods and natural remedies includes garlic as a potent aid in managing cholesterol levels. It is recommended to incorporate garlic into the diet regularly, either through raw garlic or garlic supplements, to achieve these cholesterol-lowering benefits.

Blood Pressure Reduction with Garlic

In addition to its cholesterol-lowering properties, garlic is also effective in reducing blood pressure, another major risk factor for cardiovascular diseases. High blood pressure, or hypertension, forces the heart to work harder to pump blood, which can weaken the heart and damage blood vessels over time. Garlic's ability to relax blood vessels and improve circulation helps to lower blood pressure naturally, reducing strain on the cardiovascular system.

Garlic achieves this through its impact on **nitric oxide production**, which helps dilate blood vessels and improves blood flow. This vasodilating effect not only helps to lower blood pressure but also reduces the risk of hypertension-related complications. Including garlic in the diet or taking garlic supplements is a simple and effective way to support healthy blood pressure levels.

Natural Blood Thinner and Clot Prevention

Another important benefit of garlic is its role as a natural blood thinner. Blood clots can form in the arteries, blocking the flow of blood to vital organs like the heart and brain. Garlic helps to prevent the formation of clots by reducing the stickiness of platelets, the cells responsible for clotting. This anticoagulant property is essential for reducing the risk of heart attacks and strokes.

For individuals at risk of clotting disorders, consuming garlic regularly can help support the body's natural defenses against dangerous blockages in the arteries.

Chapter 3: Lowering Cholesterol and Blood Pressure Naturally

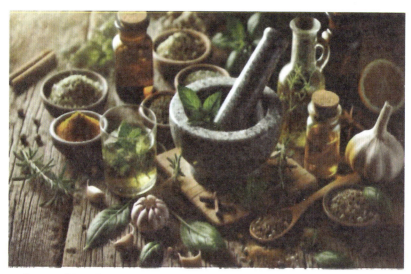

3.1 Understanding the Dangers of High Cholesterol

High levels of low-density lipoprotein (LDL) cholesterol, commonly referred to as "bad" cholesterol, pose significant risks to cardiovascular health. When LDL cholesterol accumulates in the bloodstream, it can lead to plaque buildup along the walls of the arteries, a condition known as atherosclerosis. This narrowing and hardening of the arteries increases the risk of heart attacks and strokes by restricting blood flow and making it more difficult for oxygen-rich blood to reach vital organs.

Elevated LDL cholesterol levels are often linked to an unhealthy diet rich in saturated fats, trans fats, and refined sugars. Consuming these types of foods contributes to increased cholesterol production in the liver, leading to higher levels of LDL in the bloodstream. In addition, poor lifestyle habits, such as physical inactivity, smoking, and chronic stress, exacerbate the problem by further damaging the cardiovascular system and increasing the likelihood of plaque formation.

Diet plays a crucial role in cholesterol management. A diet high in processed and fried foods, animal fats, and refined carbohydrates can significantly elevate LDL cholesterol levels. Conversely, a clean, nutrient-dense diet has the power to lower cholesterol naturally by supporting the body's ability to process and eliminate excess cholesterol. Whole foods, particularly those rich in fiber and healthy fats, help reduce LDL cholesterol and improve overall cardiovascular health.

3.2 Plant-Based Diet for Heart Health

A whole-food, plant-based diet is essential for maintaining optimal heart health, as it provides the body with vital nutrients that protect the cardiovascular system. A diet rich in natural, unprocessed foods such as fruits, vegetables, whole grains, and healthy fats is fundamental for reducing cholesterol levels and supporting overall heart function.

Whole-Food, Plant-Based Diet for Cholesterol Reduction

A key component of heart health is managing cholesterol levels. High cholesterol, particularly LDL (low-density lipoprotein), is a major risk factor for heart disease, as it can lead to the buildup of plaque in the arteries, restricting blood flow and increasing the risk of heart attack and stroke. A plant-based diet, rich in fiber and antioxidants, helps to reduce LDL cholesterol levels naturally. Foods such as **oats, beans, and legumes** are particularly effective in lowering cholesterol, as they contain soluble fiber that binds to cholesterol in the digestive tract and helps to remove it from the body.

Leafy greens, such as **kale, spinach, and arugula**, are also powerful allies in reducing cholesterol levels. These vegetables are rich in nitrates, which help to relax blood vessels and improve circulation. Additionally, they are high in fiber and antioxidants, which contribute to lowering cholesterol and protecting the heart from oxidative stress.

Supporting the Cardiovascular System with Nutrient-Dense Foods

A whole-food, plant-based diet offers a wide range of nutrients that are vital for maintaining heart health. **Fruits and vegetables**, particularly those high in antioxidants like berries, tomatoes, and carrots, help to neutralize free radicals in the body, reducing oxidative stress on the cardiovascular system. This is essential for preventing the damage to blood vessels that can lead to heart disease.

Whole grains, such as quinoa, brown rice, and barley, are another key component of a heart-healthy diet. These grains provide complex carbohydrates that help maintain steady blood sugar levels, reducing the risk of insulin resistance, which is linked to heart disease. Whole grains are also high in fiber, which further aids in lowering cholesterol and supporting healthy digestion, both of which are crucial for cardiovascular health.

3.3 Reducing Blood Pressure with Natural Remedies

High blood pressure is a leading risk factor for heart disease, but it can be managed and reduced through natural methods. Rather than relying solely on medications, lifestyle adjustments and specific natural remedies can effectively lower blood pressure and promote cardiovascular health.

Magnesium-Rich Foods and Their Benefits

Magnesium is a vital mineral that plays a significant role in regulating blood pressure. It helps relax the blood vessels, which in turn reduces the resistance the heart must overcome to pump blood. Foods that are rich in magnesium can be easily incorporated into the diet to support heart health and naturally lower blood pressure. Some of the best sources of magnesium include leafy green vegetables, nuts, seeds, and whole grains.

Dark leafy greens such as spinach and kale are particularly high in magnesium and provide additional nutrients that benefit overall cardiovascular health. Nuts like almonds and seeds, including pumpkin seeds and sunflower seeds, offer not only magnesium but also healthy fats that support blood vessel flexibility. Whole grains, such as quinoa and brown rice, are also excellent choices to maintain optimal blood pressure levels.

Consuming these magnesium-rich foods daily helps to maintain normal blood pressure levels by promoting relaxation in the arteries and preventing the constriction that leads to elevated blood pressure.

Herbs to Support Blood Pressure Reduction

Several herbs are known for their ability to lower blood pressure naturally. Hibiscus is one of the most well-known herbs for managing hypertension. Its natural compounds act as ACE inhibitors, similar to some pharmaceutical blood pressure medications, helping to relax blood vessels and reduce pressure.

Another beneficial herb is dandelion, which has natural diuretic properties. By promoting increased urination, dandelion helps the body eliminate excess fluids and sodium, which are common contributors to high blood pressure. Reducing fluid retention relieves the pressure on the blood vessels, supporting healthier blood pressure levels.

Incorporating these herbs into daily routines, whether through herbal teas or supplements, offers a natural approach to managing blood pressure without the side effects often associated with conventional medications.

Chapter 4: The Role of Exercise in Preventing Heart Disease

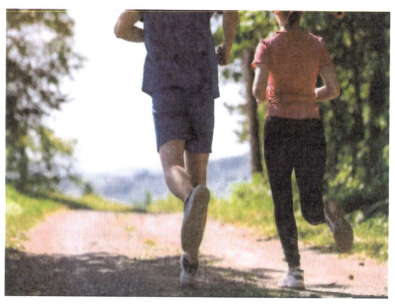

Exercise: A Key Component of Cardiovascular Wellness

Regular physical activity is essential for maintaining heart health, but not all exercises are suitable for everyone. For those seeking to improve cardiovascular health without placing excessive strain on the body, low-impact exercises are highly effective. These types of exercises are gentle on the joints and muscles, yet still provide significant benefits for the cardiovascular system.

The Benefits of Low-Impact Exercises

Low-impact exercises, such as walking and yoga, are particularly recommended for individuals who want to strengthen their heart without the risks associated with high-intensity activities. These exercises promote cardiovascular health by improving circulation, lowering blood pressure, and enhancing overall endurance. Walking, for instance, is a simple yet powerful way to support heart function. It helps to increase heart rate in a controlled manner, which strengthens the heart muscles over time. Additionally, walking promotes better blood flow, reducing the risk of blood clots and improving the delivery of oxygen throughout the body.

Another advantage of low-impact exercises is that they minimize the risk of injury. For individuals with joint problems, arthritis, or other physical limitations, these exercises provide a safer alternative to more strenuous forms of exercise. The reduced impact on the knees, hips, and ankles allows for consistent physical activity without the concern of exacerbating existing conditions.

Walking for Cardiovascular Health

Walking is one of the most accessible and effective exercises for improving heart health. It can be adapted to suit various fitness levels, making it ideal for beginners or those with physical limitations. Walking at a moderate pace for 30 minutes a day has been shown to lower blood pressure, reduce bad cholesterol (LDL), and increase good cholesterol (HDL). These improvements in cholesterol levels directly contribute to better heart health by preventing the buildup of plaque in the arteries, which can lead to heart disease.

Regular walking also helps regulate body weight, which is crucial for maintaining a healthy heart. Excess weight places additional strain on the heart, increasing the risk of cardiovascular conditions such as hypertension and heart attack. By incorporating walking into a daily routine, individuals can improve heart efficiency and reduce the overall workload on the cardiovascular system.

Yoga and Heart Health

Yoga, another low-impact exercise, offers a holistic approach to heart health by combining physical movement with mental relaxation. Yoga is particularly beneficial for reducing stress, a major contributor to heart disease. Through its focus on deep breathing and controlled movements, yoga helps to calm the nervous system, reducing the production of stress hormones like cortisol and adrenaline. This relaxation effect lowers blood pressure and promotes a steady heart rate, which is essential for long-term heart health.

In addition to its stress-relieving benefits, yoga also strengthens the muscles that support the cardiovascular system. Certain poses, such as **Mountain Pose** or **Warrior Pose**, engage large muscle groups, promoting better circulation and enhancing heart function. The stretching and lengthening movements in yoga improve flexibility and reduce tension in the body, which can further alleviate strain on the heart.

For individuals looking to incorporate yoga into their heart-health routine, practices such as **Hatha yoga** or **restorative yoga** are excellent choices. These forms of yoga focus on slow, deliberate movements and deep breathing, making them suitable for people of all fitness levels. Over time, consistent yoga practice helps improve heart function by lowering heart rate variability and supporting the body's natural ability to maintain cardiovascular balance.

Combining Walking and Yoga

For optimal heart health, combining walking and yoga can be particularly effective. While walking provides cardiovascular endurance and promotes healthy circulation, yoga complements this by enhancing flexibility, reducing stress, and improving overall body alignment. This combination allows for a well-rounded approach to heart health that targets both the physical and mental aspects of wellness.

Chapter 5: 10 Natural Remedies for Heart Health

The appendix provides more details for each remedy.

1. Hawthorn Berry Tincture
2. Flaxseed Oil
3. Garlic Capsules
4. Cayenne Pepper Supplement
5. Turmeric Capsules
6. Hibiscus Tea
7. Magnesium Supplement
8. Omega-3 Fish Oil
9. Dandelion Leaf Tea
10. Ginger Tea

Part 13:
Bone and Joint
Health with Natural
Solutions

Chapter 1: Strengthening Bones and Joints with Natural Remedies

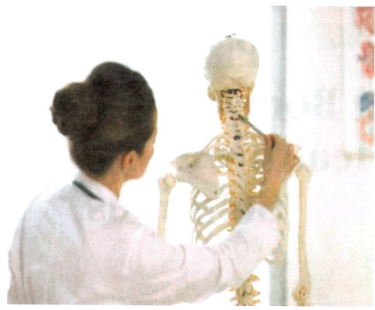

1.1 The Importance of Bone and Joint Health

Bone and joint health plays a critical role in maintaining overall well-being, particularly as we age. Barbara O'Neill emphasizes that it is easy to overlook the importance of these systems until we begin to experience issues such as osteoporosis, arthritis, or chronic joint pain. These conditions often emerge as a result of poor nutritional and lifestyle habits accumulated over time. By focusing on prevention through proper care, it is possible to maintain strong bones and flexible joints well into later years.

Preventing Joint Degeneration

Joint health is closely tied to flexibility and mobility, and it is important to prevent the degeneration of cartilage, which cushions joints and allows for smooth movement. One of the main causes of joint pain is the breakdown of this cartilage, which leads to conditions such as osteoarthritis. To protect joints, maintaining a diet rich in anti-inflammatory foods is essential. Inflammation contributes to joint pain and stiffness, so reducing inflammatory foods like processed sugars and refined grains can have a significant impact on joint health.

Omega-3 fatty acids, which are found in foods like flaxseeds, chia seeds, and fatty fish, are known for their anti-inflammatory properties. Incorporating these into a daily diet helps to reduce inflammation in the joints and may slow down the progression of arthritis. Omega-3s also support overall joint lubrication, which is important for maintaining flexibility and reducing pain during movement.

Collagen, a protein that makes up a large portion of cartilage, is another key element in joint health. Foods rich in collagen, such as bone broth, help to support the repair and maintenance of joint tissues. This is particularly beneficial for individuals experiencing wear and tear on their joints due to age or physical activity.

The Impact of Lifestyle on Bone and Joint Health

In addition to nutrition, lifestyle factors play a crucial role in maintaining strong bones and healthy joints. Regular physical activity, particularly weight-bearing exercises, is essential for preserving bone density. Activities such as walking, hiking, and strength training put stress on the bones, prompting them to maintain or increase their density to support the body. This is especially important as we age, as bone density naturally declines over time, increasing the risk of fractures.

For joint health, maintaining an active lifestyle is equally important. Exercises that promote flexibility, such as yoga and stretching, keep the joints limber and prevent stiffness. Additionally, low-impact exercises like swimming or cycling are excellent for maintaining mobility without putting excessive strain on the joints. Regular movement helps to keep the synovial fluid, which lubricates the joints, flowing, allowing for smoother and pain-free motion.

Another critical lifestyle factor is maintaining a healthy weight. Excess weight puts additional strain on the joints, particularly those in the lower body such as the knees and hips. Over time, this can lead to the accelerated breakdown of cartilage, contributing to joint pain and conditions like osteoarthritis. By maintaining a healthy weight through balanced nutrition and regular exercise, it is possible to reduce the stress placed on the joints and prevent long-term damage.

1.2 The Body's Self-Healing Mechanism for Bones

Bones are living tissues that constantly regenerate, a process essential for maintaining strength and density. According to Barbara O'Neill, the body's natural ability to heal and strengthen itself relies heavily on providing the right nutrients and support. Without these, the bones cannot maintain their optimal health, leading to issues like osteoporosis and fractures.

Bone Regeneration and Essential Nutrients

Bone regeneration is a continuous process, where old bone cells are broken down, and new cells are formed. This renewal process is known as **bone remodeling**, and it ensures that bones remain strong and resilient throughout a person's life. However, for this to happen effectively, the body requires an adequate supply of essential minerals, most notably **calcium, magnesium**, and **vitamin D**.

Calcium is the primary mineral responsible for bone density. It is stored in the bones and provides the structural support they need to remain strong. Without sufficient calcium, bones can become weak and brittle, increasing the risk of fractures. Magnesium plays a complementary role by aiding in the absorption of calcium into the bones. It also contributes to the structural matrix of the bone, ensuring that calcium is used effectively within the body. Inadequate magnesium levels can lead to improper calcium absorption, causing imbalances that weaken bone tissue over time.

Vitamin D is equally crucial for bone health. It facilitates the absorption of calcium from the diet into the bloodstream and helps deposit it into the bones. Without sufficient vitamin D, the body cannot absorb calcium effectively, no matter how much is consumed through food or supplements. In addition to supporting calcium absorption, vitamin D also plays a role in maintaining bone density and preventing conditions like osteoporosis. O'Neill stresses the importance of regular sun exposure or supplementation to ensure adequate levels of vitamin D in the body.

Chapter 2: Anti-Inflammatory Herbs for Joint Pain

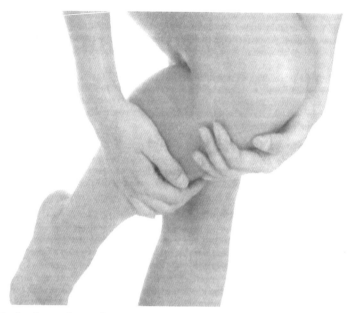

2.1 Reducing Joint Inflammation Naturally

Inflammation is at the core of most joint pain, whether caused by arthritis, injury, or the natural wear and tear of aging. Addressing inflammation directly is essential for reducing discomfort and restoring joint mobility. By managing inflammation, not only can pain be alleviated, but further damage to the joints can also be prevented.

One of the primary recommendations for reducing inflammation is the use of **anti-inflammatory herbs**. Among the most powerful are **Boswellia, ginger**, and **turmeric**. These herbs have been extensively studied for their ability to reduce swelling and pain in the joints. Boswellia, sometimes referred to as frankincense, is known for its anti-inflammatory properties, particularly in conditions such as arthritis. It works by inhibiting enzymes that contribute to inflammation in the body, making it a potent tool for managing chronic joint pain.

Ginger is another highly effective herb for reducing inflammation. It has been used for centuries in traditional medicine for its warming and pain-relieving properties. Ginger works by reducing the production of inflammatory cytokines, proteins that play a key role in triggering inflammation in the joints. Additionally, it supports circulation, which can help improve mobility and reduce stiffness.

Turmeric is perhaps one of the most well-known anti-inflammatory herbs, thanks to its active compound **curcumin**. Curcumin has been shown to inhibit inflammatory pathways and reduce the production of pro-inflammatory substances in the body. Turmeric's ability to combat oxidative stress, which often accompanies inflammation, makes it a valuable remedy for those suffering from joint pain due to conditions like osteoarthritis.

These herbs can be consumed in various forms, including **teas, supplements**, or **topical balms**. Drinking ginger or turmeric tea, for example, provides a gentle and effective way to introduce these herbs into your daily routine. Many people also find relief by applying topical balms containing Boswellia, ginger, or turmeric directly to the affected areas. These balms penetrate the skin and deliver the anti-inflammatory properties of the herbs directly to the joints, providing targeted relief.

While these herbs can provide significant benefits, it is also important to address lifestyle factors that contribute to chronic inflammation. **Diet** plays a crucial role in managing inflammation in the body. Reducing the intake of processed foods, refined sugars, and trans fats can lower overall inflammation levels, while incorporating more whole, plant-based foods supports the body's natural healing processes. **Regular movement** and gentle exercise are also key to maintaining joint flexibility and reducing stiffness, which often accompanies chronic inflammation.

2.2 The Role of Omega-3 Fatty Acids in Reducing Inflammation

In addition to anti-inflammatory herbs, **Omega-3 fatty acids** are essential for managing inflammation in the body, particularly in the joints. These healthy fats, found primarily in **flaxseed oil** and **fish oil**, play a critical role in reducing joint pain and stiffness. Omega-3s work by decreasing the production of inflammatory molecules known as eicosanoids and cytokines, which are responsible for much of the inflammation in conditions like arthritis.

Omega-3 fatty acids not only reduce inflammation, but they also provide essential support for **joint lubrication**. This is particularly important in reducing wear and tear on the cartilage, the tissue that cushions joints. Over time, the degradation of cartilage can lead to conditions like osteoarthritis, where bones begin to rub against each other, causing pain and reduced mobility. By ensuring that the joints are well-lubricated, Omega-3s help to protect the cartilage and reduce the friction that leads to further damage.

Barbara O'Neill recommends incorporating **flaxseeds** and **fish oil** into the diet as effective ways to increase Omega-3 intake. Flaxseeds, in particular, are an excellent plant-based source of Omega-3s and can easily be added to smoothies, salads, or baked goods. Fish oil, derived from fatty fish such as salmon, mackerel, and sardines, provides a concentrated source of Omega-3s and can be taken as a supplement to ensure consistent intake.

Including Omega-3s in the diet can also improve overall joint flexibility and help reduce morning stiffness, a common symptom for those with chronic joint pain. This is particularly beneficial for individuals suffering from rheumatoid arthritis, an autoimmune condition characterized by joint inflammation. Omega-3s have been shown to reduce the duration of morning stiffness and improve joint mobility throughout the day.

Incorporating **anti-inflammatory foods** into the diet is another important step in managing joint health. Foods rich in Omega-3s, such as **chia seeds**, **walnuts**, and **leafy greens**, can complement the benefits of flaxseed oil and fish oil, further supporting the body's natural ability to manage inflammation. Avoiding inflammatory foods, such as processed meats, refined carbohydrates, and unhealthy oils, is equally important for maintaining healthy joints.

In addition to dietary changes, certain **lifestyle adjustments** can enhance the benefits of Omega-3s. Regular exercise, particularly low-impact activities such as swimming, cycling, or walking, helps to keep the joints mobile and reduces stiffness. Gentle stretching and strengthening exercises can also improve joint flexibility, helping to alleviate the discomfort associated with joint inflammation.

Chapter 3: Natural Supplements for Bone Density

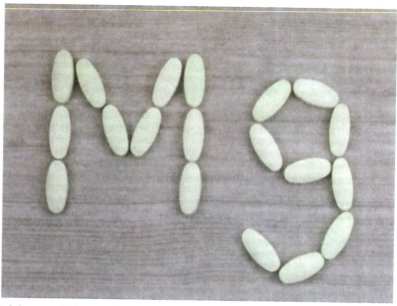

3.1 Calcium and Magnesium: Essential for Bone Strength

Calcium and magnesium are two minerals that play a central role in maintaining strong and healthy bones. Calcium serves as the primary building block of bones, forming the structure and density that ensures skeletal strength. Without adequate calcium intake, bones can become brittle and weak, increasing the risk of fractures and osteoporosis. However, calcium doesn't work alone in supporting bone health; it requires magnesium to be fully effective. Magnesium regulates calcium levels in the body and aids in its absorption, ensuring that calcium reaches the bones where it is needed most.

One of the key dietary recommendations is to consume foods rich in calcium, such as leafy greens, sesame seeds, and fortified plant-based milks. Leafy greens, particularly kale, collard greens, and spinach, are packed with bioavailable calcium that the body can readily absorb. Sesame seeds are another excellent source, providing not only calcium but also other minerals like zinc and phosphorus, which further support bone density. For those who follow a plant-based diet or avoid dairy, fortified plant-based milks, such as almond, soy, or oat milk, are a good alternative to ensure adequate calcium intake.

Magnesium-rich foods are just as important in maintaining bone strength. Nuts, seeds, and whole grains are excellent sources of this vital mineral. Almonds, pumpkin seeds, and sunflower seeds are particularly rich in magnesium, helping to regulate calcium levels and support bone health. Whole grains, such as quinoa, brown rice, and oats, not only provide magnesium but also offer a range of other nutrients that contribute to overall well-being. Including these foods in daily meals ensures that both calcium and magnesium are present in the diet, working together to strengthen bones.

3.2 Vitamin D: The Bone Health Enhancer

Vitamin D is another critical component of bone health because it facilitates the absorption of calcium. Without sufficient vitamin D, even a calcium-rich diet may not be enough to maintain strong bones, as the body cannot properly absorb the calcium ingested. Vitamin D acts as a regulator, ensuring that calcium is transported from the digestive system into the bloodstream and then to the bones, where it is needed for bone formation and maintenance.

The most effective way to boost vitamin D levels is through sun exposure. Barbara emphasizes the importance of spending time outdoors, especially in the morning or late afternoon when the sun is less intense. The skin produces vitamin D when exposed to sunlight, and this natural production is often more efficient than relying solely on dietary sources or supplements. However, O'Neill also acknowledges that sun exposure can be limited during the winter months or in areas where sunlight is scarce, making it difficult to maintain adequate vitamin D levels year-round.

For those who cannot get enough sunlight, O'Neill suggests considering vitamin D supplementation. She advises that it is particularly important for people living in colder climates or those with limited sun exposure to monitor their vitamin D levels and supplement as needed. Along with supplements, dietary sources of vitamin D, such as fortified plant-based milks and certain types of mushrooms, can provide additional support during the months when sun exposure is minimal. Ensuring sufficient vitamin D is essential for calcium absorption and the overall process of bone regeneration.

3.3 The Role of Silica and Boron in Bone Health

While calcium, magnesium, and vitamin D are well-known for their roles in bone health, the trace minerals silica and boron also play significant but often overlooked roles in maintaining bone strength. These elements work in synergy with calcium to enhance its absorption and utilization in the body, supporting both bone density and flexibility.

Silica, a mineral found abundantly in the earth, is crucial for the production of collagen, the protein that forms the framework of bones and connective tissues. Collagen is necessary for bone elasticity and strength, helping to reduce the risk of fractures. In addition to supporting collagen formation, silica aids in the mineralization of bones by improving the deposition of calcium and other minerals. Without sufficient silica, bones may become more prone to damage and lose their ability to repair themselves effectively.

Foods that are rich in silica include cucumbers, bell peppers, and other vegetables that have high water content. Cucumbers, in particular, are an excellent source of bioavailable silica, which can easily be absorbed by the body. Bell peppers not only provide silica but also contain vitamin C, which is essential for collagen synthesis, further promoting bone health. Including these foods in a regular diet ensures that the body receives enough silica to support both bone strength and flexibility.

Boron is another trace mineral that is often overlooked but is essential for the maintenance of bone health. Boron helps regulate the metabolism of calcium, magnesium, and vitamin D, making it a key player in the prevention of bone-related diseases like osteoporosis. Boron also influences the balance of hormones such as estrogen and testosterone, both of which are involved in maintaining bone density, particularly in older adults. By supporting the metabolism of these hormones, boron contributes to the preservation of bone mass as individuals age.

Foods that are rich in boron include nuts, seeds, and dried fruits. Almonds, walnuts, and hazelnuts are particularly high in boron, making them an ideal snack for promoting bone health. Dried fruits, such as prunes, raisins, and apricots, are also excellent sources of boron and provide the added benefit of being rich in other bone-supporting nutrients like potassium and magnesium.

Chapter 4: Exercises and Stretches for Maintaining Bone and Joint Health

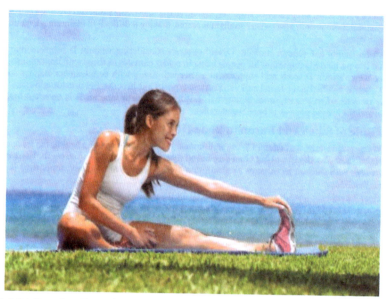

4.1 Weight-Bearing Exercises for Bone Density

Weight-bearing exercises are critical for maintaining and improving bone density, particularly as the body ages. The process of strengthening bones occurs when mechanical stress is applied to them, prompting bone-forming cells, called osteoblasts, to work harder. This is especially important in reducing the risk of conditions like osteoporosis, which weakens bones and makes them more prone to fractures. Weight-bearing activities, such as walking, hiking, and resistance training, place the necessary strain on bones to keep them strong and healthy.

Simple activities like walking or hiking are effective forms of weight-bearing exercise. When the body moves against gravity, the bones in the legs, hips, and spine are stimulated to grow stronger. Hiking, with its varied terrain, provides additional challenges that further promote bone strength by requiring the body to adapt to different angles and pressures. Regular walking or hiking can help slow the natural bone loss that occurs with age, keeping the skeletal structure robust and resilient.

In addition to walking, resistance training is another excellent method for building bone density. Utilizing weights or resistance bands, among other forms of external resistance, resistance training challenges the bones and muscles. This type of exercise not only strengthens the muscles but also promotes the development of stronger bones by applying stress to the skeletal system. Simple strength-training exercises can be done at home using resistance bands or light weights, making it accessible to people of all fitness levels. Squats, lunges, and bicep curls are just a few examples of exercises that target major muscle groups while also benefiting bone health.

Barbara emphasizes that incorporating these exercises into a regular fitness routine is key to preventing conditions like osteoporosis and ensuring long-term bone health. Consistency is essential, as bones need frequent stimulation to remain strong. By regularly engaging in weight-bearing and resistance exercises, individuals can effectively support both their bone and muscle health.

4.2 Stretching for Joint Flexibility

Flexibility is another essential aspect of maintaining musculoskeletal health, particularly when it comes to joint function. Joints, the connection points between bones, are responsible for enabling a wide range of movements, but they can become stiff or limited in motion if not properly maintained. Stretching is one of the most effective ways to keep joints flexible and reduce stiffness, allowing for smooth, pain-free movement.

Daily stretching routines can greatly improve joint flexibility by increasing the range of motion and reducing the risk of injury. Stretching helps maintain the elasticity of muscles and tendons that support the joints, making it easier to move without strain. Over time, lack of flexibility can lead to joint stiffness, discomfort, or even injury, particularly in the hips, knees, and lower back, which are commonly affected areas.

Yoga and Pilates are highly effective practices for improving joint mobility, as they combine stretching with strength-building exercises. Yoga, in particular, focuses on slow, controlled movements that stretch and strengthen muscles around the joints. Poses like the forward bend or downward-facing dog help increase flexibility in the hips and lower back, while also reducing stiffness in the knees. Pilates also focuses on core strength and joint flexibility, with exercises that target specific areas of the body to improve mobility and alignment.

4.3 The Importance of Posture and Alignment

Proper posture and body alignment play a significant role in maintaining joint health and preventing injury. When the body is aligned correctly, weight is evenly distributed across the joints, reducing unnecessary strain and preventing wear and tear. On the other hand, poor posture places undue stress on specific joints, which can lead to pain, discomfort, and even long-term damage.

For instance, slouching while sitting or standing can cause misalignment in the spine, which, in turn, affects the hips and knees. Over time, poor posture can lead to chronic pain in the back, neck, and shoulders as the joints and muscles are forced to compensate for the body's imbalance. Correcting posture and maintaining proper alignment can significantly reduce these issues and improve overall joint function.

Barbara highlights simple changes that can make a significant difference in posture. For example, sitting up straight with the shoulders back and feet flat on the floor can help distribute weight evenly across the hips and spine, reducing the strain on these areas. Similarly, standing with the shoulders aligned over the hips and the knees slightly bent can prevent pressure from building up in the lower back and knees.

In addition to proper sitting and standing habits, exercises that focus on improving core strength can further support good posture. The core muscles—those in the abdomen, back, and pelvis—play a vital role in stabilizing the body and maintaining alignment. Strengthening these muscles can help keep the spine in its natural curve, which in turn supports better posture. Activities like Pilates and yoga are particularly effective at building core strength and improving alignment.

To further support posture, regular stretching and strength training exercises that target the back, shoulders, and hips can help correct imbalances that may contribute to poor alignment. Stretching the hip flexors, hamstrings, and chest muscles can release tightness that often causes misalignment, while strengthening the back and abdominal muscles provides the stability needed to maintain proper posture throughout the day.

Chapter 5: 12 Natural Remedies for Bone and Joint Health

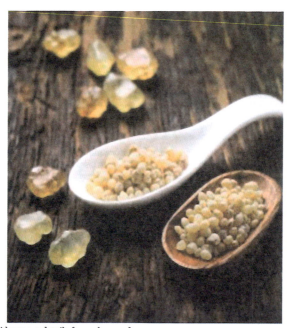

The appendix provides more details for each remedy.

1. Boswellia Extract

2. Turmeric Capsules

3. Ginger Tea

4. Magnesium Oil

5. Flaxseed Oil

6. Calcium Supplement

7. Vitamin D3 Supplement

8. Silica Powder

9. Boron Capsules

10. Epsom Salt Bath

11. Comfrey Root Balm

12. Willow Bark Extract

Part 14:
Skin Health –
Natural Remedies
for Radiant Skin

Chapter 1: Maintaining Healthy Skin with Natural Ingredients

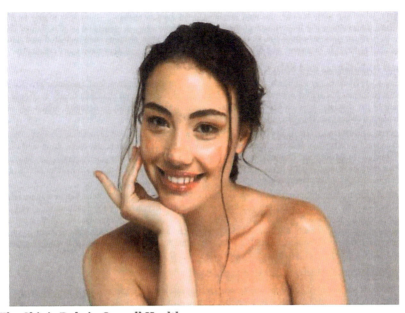

1.1 The Skin's Role in Overall Health

The skin, as the body's largest organ, serves multiple critical functions beyond its role as a physical barrier. Barbara O'Neill highlights the skin's importance not only in protecting the body from external threats but also in detoxification, temperature regulation, and reflecting the body's internal health. Through her holistic approach to wellness, she emphasizes that healthy skin is a sign of a well-functioning body, and many skin issues stem from imbalances within.

Skin as a Protective Barrier and Detoxification Organ

The primary role of the skin is to act as a protective barrier, shielding the body from harmful environmental elements such as bacteria, toxins, and pollutants. However, its functions extend far beyond protection. The skin plays an active role in the body's detoxification processes. Through sweat, the skin helps to eliminate toxins, thereby reducing the toxic load that the liver and kidneys must process. This detoxification process is especially important in modern times, where exposure to environmental pollutants, chemicals in food, and synthetic materials can overwhelm the body's internal detox systems.

Barbara O'Neill explains that when the body's detox pathways—such as the liver and kidneys—are overloaded, the skin often takes on a greater role in toxin elimination. This increased demand on the skin can lead to skin problems such as rashes, acne, and other inflammatory conditions. These outward manifestations are signs that the body is trying to rid itself of internal toxins. By supporting the skin's detoxification role through proper nutrition, hydration, and the use of natural skincare products, the skin can function more effectively, and its appearance will improve as a result.

Temperature Regulation and Skin Health

The skin also plays a vital role in regulating the body's temperature. Through processes such as sweating and vasodilation, the skin helps maintain a stable internal environment, even when external temperatures fluctuate. This function is critical in preventing overheating or excessive cooling, which can stress the body and lead to various health complications.

When the body overheats, the sweat glands in the skin release moisture, which evaporates and cools the body. Conversely, when the body is cold, the skin restricts blood flow to conserve heat. This ability to regulate temperature underscores the importance of maintaining healthy skin, as damaged or dehydrated skin can struggle to perform these essential functions. Ensuring that the skin remains well-hydrated and nourished with essential fatty acids, vitamins, and minerals helps it perform its regulatory roles more efficiently.

Internal Imbalances and Skin Conditions

According to O'Neill, many common skin conditions such as acne, eczema, and psoriasis are not simply superficial problems but reflect deeper internal imbalances. She points out that skin health is closely tied to the health of the digestive system, hormonal balance, and the body's ability to detoxify. When any of these systems are out of balance, the skin often exhibits signs of distress.

Acne, for example, is frequently linked to poor digestion and the accumulation of toxins in the body. When the digestive system is sluggish or overwhelmed by processed foods, it cannot efficiently break down and eliminate waste, leading to toxin buildup. These toxins may then be expelled through the skin, resulting in clogged pores and inflammation. Supporting the digestive system with a clean, whole-food diet, rich in fiber and probiotics, is one of the ways to address the root cause of acne.

Eczema and psoriasis are other conditions that Barbara O'Neill associates with internal issues, often related to the immune system and inflammation. Eczema is commonly triggered by food sensitivities, stress, and exposure to environmental allergens, which lead to an overactive immune response. Psoriasis, on the other hand, is an autoimmune condition where the body mistakenly attacks its own skin cells, leading to rapid cell turnover and inflammation. Both conditions benefit from a holistic approach that includes reducing inflammation through diet, avoiding triggers, and supporting the immune system.

1.2 Nourishing the Skin from the Inside Out

Healthy, radiant skin is not just a matter of external treatments; it is a reflection of what we nourish our bodies with internally. A nutrient-dense, plant-based diet plays a vital role in supporting skin health, and Barbara O'Neill emphasizes that beautiful skin begins from within. By providing the skin with essential vitamins, minerals, and hydration, we can support collagen production, enhance skin elasticity, and promote cellular repair.

Chapter 2: Remedies for Common Skin Conditions – Acne, Eczema, and Psoriasis

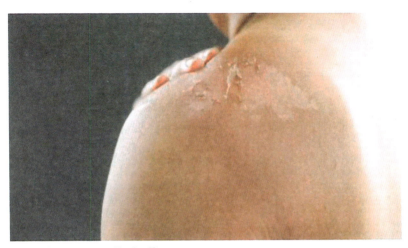

2.1 Addressing Acne Holistically

Acne is a skin condition that is often tied to several internal and external factors. Hormonal imbalances, a poor diet, and clogged pores are some of the most common contributors to this problem. According to Barbara O'Neill, the key to addressing acne lies in approaching it holistically—balancing internal health through detoxification while also using natural topical remedies to treat the skin. One of the major factors involved in acne is hormonal fluctuation. When hormones such as androgens increase, they can stimulate the skin's sebaceous glands to produce excess oil, leading to clogged pores and the development of pimples. For this reason, balancing hormones through diet and lifestyle changes is essential in treating acne from the inside out.

Detoxification is central to clearing up acne. Barbara emphasizes the importance of internal cleansing, which involves supporting the liver and digestive system to remove toxins from the body. A congested liver may struggle to process hormones efficiently, leading to hormone imbalances that contribute to acne. To support the liver, she recommends consuming foods rich in antioxidants and liver-friendly herbs such as dandelion root and milk thistle. These ingredients help to cleanse the liver, improve its function, and promote hormone balance, which can, in turn, reduce the occurrence of acne.

Diet plays a significant role in managing acne. Poor dietary choices, especially those high in processed foods and sugars, can exacerbate acne by increasing inflammation and contributing to hormonal imbalances. O'Neill advises reducing or eliminating foods that are known to trigger acne, such as dairy, refined sugars, and processed carbohydrates. Instead, she suggests focusing on whole, nutrient-dense foods that promote clear skin. For example, zinc-rich foods like pumpkin seeds, oysters, and chickpeas are recommended due to zinc's ability to regulate oil production in the skin and reduce the severity of acne. Zinc is also known for its anti-inflammatory properties, which help to calm inflamed skin and prevent further breakouts.

In addition to dietary changes, topical treatments are an important part of acne management. Barbara highlights the use of **tea tree oil**, which is known for its antibacterial and anti-inflammatory properties. Tea tree oil can be applied directly to blemishes to kill acne-causing bacteria and reduce redness. It is considered a gentler alternative to harsh chemical treatments commonly used in acne medications, making it suitable for those with sensitive skin.

Another effective topical remedy for acne is **aloe vera**, which can be used to soothe irritated skin, reduce inflammation, and promote healing. Aloe vera is particularly beneficial for reducing the appearance of acne scars, as it helps to stimulate skin regeneration and repair damaged tissue. Barbara recommends using fresh aloe vera gel directly from the plant for the best results.

For those struggling with cystic acne or deeper breakouts, **clay masks** can be beneficial. Clay, especially bentonite clay, has the ability to draw out impurities from the skin and reduce oil production, which helps to prevent clogged pores. Applying a clay mask once or twice a week can aid in detoxifying the skin and calming inflammation, leading to fewer breakouts over time.

2.2 Eczema: Calming Inflammation

Eczema, also known as atopic dermatitis, is another skin condition that can be influenced by internal and external factors. It is typified by skin spots that are irritated, itching, and occasionally seeping. In Barbara O'Neill's approach, eczema is often tied to internal imbalances such as food intolerances, stress, and poor gut health. She suggests that by addressing these underlying issues, it is possible to reduce flare-ups and manage eczema more effectively.

One of the first steps in treating eczema holistically is identifying and eliminating potential food triggers. Many individuals with eczema have sensitivities to certain foods, with common culprits including dairy, gluten, and processed foods. These foods can contribute to inflammation in the body, which can manifest as eczema on the skin. Barbara recommends conducting an elimination diet to identify specific food intolerances. This involves removing suspected trigger foods from the diet for several weeks and then gradually reintroducing them while monitoring the skin's reaction. Eliminating or reducing these foods can often lead to significant improvements in eczema symptoms.

In addition to dietary adjustments, managing stress is crucial for reducing eczema flare-ups. Stress has a direct impact on the immune system and can exacerbate inflammatory conditions like eczema. Incorporating stress-reducing techniques such as meditation, deep breathing, and regular physical activity can help to calm the body's inflammatory response. Barbara encourages the use of natural relaxation practices to keep stress levels in check, which in turn helps to minimize the occurrence of eczema.

Herbal remedies play an essential role in soothing the symptoms of eczema. Anti-inflammatory herbs such as **chamomile** and **calendula** are highly effective in calming irritated skin. Chamomile, known for its gentle anti-inflammatory and soothing properties, can be used both internally and externally. Drinking chamomile tea helps to reduce internal inflammation, while applying chamomile-infused oils or creams directly to the affected areas can provide immediate relief from itching and irritation. Calendula, another powerful herb, often used in salves and creams for its ability to speed up the healing process and calm inflamed skin. Barbara recommends using calendula-based lotions or oils to moisturize dry, irritated skin and promote healing.

In more severe cases of eczema, **oatmeal baths** are a traditional remedy that can provide significant relief. Oatmeal has natural anti-inflammatory properties and helps to lock in moisture, making it ideal for soothing dry, itchy skin. Adding colloidal oatmeal to a warm bath can calm flare-ups and reduce the itching associated with eczema. It also forms a protective barrier over the skin, which helps to prevent further irritation.

Another key recommendation for managing eczema is the use of **coconut oil**. Coconut oil is a natural moisturizer with antibacterial and anti-inflammatory properties, making it an excellent choice for soothing dry, irritated skin. Applying coconut oil to the affected areas helps to hydrate the skin and reduce inflammation, which is essential for preventing eczema flare-ups.

For individuals who suffer from eczema on the face or delicate areas of the body, **honey** can be an effective treatment. Honey, particularly raw or Manuka honey, has been shown to have both antibacterial and anti-inflammatory properties making it beneficial for reducing the risk of infection and calming irritated skin. Applying a thin layer of honey to the affected areas and leaving it on for 15-20 minutes can provide relief from itching and promote skin healing. Honey can also be combined with other soothing ingredients, such as aloe vera, for an even more effective treatment.

Addressing eczema holistically involves treating the skin externally while also focusing on internal factors like diet, stress, and gut health. Barbara emphasizes that by taking a comprehensive approach, it is possible to reduce inflammation and manage eczema more effectively.

2.3 Psoriasis: Supporting Detox and Skin Regeneration

Psoriasis is a chronic autoimmune condition characterized by rapid skin cell turnover and inflammation. The skin becomes red, scaly, and often itchy due to the accumulation of dead skin cells that the body is unable to shed effectively. Addressing psoriasis from a holistic perspective involves not only treating the external symptoms but also supporting internal systems such as the liver, which plays a critical role in detoxification. When the liver is functioning optimally, it helps to remove toxins from the body that might otherwise exacerbate skin conditions like psoriasis.

One of the herbal remedies frequently suggested to support liver detoxification is **burdock root**. Burdock root is known for its blood-purifying properties and its ability to improve liver function. This herb helps to cleanse the blood, which in turn reduces the toxic load on the skin. It acts as a diuretic, helping to eliminate excess fluids and toxins through the urine, and promotes clearer, healthier skin by addressing the internal imbalances that contribute to psoriasis.

Another important herb for liver support is **milk thistle**. Milk thistle contains an active compound called silymarin, which has been shown to protect and regenerate liver cells. It works by shielding the liver from toxins while also promoting the production of new, healthy liver cells. This is particularly important for individuals with psoriasis, as a well-functioning liver is crucial for effective detoxification. By incorporating milk thistle into a detoxification program, individuals can reduce the toxic burden on their skin and support its natural healing process.

For soothing the external symptoms of psoriasis, **aloe vera** is highly recommended. Aloe vera has long been used for its anti-inflammatory and skin-healing properties. When applied topically, aloe vera gel can help to calm inflamed skin, reduce itching, and promote the regeneration of healthy skin cells. It is particularly effective for soothing the red, irritated patches that are common in psoriasis. Aloe vera is also known for its hydrating properties, which can help to alleviate the dryness and scaling often associated with the condition.

Chapter 3: DIY Skincare Recipes for Glowing, Youthful Skin

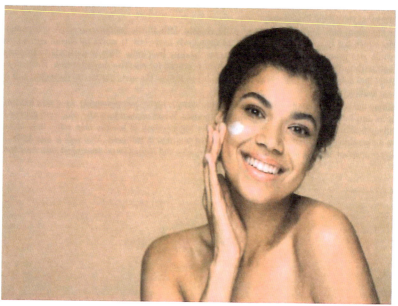

3.1 Using Natural Ingredients in Skincare

Maintaining healthy skin requires the use of products that are free from harsh chemicals and synthetic ingredients, which can aggravate skin conditions like psoriasis. Natural skincare is not only gentler on the skin but also supports its natural ability to heal and regenerate. Barbara O'Neill advocates for using **natural skincare products** that are made from simple, organic ingredients, as the skin readily absorbs what is applied to it. Harsh chemicals found in many commercial skincare products can disrupt the skin's barrier function and exacerbate inflammation, making conditions like psoriasis worse.

One of the key ingredients promoted for natural skincare is **aloe vera**, which can be used in its pure form to hydrate and soothe the skin. Aloe vera is rich in vitamins, minerals, and antioxidants, making it an excellent choice for repairing damaged skin and maintaining overall skin health. Its anti-inflammatory properties also make it ideal for individuals with sensitive skin or those prone to irritation.

Coconut oil is another popular natural ingredient that offers a range of benefits for the skin. Rich in moisture, coconut oil aids in the restoration of the skin's natural lipid barrier. This is particularly beneficial for individuals with dry or flaky skin, as it helps to lock in moisture and prevent further dryness. Coconut oil also contains antimicrobial properties, which can help to protect the skin from infections that might arise due to broken or inflamed skin. When used consistently, coconut oil can improve skin texture and leave the skin feeling soft and nourished.

In addition to these basic ingredients, **essential oils** are often included in natural skincare formulations for their therapeutic properties. Oils such as **lavender**, **tea tree**, and **chamomile** are commonly used to promote healing and reduce inflammation. Lavender oil, for instance, is known for its calming and soothing effects on the skin. It can help reduce redness and irritation, making it a great choice for sensitive or inflamed skin. Tea tree oil, on the other hand, is valued for its antibacterial and antifungal properties, making it particularly useful for treating acne-prone skin or preventing infections.

Barbara emphasizes the importance of using **pure, organic ingredients** in skincare products, as the skin absorbs what is applied to it. This means that any harmful chemicals present in skincare products can potentially enter the bloodstream, leading to further health complications. By choosing products made from natural, non-toxic ingredients, individuals can ensure that they are supporting their skin's health rather than harming it. Additionally, many natural ingredients, such as coconut oil and aloe vera, are not only safe for the skin but also offer a range of healing and protective benefits.

For those who wish to create their own skincare products, **DIY skincare solutions** are an excellent option. Simple recipes using ingredients like aloe vera, coconut oil, and essential oils can be made at home to cater to specific skin needs. For example, a basic moisturizer for dry skin can be made by combining coconut oil with a few drops of lavender essential oil. This type of product not only hydrates the skin but also helps to soothe any irritation or redness. Similarly, a soothing face mask for inflamed skin can be made by mixing aloe vera gel with a few drops of tea tree oil. These DIY solutions are customizable and allow individuals to control exactly what they are putting on their skin.

3.2 DIY Cleansing and Exfoliating Recipes

Exfoliation is an essential part of maintaining healthy, glowing skin. By removing dead skin cells, regular exfoliation helps to promote cell regeneration, improve skin texture, and reduce the appearance of blemishes and fine lines. Barbara O'Neill recommends using gentle, natural exfoliants, as they effectively cleanse the skin without causing irritation or stripping it of its natural oils. Among her preferred ingredients for DIY exfoliating recipes are oatmeal and sugar, both of which are readily available and provide excellent results for various skin types.

One of the most notable benefits of using **oatmeal** as an exfoliant is its soothing properties. Oatmeal is particularly effective for sensitive or inflamed skin, as it gently removes dead skin cells while calming irritation. It is rich in anti-inflammatory compounds and antioxidants, which help to protect the skin from environmental stressors. Additionally, oatmeal can help maintain the skin's moisture barrier, ensuring that the exfoliation process does not lead to dryness or discomfort. Barbara advises mixing finely ground oatmeal with water to form a paste that can be gently massaged onto the skin in circular motions. This simple yet effective method not only exfoliates but also provides hydration.

For a more invigorating exfoliation experience, **sugar** is another natural exfoliant that Barbara recommends. Sugar granules are slightly rougher than oatmeal, making them ideal for removing stubborn dead skin cells and encouraging blood circulation to the skin's surface. The natural glycolic acid present in sugar helps to break down the bond between dead skin cells, allowing them to be easily removed. Barbara often suggests combining sugar with a natural oil, such as coconut oil, to create a moisturizing exfoliant. This combination sloughs off dead skin while simultaneously nourishing the skin, leaving it smooth and supple.

One of Barbara's favored DIY exfoliating recipes is a **honey and oatmeal face scrub**. Honey is a natural humectant, meaning it draws moisture into the skin, while its antibacterial properties help prevent acne and other skin infections. When combined with the soothing and exfoliating properties of oatmeal, this scrub not only removes dead skin cells but also hydrates and protects the skin. To make this scrub, mix one tablespoon of honey with two tablespoons of finely ground oatmeal and a small amount of water to form a paste. Gently massage the mixture onto the face for a few minutes before rinsing it off with warm water. All skin types can use this formula, however those with dry or sensitive skin should use it especially.

Exfoliating once or twice a week is typically enough to maintain healthy skin, though this frequency can be adjusted depending on individual skin needs. Over-exfoliating can lead to irritation and compromise the skin's natural barrier, so it is important to balance exfoliation with proper hydration and moisturizing practices.

3.3 Moisturizing with Oils

After exfoliation, it is crucial to replenish the skin's moisture to maintain its elasticity, smoothness, and overall health. Barbara recommends natural oils such as **coconut, almond**, and **jojoba** for deeply hydrating the skin while helping to balance sebum production. These oils are rich in essential fatty acids, vitamins, and antioxidants, which support the skin's natural barrier and promote healing.

Coconut oil is a favorite due to its ability to penetrate deeply into the skin, providing long-lasting hydration without clogging pores. It contains medium-chain fatty acids that help reduce inflammation and improve skin elasticity, making it an ideal moisturizer for dry or damaged skin. Additionally, coconut oil's antibacterial and antifungal properties help protect the skin from infections and promote healing of minor cuts or irritations. For application, Barbara suggests warming a small amount of coconut oil in the palms of your hands before gently massaging it into the skin. This not only moisturizes but also creates a protective barrier that locks in moisture.

Almond oil is another highly recommended oil for its ability to nourish the skin while keeping it soft and supple. It is rich in vitamin E, a powerful antioxidant that helps protect the skin from free radical damage and supports the skin's natural healing processes. Almond oil is especially beneficial for people with dry or sensitive skin, as it soothes irritation and provides a lightweight moisture that absorbs quickly without leaving a greasy residue. Barbara suggests applying almond oil to damp skin after a shower or bath to seal in hydration and maintain the skin's moisture balance throughout the day.

Jojoba oil is particularly unique because it closely resembles the skin's natural sebum, making it an excellent choice for those with oily or combination skin. Jojoba oil aids in controlling sebum production, keeping the skin from getting overly dry or oily. It also contains anti-inflammatory properties that can help reduce redness and irritation, making it suitable for acne-prone skin. Barbara recommends using jojoba oil as a facial moisturizer, either alone or combined with other natural oils, for a lightweight yet effective hydrating solution.

In addition to oils, **aloe vera** is another highly effective moisturizer that Barbara often recommends for its hydrating properties without clogging pores. Aloe vera is known for its soothing and cooling effects, making it ideal for calming irritated or sun-damaged skin. It also provides a lightweight moisture that is easily absorbed by the skin, making it suitable for all skin types. Aloe vera's natural polysaccharides help to lock in moisture and promote the production of collagen, which supports skin elasticity and firmness. Barbara suggests applying pure aloe vera gel directly to the skin after cleansing or exfoliating, allowing it to fully absorb before applying any additional oils or moisturizers.

Combining natural oils with aloe vera provides a well-rounded approach to skin hydration, offering both deep moisture and soothing relief. For those looking for a more customized approach, Barbara suggests creating a DIY **moisturizing blend** using a combination of oils that cater to individual skin needs. For example, a blend of coconut and jojoba oils can be particularly beneficial for those with combination skin, while almond and aloe vera are ideal for those with dry or sensitive skin.

Maintaining proper hydration is crucial for overall skin health, and these natural ingredients provide the essential nutrients needed

Chapter 4: Detoxifying the Skin Through Diet and Hydration

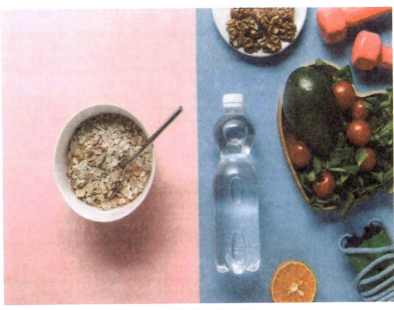

4.1 The Connection Between Diet and Skin Health

Skin health is a direct reflection of internal wellness, and what we eat plays a crucial role in maintaining clear, radiant skin. One of the core principles emphasized is that many skin conditions, such as acne, eczema, and dullness, are linked to an unbalanced diet. Consuming a diet high in processed foods, refined sugars, and unhealthy fats contributes to inflammation throughout the body, and this inflammation is often mirrored in the skin. Inflammation can cause clogged pores, increased oil production, and a lackluster complexion, as the skin struggles to cope with the body's toxic load.

In particular, foods rich in refined sugars and simple carbohydrates have a detrimental effect on the skin. These foods cause a spike in blood sugar, which in turn increases the production of insulin. High insulin levels have the ability to increase sebum production, which is the greasy material that clogs pores and causes acne outbreaks. Moreover, diets high in unhealthy fats, particularly trans fats and hydrogenated oils, promote inflammation, which can exacerbate skin conditions like rosacea and eczema.

To counteract these effects, it is recommended to adopt a diet that emphasizes whole, unprocessed foods. A clean diet rich in fruits, vegetables, whole grains, and healthy fats helps to reduce inflammation and support skin health. These nutrient-dense foods provide the body with essential vitamins, minerals, and antioxidants that promote skin regeneration and repair. For instance, **vitamin C**, found abundantly in berries, citrus fruits, and leafy greens, is a powerful antioxidant that aids in collagen production, helping to maintain the skin's elasticity and firmness.

Furthermore, **vitamin A**, present in carrots, sweet potatoes, and dark leafy greens, supports the skin's cell turnover process, helping to shed dead skin cells and reveal fresh, glowing skin underneath. Zinc, a mineral found in nuts, seeds, and legumes, is known for its ability to reduce inflammation and protect the skin from oxidative damage.

Healthy fats, such as those found in **avocados, nuts,** and **seeds**, are crucial for maintaining the skin's moisture barrier. Omega-3 fatty acids, in particular, help to keep the skin hydrated and supple by preventing the loss of water through the skin's outer layer. Foods rich in omega-3s, like flaxseeds, chia seeds, and walnuts, help to reduce inflammation and support overall skin health by improving hydration and elasticity.

Another group of beneficial foods includes **berries**, such as blueberries, raspberries, and strawberries. These fruits are rich in antioxidants, which neutralize free radicals and protect the skin from environmental damage. Antioxidants also play a role in reducing inflammation, which helps to prevent skin flare-ups and promote a clear complexion.

Whole grains are another important part of a skin-friendly diet. Unlike refined grains, which can cause spikes in blood sugar and insulin levels, whole grains like quinoa, brown rice, and oats are digested more slowly, providing a steady source of energy without causing inflammation. These grains are also rich in fiber, which supports the body's detoxification process by promoting regular bowel movements and preventing the buildup of toxins that can negatively impact the skin.

In addition to these food groups, it is essential to minimize the intake of processed foods, refined sugars, and unhealthy fats. By reducing the consumption of inflammatory foods and replacing them with nutrient-dense alternatives, it is possible to improve skin clarity, reduce breakouts, and achieve a natural, healthy glow.

4.2 Hydration for Radiant Skin

Hydration is one of the most critical factors in maintaining healthy, youthful skin. Water is essential for the body's detoxification processes, as it helps to flush out toxins and keep the skin hydrated from the inside out. When the body is properly hydrated, the skin appears plumper, smoother, and more radiant. Dehydrated skin, on the other hand, tends to look dry, flaky, and prone to fine lines and wrinkles.

Drinking at least **2-3 liters of pure water daily** is a key recommendation for promoting healthy skin. Water helps to maintain the skin's elasticity, support cell regeneration, and prevent the buildup of toxins that can lead to breakouts and other skin issues. Hydration also supports the body's lymphatic system, which plays a vital role in removing waste products and toxins from the body. When the lymphatic system is functioning optimally, the skin is more likely to remain clear and radiant.

In addition to water, **herbal teas** can play a supportive role in skin health by promoting detoxification and improving kidney and liver function. Herbal teas such as **nettle** and **dandelion** are particularly beneficial for the skin, as they help to cleanse the blood and support the body's natural detoxification pathways.

Nettle tea is rich in antioxidants and anti-inflammatory compounds, making it an excellent choice for those suffering from acne or other inflammatory skin conditions. Nettle helps to reduce redness and irritation while also providing a range of vitamins and minerals that support overall skin health. It is especially effective at helping to clear the skin by promoting kidney health, as the kidneys play a crucial role in filtering out toxins from the blood.

Dandelion tea is another powerful detoxifier that supports liver function. The liver is one of the body's primary detoxification organs, and when it is functioning optimally, the skin benefits as well. Dandelion tea helps to cleanse the liver, promoting the elimination of toxins that might otherwise contribute to skin issues like acne, eczema, or dullness. By supporting liver health, dandelion tea helps to keep the skin clear and glowing.

Peppermint tea is another option that can improve skin clarity. It has natural antimicrobial properties that can help to reduce the occurrence of acne-causing bacteria on the skin. Additionally, peppermint has a calming effect on the digestive system, which can help to reduce stress-related skin flare-ups, particularly those linked to conditions like eczema or psoriasis.

Apart from herbal teas, **hydration through foods** is another effective strategy for maintaining healthy skin. Water-rich fruits and vegetables, such as cucumbers, watermelon, and leafy greens, not only provide hydration but also supply essential vitamins and minerals that support skin health. These foods help to keep the skin hydrated and improve its overall texture and appearance.

While proper hydration is essential for all skin types, it is particularly important for individuals with dry or sensitive skin. When the skin is well-hydrated, it is better able to maintain its protective barrier, which helps to prevent irritation and inflammation. Hydration also plays a role in reducing the appearance of fine lines and wrinkles, as plump, hydrated skin appears smoother and more youthful.

Chapter 5: 12 Natural Remedies for Skin Health

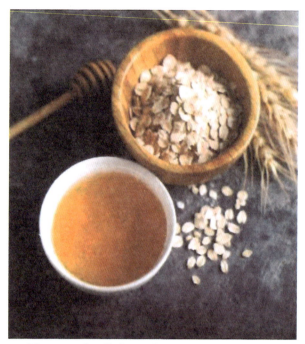

The appendix provides more details for each remedy.

1. Honey and Oatmeal Face Scrub

2. Aloe Vera Gel Moisturizer

3. Tea Tree Oil Spot Treatment

4. Calendula Balm

5. Cucumber Eye Compress

6. Chamomile Steam Facial

7. Coconut Oil Moisturizer

8. Turmeric Face Mask

9. Rose Water Toner

10. Lemon and Sugar Scrub

11. Apple Cider Vinegar Toner

12. Bentonite Clay Face Mask

Part 15:
Respiratory Health
and Herbal Support

Chapter 1: Natural Remedies for Asthma, Bronchitis, and Respiratory Issues

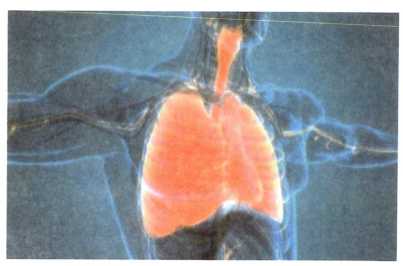

1.1 The Respiratory System: Its Vital Role in Health

The respiratory system is fundamental to sustaining life, as it is responsible for oxygenating the body and expelling carbon dioxide, both of which are essential for maintaining balance and overall vitality. When functioning optimally, the respiratory system ensures that the body receives the oxygen needed to fuel cellular energy production and supports the body's natural detoxification processes. Barbara O'Neill emphasizes the importance of a well-functioning respiratory system, noting that it plays a critical role in health and well-being.

The Respiratory System's Function in the Body's Oxygenation

Oxygen is crucial for energy production in every cell. Through the process of respiration, oxygen is taken in from the air and transported via the bloodstream to the cells, where it is used to produce energy in the form of adenosine triphosphate (ATP). ATP is the energy currency of the body and powers all biological functions. A steady supply of oxygen is necessary to maintain cellular function, metabolism, and vitality.

The respiratory system also plays a crucial role in eliminating carbon dioxide, a byproduct of cellular respiration. Carbon dioxide is carried back through the bloodstream to the lungs, where it is expelled during exhalation. The efficient removal of this waste product is essential to prevent the buildup of toxins in the body, which can lead to fatigue, brain fog, and other symptoms of poor respiratory function. A healthy respiratory system thus supports the body's overall energy levels, mental clarity, and ability to detoxify naturally.

Effects of Compromised Respiratory Health

When the respiratory system is compromised, the entire body suffers. Conditions such as asthma, bronchitis, and chronic colds can severely limit the ability of the lungs to take in oxygen and expel carbon dioxide effectively. Asthma, for example, is a condition where the airways become inflamed and constricted, making it difficult to breathe. This can lead to insufficient oxygenation of the body's tissues, resulting in low energy levels, difficulty concentrating, and weakened immunity.

Bronchitis, which involves inflammation of the bronchial tubes, can also impair lung function, causing excessive mucus production and difficulty breathing. Chronic bronchitis, often caused by exposure to environmental pollutants or smoking, can lead to long-term damage to the respiratory system, reducing lung capacity and increasing susceptibility to infections. Repeated respiratory infections or chronic colds also place a significant burden on the lungs, leading to decreased respiratory efficiency over time.

1.2 Asthma: A Holistic Approach to Management

Asthma is a chronic inflammatory condition that affects the airways, making it difficult for individuals to breathe normally. The inflammation causes the airways to become narrow, leading to symptoms such as wheezing, shortness of breath, and chest tightness. This condition is often triggered by a variety of factors, including allergens, poor diet, and exposure to environmental toxins. In her teachings, Barbara O'Neill emphasizes the importance of addressing the root causes of asthma by focusing on reducing inflammation, strengthening the immune system, and avoiding known triggers that exacerbate the condition.

Understanding Asthma as an Inflammatory Condition

Asthma, at its core, is driven by inflammation in the bronchial tubes, which is often triggered by allergens such as pollen, dust mites, mold, or animal dander. When these allergens enter the respiratory system, they provoke an immune response that leads to inflammation in the airways, making breathing difficult. While conventional treatments like inhalers aim to open the airways temporarily, they do not address the underlying inflammation, which is critical to managing asthma in the long term.

O'Neill explains that asthma can be better managed by taking a holistic approach, which focuses on reducing inflammation naturally. A major part of this strategy involves identifying and eliminating environmental triggers that may be contributing to the condition. Exposure to pollutants such as cigarette smoke, chemical cleaning products, and industrial fumes can worsen the symptoms of asthma. In addition to avoiding these external irritants, it is essential to focus on internal factors such as diet and lifestyle, which can also play a significant role in managing the inflammation that drives asthma.

Strengthening the Immune System to Manage Asthma

A strong immune system is essential for managing asthma, as it helps the body to respond to allergens and environmental triggers without overreacting. O'Neill emphasizes that by fortifying the immune system, individuals can reduce the frequency and severity of asthma attacks. One of the most effective ways to boost the immune system naturally is through diet, particularly by consuming foods rich in vitamins and minerals that support immune function. Zinc, found in foods like nuts, seeds, and legumes, plays a critical role in immune health and can help to reduce inflammation in the airways.

In addition to dietary changes, reducing stress is another important factor in strengthening the immune system. Chronic stress can weaken the body's defenses, making it more susceptible to asthma triggers. Incorporating relaxation techniques, such as deep breathing exercises and meditation, can help to reduce stress levels and promote a more balanced immune response. Regular physical activity, particularly exercises that focus on lung capacity, such as swimming and yoga, can also improve respiratory function and strengthen the immune system over time.

Avoiding Known Triggers

Managing asthma effectively requires identifying and avoiding the triggers that lead to inflammation and airway constriction. For many individuals, this includes environmental allergens such as pollen and dust, which can be minimized by keeping living spaces clean and well-ventilated. In addition, avoiding exposure to cigarette smoke, chemical fumes, and harsh cleaning products is essential in preventing asthma flare-ups.

Dietary triggers, such as processed foods, sugars, and dairy, should also be avoided to reduce inflammation in the body. By eliminating these triggers and focusing on natural remedies and lifestyle adjustments, individuals with asthma can manage their symptoms more effectively and improve their overall quality of life

1.3 Bronchitis: Addressing Inflammation and Mucus

Bronchitis is a respiratory condition that results from the inflammation of the bronchial tubes, which leads to increased mucus production and breathing difficulties. In her holistic approach to respiratory health, Barbara O'Neill addresses the root causes of bronchitis, focusing on natural methods to reduce inflammation and encourage the body to expel excess mucus. This method involves the use of specific herbs and lifestyle modifications that work in harmony with the body's self-healing mechanisms.

Understanding Inflammation and Mucus in Bronchitis

Bronchitis, whether acute or chronic, typically occurs when the lining of the bronchial tubes becomes inflamed due to an infection or irritants such as smoke and pollutants. This inflammation causes the bronchial tubes to swell and produce an excessive amount of mucus. The excess mucus not only leads to coughing and congestion but also makes it harder for the airways to function efficiently, resulting in shortness of breath and discomfort.

Chronic bronchitis, often linked to long-term exposure to environmental toxins or smoking, can lead to persistent inflammation and mucus production. This ongoing inflammation creates a cycle of irritation and swelling that weakens the respiratory system over time. One of the key principles in managing bronchitis, as highlighted in O'Neill's teachings, is reducing inflammation and helping the body clear mucus naturally.

Encouraging Mucus Expulsion Naturally

In addition to herbal remedies, natural lifestyle practices can help the body expel mucus more effectively, improving respiratory health and reducing the duration of bronchitis. Staying properly hydrated is one of the simplest but most effective ways to thin mucus, making it easier for the body to clear the airways. Drinking water, herbal teas, and broths helps to keep the mucus loose and prevents it from becoming too thick and sticky, which can exacerbate breathing difficulties.

Inhalation therapy using steam is another method O'Neill suggests for supporting mucus clearance. By adding essential oils like eucalyptus or thyme to a bowl of hot water and inhaling the steam, the airways are soothed, and the mucus is loosened, facilitating its expulsion from the lungs. This practice not only provides immediate relief from congestion but also helps to calm inflammation in the bronchial tubes, aiding in the overall healing process.

Gentle physical activity, such as walking or yoga, can also stimulate lung function and encourage the movement of mucus. Engaging in activities that promote deep breathing helps to increase oxygen flow to the lungs and supports the body's natural efforts to clear the respiratory system.

Chapter 2: Best Herbs for Lung Health

2.1 Mullein: A Soothing Herb for the Lungs

Mullein is one of the most effective herbs for supporting respiratory health. It has been traditionally used for centuries as a natural remedy to treat lung-related issues. Mullein is particularly beneficial for soothing irritated tissues in the respiratory system, especially the lungs, where it helps reduce inflammation and promote healing. It is often recommended for conditions such as bronchitis, asthma, and chronic coughs, as it helps to alleviate discomfort and calm irritation in the airways.

This herb acts as a natural expectorant, which means it encourages the expulsion of mucus from the lungs, helping to clear the respiratory tract. Mullein's ability to support the body's natural mechanisms for clearing out congestion makes it a valuable tool in managing respiratory conditions where mucus buildup is a problem. By loosening and expelling mucus, mullein facilitates better breathing and contributes to improved lung function.

One of the key ways to incorporate mullein into a daily routine is through the use of **mullein tea**. Steeping the dried leaves in hot water creates a gentle and soothing tea that can be consumed throughout the day to support lung health. Drinking mullein tea regularly helps to reduce inflammation in the lungs and eases coughing, particularly in cases of dry, unproductive coughs. The warmth of the tea also provides additional comfort by relaxing the muscles of the respiratory system and helping the body eliminate congestion.

For those who prefer a more concentrated option, **mullein tinctures** are another effective form of this herbal remedy. A tincture allows for a higher potency of the herb and can be taken in small doses for fast relief. Mullein tinctures are particularly useful for people experiencing acute respiratory issues, such as colds or bronchitis, as they deliver the benefits of the herb more quickly and efficiently. The tincture can be added to water or taken directly under the tongue for ease of use.

2.2 Eucalyptus: Clearing the Airways

Eucalyptus is another powerful herb recommended for respiratory health, especially for its ability to open up the airways and reduce congestion. It is widely known for its strong, aromatic properties, which help to clear mucus and improve breathing. Eucalyptus is particularly beneficial in conditions such as colds, sinus congestion, and bronchitis, where the airways become blocked by excess mucus or inflammation.

One of the most effective ways to use eucalyptus is through **steam inhalations**. Adding a few drops of eucalyptus essential oil to hot water and inhaling the steam helps to break up mucus and clear the sinuses. This method is especially helpful for relieving congestion in the nasal passages and lungs, making breathing easier and more comfortable. Steam inhalation not only helps to clear the airways but also provides a soothing effect on inflamed tissues, allowing for faster recovery.

Eucalyptus is also known for its **anti-inflammatory** and **antimicrobial properties**, which make it highly effective in treating respiratory infections. When inhaled, the essential oil works to reduce swelling in the bronchial tubes and fight off harmful pathogens that may be causing the infection. This dual action of clearing mucus and combating infection makes eucalyptus a powerful remedy for a wide range of respiratory conditions.

For those who suffer from chronic respiratory issues, such as asthma or chronic bronchitis, eucalyptus can be a useful addition to their daily routine. Using **eucalyptus essential oil** in a diffuser or adding it to a warm bath can help to maintain clear airways and reduce the frequency of flare-ups. Additionally, applying a diluted eucalyptus oil to the chest can provide relief from coughs and help open up the airways for better airflow.

Both mullein and eucalyptus are valuable herbs for maintaining lung health and supporting the body's natural ability to heal from respiratory conditions. These herbs can be used in combination with other natural remedies to create a comprehensive approach to respiratory wellness, ensuring that the lungs remain clear, healthy, and capable of performing their vital function of oxygen exchange.

2.3 Licorice Root: Calming Inflammation

Licorice root has been long recognized for its powerful anti-inflammatory and soothing properties. It is particularly effective in addressing respiratory conditions where inflammation is a key concern, such as asthma and bronchitis. When the airways become inflamed, breathing becomes restricted, and the body struggles to get enough oxygen, which can lead to further health complications. Licorice root works by calming this inflammation, allowing the airways to relax and expand, making breathing easier.

The herb contains compounds such as glycyrrhizin, which has been shown to reduce inflammation by inhibiting the enzymes that trigger inflammatory responses in the body. In the context of asthma, licorice root not only reduces inflammation but also helps to modulate the immune response, which is often overactive in individuals with respiratory conditions. This makes it particularly beneficial in preventing asthma attacks and managing symptoms over time.

In addition to its anti-inflammatory effects, licorice root also has soothing properties that help to protect the mucous membranes lining the respiratory tract. This is especially important in conditions like bronchitis, where persistent coughing can cause irritation and damage to these sensitive tissues. Licorice root helps to coat and protect these areas, reducing discomfort and promoting healing. Barbara O'Neill emphasizes its role in calming inflamed airways, making it easier for individuals with respiratory difficulties to breathe more comfortably.

When used in herbal formulations, licorice root is often combined with other herbs that support respiratory health, enhancing its effectiveness in treating inflammation and soothing the respiratory tract. However, it is important to note that licorice root should be used in moderation, as excessive consumption can lead to elevated blood pressure due to its glycyrrhizin content. It is always recommended to consult a healthcare provider before using licorice root, especially for individuals with pre-existing health conditions.

2.4 Thyme: A Natural Antimicrobial for Respiratory Infections

Thyme is a powerful antimicrobial herb that has been used for centuries to treat a variety of respiratory infections. Its ability to eliminate harmful pathogens from the lungs and bronchi makes it a valuable remedy for conditions such as colds, bronchitis, and pneumonia. Thyme contains essential oils, particularly thymol, which have potent antimicrobial properties capable of fighting bacteria, viruses, and fungi.

In respiratory infections, one of the primary concerns is the buildup of mucus, which can clog the airways and make breathing difficult. Thyme acts as a natural expectorant, helping to thin and loosen mucus so that it can be expelled more easily. This not only clears the airways but also helps to remove pathogens from the body, speeding up recovery. By supporting the body's natural ability to expel mucus, thyme reduces the risk of secondary infections that can develop when mucus becomes trapped in the lungs or bronchi.

Thyme's antimicrobial action is also beneficial in preventing the spread of infection within the respiratory system. It targets the underlying pathogens responsible for the infection while also supporting the immune system in its fight against illness. This dual action makes thyme particularly effective in both acute respiratory infections and in preventing recurring infections, especially in individuals with weakened immune systems.

In addition to its respiratory benefits, thyme has a warming effect on the body, which can help to relieve the discomfort associated with respiratory infections. Its warming properties stimulate circulation, which enhances the delivery of oxygen and nutrients to the tissues, supporting faster healing. Thyme can be used in a variety of forms, including teas, tinctures, and steam inhalations, to deliver its antimicrobial and expectorant benefits directly to the respiratory system.

Chapter 3: Herbal Teas, Tinctures, and Foods to Enhance Respiratory Function

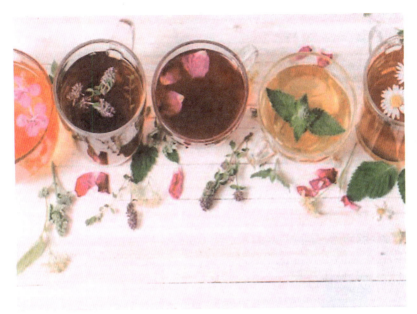

3.1 Herbal Teas for Lung Support

Herbal teas play a vital role in supporting respiratory health, especially during times of stress on the lungs, such as cold and flu season or when managing chronic respiratory conditions. Mullein, thyme, and licorice root are three herbs that Barbara O'Neill highlights as particularly beneficial for lung support. These herbs, when prepared as teas, can help soothe irritation, reduce inflammation, and promote the expulsion of mucus from the respiratory tract.

Mullein is widely known for its lung-supporting properties. This herb has been used for centuries to alleviate respiratory conditions, particularly those involving congestion. Mullein works by helping to thin mucus, making it easier for the body to expel it from the lungs. By doing so, it clears the airways, allowing for better oxygen exchange. In traditional medicine, mullein is often used for conditions such as bronchitis, asthma, and chronic coughs. Drinking mullein tea regularly, especially during cold and flu season, is an effective way to maintain lung health and keep the respiratory system functioning optimally.

Thyme is another powerful herb for supporting the lungs. It is rich in compounds like thymol, which have antiseptic and antimicrobial properties. Thyme helps to fight infections in the respiratory tract, making it particularly useful during colds and respiratory infections. Additionally, thyme has been shown to help relax the muscles of the respiratory system, easing breathing difficulties, and promoting overall lung health. Drinking thyme tea regularly can help prevent and alleviate symptoms of respiratory distress, especially in individuals prone to bronchitis or asthma attacks.

Licorice root is well-known for its soothing properties, making it a go-to herb for calming irritated airways. Licorice acts as a demulcent, forming a protective coating over the mucous membranes of the throat and lungs. This not only soothes irritation but also helps to reduce inflammation in the respiratory tract. Licorice root also has expectorant properties, encouraging the expulsion of mucus from the lungs, which is particularly beneficial during a cold or flu. Regular consumption of licorice root tea can help protect the lungs from irritation and support their healing during illness.

Barbara also emphasizes the importance of drinking warm liquids regularly, especially for those with chronic respiratory issues. Warm teas help to thin mucus, making it easier to expel, and can also soothe irritation in the throat and lungs. This is especially important during cold weather or during a respiratory infection when mucus can become thick and difficult to expel. Regular consumption of warm herbal teas not only provides the body with lung-supportive herbs but also keeps the respiratory system hydrated and functioning efficiently.

3.2 Using Tinctures for Fast Relief

In addition to herbal teas, tinctures offer a concentrated and fast-acting way to support lung health. Tinctures are alcohol-based extracts of herbs that allow for quick absorption into the bloodstream, providing rapid relief for acute respiratory issues. When dealing with conditions like bronchitis, asthma attacks, or severe respiratory discomfort, tinctures of herbs such as eucalyptus and thyme can offer quick and effective support.

Eucalyptus is well-known for its ability to open up the airways and support respiratory function. It contains a compound called eucalyptol, which acts as an expectorant and decongestant, making it easier for the body to expel mucus. Eucalyptus also has anti-inflammatory properties, reducing swelling in the respiratory tract and allowing for easier breathing. A few drops of eucalyptus tincture in water or tea can provide fast relief from congestion and help to clear the airways. Eucalyptus tincture is especially useful during an asthma attack or when experiencing bronchial congestion, as it works quickly to open up the airways and reduce discomfort.

Thyme tincture is another powerful remedy for respiratory issues. As mentioned earlier, thyme contains thymol, a compound with antimicrobial properties that can help fight infections in the respiratory tract. In tincture form, thyme provides a concentrated dose of this powerful herb, making it particularly useful for acute conditions like bronchitis or severe colds. Thyme tincture can help reduce coughing and clear mucus from the lungs, allowing for better breathing and faster recovery from respiratory infections.

Tinctures are particularly beneficial because they offer a more potent form of the herbs, providing relief more quickly than teas or capsules. The alcohol base in tinctures allows the medicinal compounds of the herbs to be absorbed rapidly into the bloodstream, making them ideal for situations where immediate relief is needed. For those dealing with chronic respiratory issues, keeping tinctures of lung-supportive herbs on hand can be an effective way to manage symptoms and support lung health during flare-ups.

In summary, herbal teas and tinctures made from lung-supportive herbs like mullein, thyme, licorice root, and eucalyptus offer powerful, natural support for respiratory health. Whether used to maintain lung function during cold and flu season or to provide fast relief during acute respiratory discomfort, these herbal remedies help keep the respiratory system healthy and functioning optimally.

3.3 Foods that Support Lung Health

Diet plays a significant role in maintaining respiratory health. Certain foods, particularly those with anti-inflammatory and antimicrobial properties, are especially effective in supporting lung function and protecting the respiratory system from infections and inflammation. Garlic and onions, two common ingredients in many cuisines, are particularly valuable for their lung-protective benefits.

Garlic is rich in compounds like allicin, which has strong antimicrobial properties. This makes it effective in fighting infections, including those that can affect the respiratory system. Consuming garlic regularly helps to protect the lungs from bacteria and viruses, which can cause illnesses like bronchitis and pneumonia. Additionally, garlic has been shown to reduce inflammation in the lungs, which is crucial for individuals suffering from chronic conditions such as asthma or chronic obstructive pulmonary disease (COPD). By lowering inflammation, garlic helps improve breathing and reduces the risk of respiratory flare-ups.

Onions, like garlic, also contain powerful anti-inflammatory and antimicrobial properties. They are high in sulfur compounds, which not only help fight infections but also support the detoxification process in the lungs. Onions assist the body in expelling toxins, particularly those that accumulate from environmental pollutants like smoke and chemicals. This detoxification process is essential for maintaining lung health in modern environments where air quality is often compromised. Onions can also thin mucus, making it easier for the body to expel it, which is beneficial for clearing the airways and improving breathing.

Another food that Barbara emphasizes for lung health is ginger. Known for its warming properties, ginger is particularly effective in breaking up mucus and clearing the respiratory pathways. When mucus builds up in the lungs, it can create an environment where bacteria and viruses thrive, leading to infections. By reducing mucus buildup, ginger helps prevent these infections and promotes better lung function. Ginger's anti-inflammatory properties also contribute to reducing inflammation in the respiratory system, helping individuals with conditions such as asthma or allergies breathe more easily.

In addition to its ability to reduce mucus, ginger improves circulation throughout the body, including the lungs. Better circulation ensures that the lungs receive a sufficient supply of oxygen and nutrients, which are necessary for optimal function. Incorporating ginger into the diet, whether in teas, soups, or other meals, is a simple and effective way to enhance lung health and support the body's natural defenses against respiratory issues.

Chapter 4: Natural Methods to Combat Infections and Support Long-Term Immune Health

4.1 Steam Inhalations for Congestion

Steam inhalation is one of the most effective natural remedies for clearing the airways and relieving congestion. By inhaling steam, the warmth helps to loosen mucus, making it easier to expel, while the moisture soothes irritated respiratory tissues. Barbara advocates the use of steam inhalation with essential oils such as eucalyptus, peppermint, and thyme for maximum effectiveness.

Eucalyptus oil is particularly well-known for its ability to relieve respiratory issues. Its main active ingredient, eucalyptol, has been shown to have anti-inflammatory, decongestant, and antimicrobial properties. Inhaling eucalyptus-infused steam helps to open up the airways, reduce mucus buildup, and soothe inflamed respiratory tissues. This makes it an excellent remedy for colds, sinus infections, and other respiratory conditions that cause congestion. The antimicrobial properties of eucalyptus also help in fighting off infections, making it not only a treatment for symptoms but also a preventative measure.

Peppermint oil is another powerful essential oil used in steam inhalations for respiratory health. It contains menthol, a compound that provides a cooling sensation and helps to relax the muscles of the respiratory system. This relaxation effect makes breathing easier and can provide relief for individuals experiencing difficulty due to congestion. Peppermint also has antiviral and antibacterial properties, which help to address the underlying infections that may be causing the congestion. When added to steam, peppermint oil works to break up mucus and open the airways, providing quick relief from blocked nasal passages and facilitating better airflow.

Thyme oil is often recommended for its strong antimicrobial properties. It contains compounds like thymol, which have been shown to effectively combat bacteria and viruses that can cause respiratory infections. Thyme oil also acts as an expectorant, helping to loosen and expel mucus from the lungs and airways. When used in steam inhalation, thyme oil not only helps clear congestion but also boosts the body's ability to fight off the infection causing the congestion in the first place. Thyme's anti-inflammatory properties further contribute to reducing swelling in the respiratory system, allowing for easier breathing.

To perform a steam inhalation, Barbara recommends using a bowl of hot water with a few drops of essential oil added to it. By leaning over the bowl, covering the head with a towel, and inhaling deeply, the steam infused with essential oils enters the respiratory system, providing immediate relief from congestion. This simple and natural remedy can be repeated several times a day to ensure that the airways remain clear and breathing improves.

Additionally, steam inhalation can be used as a preventative measure during cold and flu season. Regular use of essential oils like eucalyptus and peppermint in steam treatments helps to keep the respiratory system clear of mucus and supports overall lung health by preventing infections from taking hold.

4.2 Boosting Immunity to Prevent Respiratory Illnesses

Maintaining a strong immune system is crucial in the prevention of respiratory illnesses, especially during the colder months when flu and colds are more prevalent. The body's immune system is its first line of defense against harmful pathogens, and when it is functioning optimally, it can ward off infections before they take hold. Stress, poor diet, and lack of sleep can all compromise immunity, making the body more susceptible to respiratory infections. To strengthen the immune system, it is essential to adopt a holistic approach that includes herbal remedies, dietary changes, and lifestyle modifications.

One of the most effective ways to support the immune system is through the use of herbs. Barbara O'Neill emphasizes the power of herbs such as **echinacea** and **elderberry** in boosting immune function, particularly during cold and flu season. Echinacea is a well-known herb for its immune-enhancing properties. It works by stimulating the production of white blood cells, which are the body's primary defense against infections. When taken as a tincture, tea, or supplement, echinacea is especially beneficial when taken right as cold symptoms are starting. Regular use during flu season can help reduce the severity and duration of respiratory illnesses.

Elderberry, another potent immune-boosting herb, is rich in antioxidants and vitamins that support immune function. It has been traditionally used to treat colds, flu, and other respiratory infections. Elderberry works by preventing viruses from attaching to and entering the body's cells, thereby reducing the likelihood of infection. In addition to its antiviral properties, elderberry is also anti-inflammatory, helping to reduce swelling in the mucous membranes of the respiratory tract, which can alleviate symptoms such as a sore throat and congestion. Elderberry syrup is a popular and convenient form of consumption, especially for children during the winter months.

In addition to echinacea and elderberry, **garlic** is another natural remedy that can help boost the immune system. Garlic has powerful antimicrobial and antiviral properties that make it an effective defense against respiratory infections. It is rich in compounds such as allicin, which helps to boost the immune response and fight off infections. Garlic can be consumed raw, in supplements, or added to food as a preventive measure during cold and flu season.

Dietary changes also play a significant role in strengthening the immune system. Consuming a diet rich in **vitamin C** and **zinc** is essential for supporting immune function. Foods like citrus fruits, bell peppers, broccoli, and spinach are excellent sources of vitamin C, while zinc can be found in nuts, seeds, and legumes. These nutrients are critical for the proper functioning of immune cells and help the body fight off infections more effectively. Additionally, staying hydrated by drinking plenty of water and herbal teas helps to keep the mucous membranes moist, which is important for preventing respiratory infections.

Another important aspect of maintaining a strong immune system is **getting adequate sleep**. The body repairs and regenerates itself during sleep, and the immune system is no exception. Lack of sleep can weaken the immune system, making it less effective at fighting off infections. Ensuring that the body gets at least seven to eight hours of restful sleep each night can significantly improve immune function.

4.3 Breathing Exercises for Lung Health

Breathing is a fundamental function of life, but it is often something that people take for granted until respiratory issues arise. The lungs play a critical role in oxygenating the blood and removing carbon dioxide from the body. When lung function is compromised due to respiratory illnesses or chronic conditions like asthma, it can significantly impact overall health and well-being. Barbara O'Neill emphasizes the importance of **breathing exercises** as a natural way to improve lung capacity and support respiratory health. These exercises not only strengthen the lungs but also promote relaxation, which can help manage stress-related breathing conditions.

One of the key benefits of deep breathing exercises is that they help to **increase lung capacity**. Many people do not use their lungs to their full potential, often taking shallow breaths that only engage the upper part of the lungs. Over time, this can reduce lung efficiency and make the body more susceptible to respiratory issues. Deep breathing exercises, such as diaphragmatic breathing, encourage the use of the diaphragm and the lower parts of the lungs, which helps to improve lung function and oxygen exchange. Practicing deep breathing regularly can enhance lung capacity and make it easier to breathe deeply and efficiently.

In addition to improving lung capacity, breathing exercises can help to **relieve stress and anxiety**, which are often linked to respiratory conditions like asthma. Stress triggers the release of stress hormones like cortisol, which can lead to tightness in the chest and difficulty breathing. For individuals with asthma or other stress-related breathing issues, this can exacerbate symptoms and make it harder to manage flare-ups. Deep breathing exercises activate the parasympathetic nervous system, which promotes relaxation and helps to counteract the body's stress response. By practicing breathing exercises regularly, individuals can reduce stress and improve their ability to manage asthma symptoms.

The 4-7-8 breathing technique is a basic and efficient breathing exercise that entails four counts of inhalation, seven counts of holding the breath, and eight counts of leisurely exhalation. This technique helps to calm the nervous system and can be particularly useful during times of stress or anxiety. Another beneficial exercise is **alternate nostril breathing**, which is commonly used in yoga and meditation practices. Using this method, you close one nostril and inhale through the other, then swap your nostrils to exhale. It helps to balance the body's energy and can promote a sense of calm and relaxation, making it ideal for individuals dealing with respiratory issues.

For individuals with chronic respiratory conditions like **asthma**, regular practice of breathing exercises can help improve lung function and reduce the severity of symptoms. In addition to the physical benefits, the mental relaxation that comes from deep breathing can make it easier to cope with the stress that often accompanies chronic illness. Simple breathing exercises, when practiced consistently, can make a significant difference in overall lung health and quality of life.

Finally, maintaining an environment that supports lung health is equally important. Reducing exposure to **pollutants**, such as tobacco smoke, dust, and chemicals, can prevent further damage to the lungs. Keeping indoor air clean by using air purifiers and ventilating the home properly is also essential

Chapter 5: 12 Natural Remedies for Respiratory Health

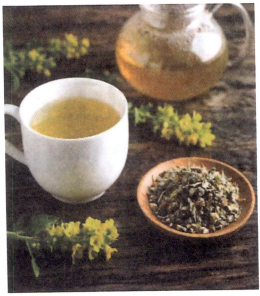

The appendix provides more details for each remedy.

1. Mullein Tea

2. Eucalyptus Steam Inhalation

3. Licorice Root Tincture

4. Thyme

5. Garlic Syrup

6. Onion Poultice

7. Peppermint Oil Steam

8. Elderberry Syrup

9. Ginger Tea

10. Cayenne Pepper and Honey Cough Syrup

11. Hot Lemon and Honey Drink

12. Marshmallow Root Tea

Part 16:
Gut Health and
Digestive Wellness

Chapter 1: Maintaining a Healthy Digestive System

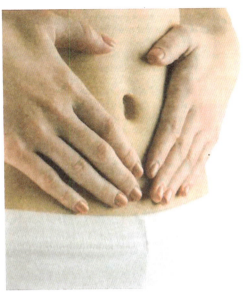

The Importance of Gut Health in Overall Wellness

Gut health is fundamental to overall wellness, as the digestive system plays a crucial role not only in nutrient absorption but also in maintaining the immune system and preventing inflammation. The gut, often referred to as the body's "second brain," is home to trillions of microorganisms, including bacteria, yeast, and fungi, that collectively make up the gut flora. When in balance, these microorganisms support digestion, protect the body from harmful pathogens, and promote overall health. However, when the balance is disrupted, it can lead to a wide range of health issues, from digestive problems to more systemic conditions such as autoimmune disorders and skin problems.

The Role of the Gut in Nutrient Absorption and Immunity

The digestive system is responsible for breaking down the food we eat and extracting the nutrients needed for energy, repair, and growth. A healthy gut lining allows for the efficient absorption of these nutrients, ensuring that the body gets what it needs to function properly. Without proper nutrient absorption, deficiencies can develop, which may lead to a weakened immune system and a variety of other health issues.

One of the most critical aspects of gut health is its connection to the immune system. The gut is home to a significant portion of the body's immune cells, and the health of the gut lining determines how well these cells can function. When the gut is in good condition, it acts as a barrier, preventing harmful substances like pathogens and toxins from entering the bloodstream. Additionally, the beneficial bacteria in the gut help train the immune system, teaching it to recognize and fight off harmful invaders while tolerating harmless substances, such as food and environmental particles. This balance is essential in reducing inflammation and preventing autoimmune responses, where the immune system mistakenly attacks the body's own tissues.

Inflammation is a natural response of the immune system to injury or infection. However, chronic inflammation, which can result from poor gut health, is linked to a variety of chronic diseases, including heart disease, diabetes, and autoimmune disorders. The digestive system's role in regulating inflammation highlights the importance of maintaining gut health as part of an overall strategy for disease prevention.

Gut Health and Chronic Conditions

When the gut microbiome is out of balance, it can lead to a host of health problems beyond digestive discomfort. Skin issues, such as acne, eczema, and psoriasis, are often linked to poor gut health. The connection between the gut and the skin, sometimes referred to as the "gut-skin axis," highlights how an unhealthy gut can manifest in external symptoms. For example, a leaky gut can allow inflammatory substances to enter the bloodstream, which can exacerbate skin conditions and cause flare-ups.

Autoimmune disorders, in which the immune system attacks the body's own cells, are also closely connected to gut health. Research suggests that a damaged gut lining and an imbalanced microbiome can trigger autoimmune reactions by allowing foreign substances to enter the bloodstream and stimulate the immune system. When this happens repeatedly, it can lead to chronic inflammation and contribute to the development of autoimmune diseases such as rheumatoid arthritis, lupus, and multiple sclerosis.

Digestive disorders, including IBS and IBD, are perhaps the most direct consequences of poor gut health. These conditions are often associated with dysbiosis and chronic inflammation in the gut. Managing gut health through dietary changes, stress reduction, and the use of probiotics can be an effective strategy for alleviating symptoms and improving overall digestive function.

Chapter 2: Herbal Remedies for Digestive Issues

2.1 Peppermint for Soothing the Digestive Tract

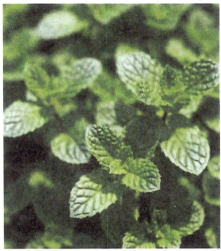

Peppermint is widely recognized for its ability to soothe the digestive system, and it has been used as a natural remedy for centuries to address a range of GI issues. Barbara O'Neill recommends peppermint as an effective treatment for individuals suffering from IBS, bloating, or cramping, noting that it works by relaxing the muscles of the GI tract. This relaxing effect helps to ease discomfort associated with digestive distress.

Peppermint contains menthol, which has antispasmodic properties. These properties allow peppermint to calm the muscles in the intestines, reducing cramping and promoting smoother digestion. For individuals with IBS, peppermint can help alleviate symptoms by preventing spasms in the colon that cause pain and discomfort. By relaxing the muscles, it helps to reduce the frequency of painful episodes, allowing for better digestion and a reduction in bloating.

One of the simplest ways to incorporate peppermint into a daily routine is through peppermint tea. Drinking peppermint tea after meals can help stimulate digestion and prevent bloating or gas that may result from improper digestion. For those who prefer a more concentrated form, peppermint essential oil capsules are another option. These capsules are particularly effective for IBS as they release peppermint oil directly into the GI tract, where it can have a direct soothing effect on the muscles.

Peppermint is also useful for alleviating the discomfort associated with indigestion. It can help reduce feelings of fullness and bloating that occur after meals by improving the flow of bile, which is essential for digesting fats. This increase in bile flow helps the body break down food more efficiently, preventing indigestion and reducing the buildup of gas in the intestines. Whether consumed as tea, capsules, or even inhaled through steam, peppermint is a versatile remedy for maintaining digestive health.

While peppermint is highly effective, it is important to use it appropriately. Peppermint may relax the lower esophageal sphincter in certain people, particularly those who have gastroesophageal reflux disease (GERD), which could exacerbate symptoms by allowing stomach acid to reflux back up into the esophagus. Therefore, individuals with GERD should consult with a healthcare provider before using peppermint in large amounts.

2.2 Fennel for Reducing Bloating and Gas

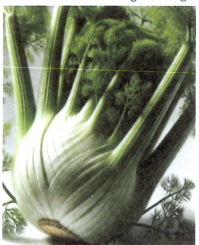

Fennel is another powerful herb frequently suggested for digestive wellness. Known for its ability to relieve gas, bloating, and indigestion, fennel has been used for centuries as a natural digestive aid. The seeds, in particular, contain compounds that help to relax the muscles of the digestive tract and reduce the buildup of gas, making it an ideal remedy for individuals who experience bloating or discomfort after eating.

Fennel works by stimulating the production of gastric enzymes, which are essential for breaking down food. When these enzymes are produced in sufficient quantities, digestion becomes more efficient, and the likelihood of bloating or gas is reduced. Barbara often points out that poor digestion can lead to the fermentation of food in the intestines, which in turn causes gas to build up. By supporting proper digestion, fennel helps to prevent this process, reducing both gas and bloating.

Fennel can be consumed in several forms to aid digestion. One of the most common methods is to chew fennel seeds after meals. This simple practice helps stimulate the digestive system and reduce the risk of bloating or gas. Fennel seeds can also be used to make a soothing tea. Drinking fennel tea after meals is particularly effective for those who experience regular bloating or indigestion, as it promotes smoother digestion and helps relieve discomfort in the abdomen.

The anti-inflammatory properties of fennel make it useful for individuals suffering from indigestion related to inflammation in the digestive tract. In addition to reducing gas and bloating, fennel can soothe the lining of the intestines, helping to alleviate symptoms of indigestion or discomfort. For individuals dealing with chronic digestive issues, fennel provides a gentle yet effective solution that can be incorporated into daily routines without causing side effects.

In addition to its benefits for digestion, fennel is also recognized for its ability to promote overall gut health. It helps maintain a healthy balance of gut flora, which is essential for efficient digestion and overall wellness. By supporting the microbiome, fennel can help prevent digestive issues from becoming chronic and maintain a healthy digestive system over time.

For those who prefer a more potent form of fennel, fennel essential oil can be used. A few drops of fennel oil can be added to water and consumed after meals to relieve bloating and discomfort. The oil works similarly to fennel seeds, promoting digestion and easing the tension in the digestive muscles. However, it is important to use fennel essential oil in moderation, as it is highly concentrated.

Fennel is a versatile and powerful remedy for digestive health, offering relief from bloating, gas, and indigestion. Whether consumed as seeds, tea, or essential oil, it provides a natural and effective way to support the digestive system and promote smoother, more comfortable digestion. Incorporating fennel into a daily routine is a simple yet impactful way to improve digestive wellness and maintain a balanced gut.

2.3 Chamomile for Calming the Stomach

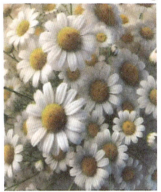

Chamomile is one of the most widely recognized herbs for calming the digestive system, particularly effective in reducing inflammation and soothing the lining of the stomach. Chamomile works by reducing the irritation and inflammation that often accompany digestive issues like gastritis or acid reflux. This herb contains anti-inflammatory properties that help ease discomfort in the stomach lining, allowing it to heal more effectively. It's especially useful for people who experience bloating, cramping, or indigestion after meals. Chamomile's calming effect on the stomach is often attributed to its ability to relax the muscles in the digestive tract, thereby improving overall digestion.

In addition to its direct effects on the stomach, chamomile also helps in reducing stress and anxiety, which are often linked to digestive problems. By calming the nervous system, chamomile indirectly supports the digestive system, as stress and anxiety can exacerbate conditions such as acid reflux and gastritis. Drinking chamomile tea, particularly before bed, not only aids in digestion but also promotes relaxation and better sleep, which are crucial for the body's healing processes.

Chapter 3: Foods and Supplements to Support Gut Health

3.1 Probiotic-Rich Foods for a Healthy Microbiome

Fermented foods are some of the best sources of probiotics. Yogurt, for example, contains live cultures that help replenish beneficial bacteria in the gut. Choosing a high-quality yogurt that is unsweetened and made from organic milk ensures that you're getting the most health benefits without added sugars, which can disrupt the gut flora. Kefir, a fermented milk drink, is another excellent source of probiotics. It contains a wider variety of bacterial strains than yogurt, making it particularly beneficial for gut health. Kefir is also easier to digest than regular milk, making it suitable for people who are lactose intolerant.

Other probiotic-rich foods include sauerkraut, kimchi, and kombucha. Sauerkraut, a fermented cabbage dish, is rich in beneficial bacteria like lactobacillus, which can help improve digestion and reduce bloating. Kimchi, a traditional Korean fermented vegetable dish, not only contains probiotics but is also high in fiber, which supports regular bowel movements and overall gut function. Kombucha, a fermented tea, is another excellent source of probiotics and enzymes that aid in digestion. Drinking kombucha regularly can help balance the gut microbiome and promote better digestive health.

The timing of taking probiotics is also important. Probiotics are most effective when taken with or after meals, as food helps protect the live bacteria as they pass through the digestive system. Consistent use of probiotic supplements, especially after antibiotic use or during periods of digestive distress, can significantly improve gut health and prevent further complications.

In addition to fermented foods and probiotics, other dietary changes can support gut health. Consuming prebiotic-rich foods, such as garlic, onions, bananas, and asparagus, provides nourishment for the beneficial bacteria in the gut, helping them thrive. Prebiotics are indispensible components of a diet that supports gut health since they are non-digestible fibers that serve as food for probiotics. By incorporating both probiotics and prebiotics into your diet, you can create an environment in the gut that supports a diverse and healthy microbiome.

3.2 The Role of Fiber in Digestive Health

Fiber plays a vital role in maintaining a healthy digestive system. It is essential for the efficient movement of food through the digestive tract, supporting regular bowel movements and preventing constipation. Dietary fiber comes in two forms: soluble and insoluble, both of which are necessary for optimal digestive health. Soluble fiber dissolves in water and forms a gel-like substance, which can help to slow digestion and promote the absorption of nutrients. Insoluble fiber, on the other hand, adds bulk to the stool and facilitates the movement of food through the intestines, helping to prevent blockages and promoting regularity.

Fruits, vegetables, whole grains, and legumes are rich sources of dietary fiber. These foods not only contribute to the bulk of the stool but also support the health of the gut microbiome. Fiber serves as a food source for beneficial bacteria in the gut, encouraging their growth and activity. A healthy balance of gut bacteria is crucial for digestive health, as these microorganisms play a key role in breaking down food, synthesizing vitamins, and protecting the body from harmful pathogens. Without sufficient fiber in the diet, the beneficial bacteria in the gut may decline, leading to digestive issues such as bloating, gas, and irregular bowel movements.

3.3 Digestive Enzymes for Better Nutrient Absorption

Digestive enzymes are essential for breaking down food into the nutrients the body needs to function properly. Each type of enzyme has a specific role in the digestion of different macronutrients: proteases break down proteins, amylases break down carbohydrates, and lipases break down fats. Without sufficient enzyme activity, food cannot be fully digested, leading to malabsorption and digestive discomfort. Incomplete digestion can result in symptoms such as bloating, gas, and nutrient deficiencies, as the body is unable to absorb essential vitamins and minerals from food.

Some individuals may suffer from enzyme deficiencies, which can impair digestion and nutrient absorption. Factors such as aging, chronic stress, and certain medical conditions can reduce the body's ability to produce digestive enzymes. To address this, Barbara recommends the use of natural digestive enzymes, such as bromelain and papain, which are derived from pineapple and papaya, respectively. These enzymes can help to improve digestion and alleviate the symptoms of enzyme deficiencies.

Bromelain, found in pineapple, is a powerful proteolytic enzyme, meaning it helps to break down proteins into smaller peptides and amino acids. This makes bromelain particularly useful for individuals who experience difficulty digesting protein-rich foods, such as meat, dairy, and legumes. Bromelain has also been shown to have anti-inflammatory properties, which can further benefit individuals with digestive disorders that involve inflammation of the gut lining, such as gastritis or IBD.

Papain, an enzyme found in papaya, also aids in protein digestion and is known for its ability to break down tough protein fibers. In addition to promoting protein digestion, papain may help to reduce symptoms of bloating and indigestion after meals. Like bromelain, papain can be consumed through fresh papaya or taken in supplement form to support digestion, particularly for individuals with low stomach acid or enzyme deficiencies.

Both bromelain and papain can be integrated into the diet through the consumption of fresh pineapple and papaya, or they can be taken as supplements to boost enzyme activity. For individuals who struggle with chronic digestive issues, supplementing with these enzymes can significantly improve nutrient absorption and alleviate discomfort after meals. By supporting the natural digestive process, these enzymes help to ensure that the body receives the full range of nutrients from the food consumed, leading to better overall health and well-being.

Chapter 4: Recipes to Promote Gut Health and Ease Digestion

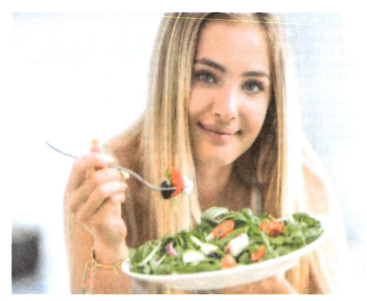

4.1 Simple, Gut-Friendly Meals

For individuals dealing with digestive issues, finding meals that are gentle on the gut while still providing essential nutrients is crucial. Barbara O'Neill emphasizes the importance of consuming simple, nutrient-dense meals that promote gut healing without causing irritation. These meals focus on ingredients that soothe the digestive system, support the repair of the gut lining, and provide the body with the necessary nutrients to facilitate healing.

Bone Broth Soup for Gut Health

One of the most recommended meals is **bone broth soup**, which is known for its gut-healing properties. Bone broth is rich in collagen and gelatin, two key components that help to repair and strengthen the gut lining. Collagen, in particular, provides the amino acids necessary for the regeneration of the intestinal walls, while gelatin works as a protective barrier within the gut, preventing the leakage of undigested food particles and toxins into the bloodstream. This is especially important for those suffering from leaky gut syndrome, a condition where the gut lining becomes permeable, allowing harmful substances to pass through.

Bone broth is also easy to digest, making it an ideal option for those with compromised digestive systems. It is packed with nutrients like glutamine, glycine, and proline, which not only support gut health but also reduce inflammation throughout the body. Incorporating bone broth into the diet regularly can significantly improve digestion and promote healing for individuals suffering from chronic digestive disorders.

Light, Nutrient-Dense Meals

Aside from bone broth, light, easily digestible meals play a key role in supporting digestive health. Meals that are low in fats and sugars but rich in essential vitamins and minerals are highly beneficial. For example, a simple meal of **steamed vegetables** accompanied by **quinoa or brown rice** provides fiber, vitamins, and minerals without overwhelming the digestive system. The fiber in vegetables helps to maintain healthy bowel movements, while quinoa and brown rice offer a gentle source of energy that doesn't irritate the gut.

O'Neill also suggests **smoothies** made with gut-friendly ingredients like leafy greens, berries, and a plant-based protein source. These smoothies are nutrient-dense but light on the stomach, making them ideal for individuals with sensitive digestion. They provide antioxidants, vitamins, and fiber in a form that is easy for the body to absorb, while also helping to balance gut flora. Adding ingredients like chia seeds or flaxseeds can enhance the fiber content, further supporting digestive health.

Incorporating Fermented Foods

Another component of a gut-friendly diet is **fermented foods**, which are rich in probiotics. These beneficial bacteria help to balance the gut microbiome, which plays a crucial role in digestive health. Probiotic-rich foods like **sauerkraut, kimchi,** and **kefir** introduce live cultures into the gut, aiding in digestion and enhancing the body's ability to absorb nutrients. Additionally, eating foods that have undergone fermentation aids in the creation of digestive enzymes, which speed up the breakdown of food and lessen the chance of bloating and discomfort.

For individuals with more severe digestive disorders, fermented foods can be particularly helpful in restoring balance to the gut flora. By improving the diversity of beneficial bacteria in the gut, these foods help to combat issues like inflammation, constipation, and diarrhea. It is important, however, to introduce fermented foods slowly into the diet, especially for those who have never consumed them before, to avoid overwhelming the system.

Soothing Herbal Teas

To complement gut-friendly meals, **herbal teas** such as **ginger, peppermint,** and **chamomile** can be used to soothe the digestive system. These teas have anti-inflammatory properties that calm the gut lining and reduce bloating and discomfort. Ginger, in particular, has been shown to improve digestion by stimulating digestive enzymes, while peppermint helps to relax the muscles of the GI tract, easing symptoms of indigestion and gas.

Herbal teas are a gentle yet effective way to support digestion, especially when consumed alongside meals. They promote the production of stomach acid and bile, which are essential for breaking down food efficiently, and they also help to prevent the buildup of gas and bloating that can result from poor digestion.

Incorporating these simple, gut-friendly meals and remedies into a daily routine can have profound effects on digestive health. By focusing on nutrient-dense, easily digestible foods, individuals can support their gut's healing process and alleviate many of the symptoms associated with digestive disorders.

4.2 Fermented Foods for Gut Healing

Fermented foods play a vital role in supporting digestive health, as they are rich in probiotics that help restore balance to the gut microbiome. Probiotics are beneficial bacteria that contribute to a healthy digestive system, and fermented foods like sauerkraut, kimchi, and kefir are excellent natural sources of these microorganisms. The inclusion of these foods in daily meals supports gut healing and enhances overall digestive function.

Sauerkraut and Gut Health

Sauerkraut, a fermented cabbage product, is one of the most powerful probiotic-rich foods. It contains a variety of beneficial bacteria, including *Lactobacillus*, which supports the digestive system by aiding the breakdown of food and the absorption of nutrients. Sauerkraut helps maintain a healthy balance of bacteria in the gut, which is essential for preventing the overgrowth of harmful microorganisms such as *Candida albicans*.

Barbara O'Neill recommends incorporating small amounts of sauerkraut into daily meals to promote digestive health. Its fermentation process not only produces probiotics but also increases the bioavailability of vitamins and minerals in cabbage, such as vitamin C and vitamin K. These nutrients contribute to gut repair and overall wellness. Regular consumption of sauerkraut can also reduce inflammation in the digestive tract, which is often linked to conditions like IBS and other GI disorders.

Kimchi for Digestive Wellness

Kimchi, a traditional Korean fermented vegetable dish, is another staple in promoting gut health. Like sauerkraut, kimchi is rich in probiotics that enhance the diversity of the gut microbiome. The presence of beneficial bacteria such as *Lactobacillus plantarum* aids in digestion and supports immune function. Kimchi is known for its anti-inflammatory properties, making it an effective food for reducing inflammation in the gut and supporting the healing of the intestinal lining.

In addition to probiotics, kimchi provides a variety of vitamins, including vitamin A and vitamin C, which play a crucial role in maintaining the health of the gut lining. The fermentation process also produces short-chain fatty acids (SCFAs) that nourish the cells of the intestinal lining, helping to maintain the integrity of the gut barrier. This makes kimchi an ideal addition to a diet focused on healing the digestive system and restoring microbial balance.

Kefir and Microbiome Restoration

Kefir, a fermented milk drink, is one of the most potent sources of probiotics available. It contains a wide range of beneficial bacteria and yeasts, which work together to support the health of the gut microbiome. Kefir's unique composition allows it to colonize the digestive tract more effectively than other fermented foods, helping to re-establish a healthy balance of microorganisms.

Kefir is particularly effective in restoring gut flora after antibiotic use, which can disrupt the balance of bacteria in the gut. The probiotics found in kefir help to repopulate the gut with beneficial bacteria, preventing the overgrowth of harmful pathogens. Additionally, kefir contains bioactive compounds that aid in digestion and improve the overall function of the GI system.

Regular consumption of kefir also promotes the production of digestive enzymes, which help break down food more efficiently, reducing symptoms of indigestion and bloating. This fermented drink is an excellent choice for anyone looking to improve gut health and support the body's natural digestive processes.

Incorporating Fermented Foods into Daily Meals

Incorporating fermented foods like sauerkraut, kimchi, and kefir into daily meals is a simple yet effective way to promote digestive wellness. By bringing good bacteria into the stomach, these meals promote gut health by keeping the microbiome in balance. Even small servings of these probiotic-rich foods can have a significant impact on the digestive system, aiding in nutrient absorption, reducing inflammation, and enhancing the body's natural ability to heal the gut.

Chapter 5: 12 Natural Remedies and Recipes for Digestive Health

The appendix provides more details for each remedy.

1. Peppermint Tea
2. Fennel Seed Chew
3. Chamomile Tea
4. Bone Broth Soup
5. Sauerkraut
6. Kefir Smoothie
7. Ginger Tea
8. Apple Cider Vinegar Tonic
9. Psyllium Husk Drink
10. Papaya Salad
11. Flaxseed Pudding
12. Golden Milk

Part 17:
Cognitive Health and Mental Clarity

Chapter 1: Supporting Cognitive Health Naturally

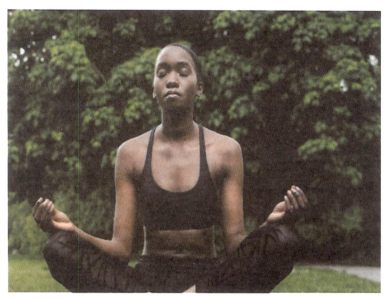

1.1 The Importance of Brain Health for Overall Wellbeing

The brain is often referred to as the command center of the body, controlling not only cognitive processes but also the regulation of essential bodily functions. According to Barbara O'Neill, the health of the brain is integral to overall well-being, as it governs everything from mental clarity to emotional balance and physical coordination. When the brain functions optimally, the entire body benefits. Conversely, when cognitive health deteriorates, it can manifest in both mental and physical symptoms that impact quality of life.

Cognitive Health and Quality of Life

Cognitive health directly influences the way individuals experience life. Memory, focus, and the ability to process information are all tied to how well the brain is functioning. When these abilities begin to decline, it is often a sign that something is out of balance in the body. Barbara O'Neill highlights that mental fog, memory loss, and difficulty focusing are not just inevitable signs of aging but can often indicate underlying health issues that need to be addressed.

When the brain is not functioning at its best, daily tasks can feel overwhelming, and decision-making becomes more difficult. This decline in cognitive function can lead to frustration, anxiety, and a diminished sense of well-being. By addressing the root causes of these cognitive impairments, it is possible to improve both mental clarity and quality of life.

Poor Diet and Brain Health

Diet plays a pivotal role in maintaining brain health. Barbara O'Neill explains that when the brain does not receive the necessary nutrients, it cannot function optimally. A diet high in processed foods, sugars, and unhealthy fats deprives the brain of the essential building blocks it needs for proper cognitive function. This type of diet can lead to inflammation, which impairs brain function and contributes to mental fog and memory issues.

In contrast, a nutrient-dense diet that includes whole foods, healthy fats, and a variety of vitamins and minerals can significantly improve brain health. Omega-3 fatty acids, in particular, are crucial for maintaining the health of brain cells. Foods rich in antioxidants, such as berries and leafy greens, help protect the brain from oxidative stress, which can damage cells and contribute to cognitive decline.

Toxicity and Its Impact on Cognitive Function

Exposure to environmental toxins is another significant factor that affects brain health. Toxins such as heavy metals, chemicals, and pollutants can accumulate in the body over time, burdening the detoxification pathways and affecting the brain's ability to function properly. Barbara O'Neill often discusses the importance of supporting the body's natural detoxification processes to prevent these toxins from interfering with cognitive health.

When the body is overloaded with toxins, it can lead to neurological symptoms such as brain fog, memory loss, and difficulty concentrating. This is because toxins disrupt neurotransmitter activity and can even damage the delicate structures of the brain. By reducing exposure to harmful substances and supporting the liver and kidneys in their detoxification roles, it is possible to alleviate some of the cognitive impairments caused by toxicity.

1.2 Inflammation and the Brain

Chronic inflammation is a key contributor to cognitive decline and the development of neurodegenerative diseases such as Alzheimer's and dementia. Inflammation in the brain can disrupt normal neurological functions, leading to issues with memory, concentration, and overall mental clarity. Several factors can trigger this inflammatory response, including poor dietary habits, exposure to environmental toxins, and chronic stress.

The Role of Diet in Brain Inflammation

Diet is one of the most significant contributors to inflammation in the brain. A diet high in processed foods, refined sugars, and unhealthy fats can lead to an overproduction of pro-inflammatory compounds in the body. These compounds, known as cytokines, travel through the bloodstream and can reach the brain, where they disrupt normal neurological activity and contribute to cognitive dysfunction.

On the other hand, adopting an anti-inflammatory diet can help reduce the risk of brain inflammation and protect cognitive health. Foods rich in omega-3 fatty acids, such as flaxseeds, chia seeds, and walnuts, are known for their anti-inflammatory properties and their ability to support brain function. Additionally, consuming antioxidant-rich fruits and vegetables helps to neutralize free radicals that contribute to inflammation.

The Impact of Toxins on Brain Inflammation

Exposure to environmental toxins is another significant factor that can trigger inflammation in the brain. Toxins such as heavy metals, pesticides, and industrial chemicals can accumulate in the body over time, leading to a toxic burden that overwhelms the body's natural detoxification processes. When these toxins reach the brain, they can cause oxidative stress and inflammation, which may contribute to cognitive decline and the development of neurodegenerative diseases.

Stress and Its Role in Brain Inflammation

Chronic stress is one of the most overlooked causes of brain inflammation. When the body is under constant stress, it produces excess cortisol, a hormone that, in large amounts, can trigger inflammation in both the body and the brain. Over time, elevated cortisol levels can lead to impaired cognitive function, memory problems, and an increased risk of developing neurodegenerative conditions like Alzheimer's.

Chapter 2: Herbs and Supplements to Enhance Memory and Focus

2.1 Ginkgo Biloba for Memory Support

Ginkgo biloba is one of the most well-known natural remedies for supporting cognitive function, particularly in relation to memory and concentration. This herb has been widely used for centuries in traditional medicine, and it remains popular due to its proven ability to enhance mental clarity and prevent cognitive decline. Ginkgo biloba works primarily by increasing blood circulation to the brain, ensuring that brain cells receive the oxygen and nutrients they need to function optimally.

Enhanced circulation to the brain is critical for maintaining cognitive performance, particularly as individuals age. As blood flow to the brain decreases, memory retention, focus, and overall cognitive sharpness can begin to decline. Ginkgo biloba helps counteract these effects by improving the delivery of oxygen to brain cells. This increased circulation allows the brain to remain alert and function at its best, even in older adults or those facing cognitive challenges.

For individuals who experience occasional lapses in concentration or memory, ginkgo biloba offers a natural way to boost mental alertness. Whether taken as a tea or in supplement form, this herb is known to help improve cognitive function, making it easier to concentrate on tasks and retain information over the long term. It can be particularly beneficial for those who are starting to notice age-related memory decline, as ginkgo biloba has been shown to support both short-term and long-term memory.

Ginkgo's effects are not limited to memory support. Its ability to improve mental clarity makes it a valuable tool for anyone looking to sharpen their focus, reduce brain fog, or enhance their cognitive performance throughout the day. Additionally, by promoting better blood flow to the brain, ginkgo biloba may help protect against certain neurodegenerative conditions that can impair cognitive abilities over time.

Regular consumption of ginkgo biloba, whether in tea or supplement form, is an effective strategy for supporting brain health. When used consistently, it can help maintain sharp mental faculties, improve concentration, and prevent the natural memory decline that often accompanies aging.

2.2 Omega-3 Fatty Acids for Brain Health

Omega-3 fatty acids are another crucial component of maintaining a healthy brain. These essential fats play a vital role in brain function and structure, and they are well known for promoting cognitive health across all stages of life. Omega-3s, particularly those found in flaxseed and fish oil, are important for supporting the brain's ability to adapt, form new neural connections, and remain flexible—a concept known as neuroplasticity.

The brain is composed largely of fat, and omega-3s are a key component of the membranes that surround brain cells. This makes these fats essential for the proper functioning of neurons, which rely on healthy membranes to send and receive signals efficiently. By maintaining the integrity of these cell membranes, omega-3 fatty acids ensure that brain cells can communicate effectively, which is critical for memory retention, learning, and overall cognitive function.

In addition to supporting the brain's structure, omega-3 fatty acids have potent anti-inflammatory properties that protect the brain from damage. Inflammation is a major contributor to cognitive decline and neurodegenerative conditions, and reducing inflammation is a key strategy for preserving brain health. Omega-3s help reduce chronic inflammation in the brain, which can protect against the gradual loss of cognitive function that often occurs with age. By lowering inflammation, omega-3s may also help prevent more serious conditions such as Alzheimer's disease and other forms of dementia.

Barbara highlights the importance of consuming omega-3-rich foods, such as flaxseeds, walnuts, and chia seeds, on a regular basis to support brain health. These foods are particularly rich in alpha-linolenic acid (ALA), a plant-based omega-3 that the body can convert into the more active forms of omega-3: eicosapentaenoic acid (EPA) and docosahexaenoic acid (DHA). DHA, in particular, is highly concentrated in the brain and is critical for maintaining the health of neural cells.

For those looking to ensure they are getting enough omega-3s, supplements such as fish oil or algae-based omega-3 supplements are also effective options. These supplements provide a direct source of EPA and DHA, the two forms of omega-3 that are most readily used by the brain. Regular consumption of these supplements can help ensure that the brain receives the omega-3s it needs to stay healthy and function optimally.

Omega-3s not only support brain health in the long term but also have immediate benefits for cognitive performance. Studies have shown that individuals who regularly consume omega-3s tend to have better memory, improved focus, and greater mental clarity. These fats are also essential for emotional health, as they play a role in regulating mood and reducing the risk of depression and anxiety, which are closely linked to brain health.

2.3 Rosemary for Mental Clarity

Rosemary is known for its powerful effects on mental clarity and focus. It has been used for centuries as a natural remedy to enhance memory and concentration. In her teachings, Barbara O'Neill includes rosemary as one of the most effective herbs for boosting mental performance. She explains that inhaling the aroma of rosemary, or using rosemary essential oil, can stimulate the brain and improve cognitive function. This stimulation occurs because the active compounds in rosemary, such as cineole, are able to interact with receptors in the brain, enhancing alertness and memory retention.

One of the simplest ways to benefit from rosemary's cognitive-enhancing properties is through aromatherapy. By inhaling the scent of rosemary oil, whether through direct application or using a diffuser, individuals can experience an immediate boost in focus and concentration. The aroma stimulates brain activity and increases blood flow to the brain, which can lead to improved mental performance, particularly in tasks requiring memory and sustained attention. This makes rosemary a popular choice for students or anyone needing to improve their cognitive performance under pressure.

Beyond its aromatic properties, rosemary can be consumed as part of the diet to support cognitive health. O'Neill highlights that rosemary tea is a gentle and effective way to incorporate the herb into daily routines. To prepare rosemary tea, a small amount of dried rosemary leaves can be steeped in hot water for several minutes. Drinking this tea regularly helps to support mental clarity and protect brain health over time. The antioxidants found in rosemary work to neutralize free radicals that can damage brain cells, further promoting long-term cognitive well-being.

In addition to using rosemary as a tea, it can be easily integrated into cooking. Fresh or dried rosemary can be added to a variety of dishes, including roasted vegetables, soups, and marinades, offering both flavor and health benefits. The herb's rich antioxidant content makes it particularly useful for protecting brain cells from oxidative stress, which is a key contributor to cognitive decline. Incorporating rosemary into meals on a regular basis can provide ongoing support for memory, focus, and overall brain health.

Chapter 3: Diet and Lifestyle Tips for Maintaining Cognitive Function

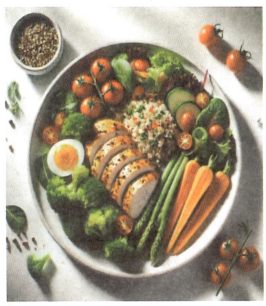

3.1 Antioxidant-Rich Foods for Brain Protection

Oxidative stress is one of the leading causes of cognitive decline and neurodegenerative diseases. Over time, the accumulation of free radicals can damage neurons, leading to issues such as memory loss and impaired cognitive function. Barbara O'Neill emphasizes the importance of including antioxidant-rich foods in the diet to protect the brain from this type of damage. Free radicals are neutralized by antioxidants, which lowers oxidative stress and improves the health of brain cells.

Berries, such as blueberries, strawberries, and raspberries, are particularly potent sources of antioxidants. These fruits contain high levels of flavonoids, which have been shown to protect neurons from oxidative damage and improve cognitive function. Regular consumption of berries is associated with slower rates of cognitive decline and a reduced risk of developing neurodegenerative diseases like Alzheimer's. Adding a variety of berries to the diet, whether in smoothies, salads, or as a snack, provides powerful protection for the brain.

Leafy greens are another essential component of an antioxidant-rich diet. Vegetables such as spinach, kale, and Swiss chard are packed with vitamins and minerals that support brain health, including vitamins C and E. These nutrients help protect the brain from oxidative stress and inflammation, which are both contributing factors to cognitive decline. Leafy greens also provide a range of phytonutrients that promote overall brain function and longevity. Incorporating leafy greens into meals, whether through salads, stir-fries, or green smoothies, offers significant benefits for cognitive protection.

Nuts, particularly walnuts, are another important source of antioxidants that support brain health. Walnuts are rich in vitamin E and omega-3 fatty acids, both of which play a crucial role in maintaining the integrity of brain cells. Studies have shown that individuals who regularly consume nuts have better cognitive function and a lower risk of developing neurodegenerative diseases. Adding a small handful of nuts to daily meals, whether as a snack or sprinkled over salads and yogurt, can provide ongoing protection against cognitive decline.

In addition to these specific foods, other antioxidant-rich options such as dark chocolate, green tea, and brightly colored vegetables like bell peppers and carrots can further enhance the brain's defenses against oxidative damage. The key is to maintain a varied diet that includes a wide range of antioxidant-rich foods. By doing so, individuals can reduce their risk of memory loss and cognitive decline, while also supporting overall brain health.

3.2 Hydration and Brain Function

Dehydration is a common yet often overlooked cause of cognitive issues such as brain fog, poor concentration, and mental fatigue. When the body lacks sufficient water, its ability to carry out essential functions, including those related to the brain, becomes impaired. The brain is made up of approximately 75% water, and even slight dehydration can have significant effects on cognitive performance. Staying hydrated is critical to maintaining optimal brain function.

Water plays a fundamental role in ensuring that nutrients are delivered to brain cells and waste products are removed. Without adequate hydration, the brain's energy levels decrease, which leads to fatigue and a reduced ability to focus. Cognitive functions such as memory, attention, and reasoning are also directly affected when the body does not have enough water. Studies have shown that dehydration as mild as 1-2% can significantly impair cognitive performance, particularly in tasks that require concentration and short-term memory.

In her teachings, Barbara O'Neill stresses the importance of drinking water consistently throughout the day to prevent dehydration and maintain mental clarity. She often emphasizes that many people mistake thirst for hunger, leading to overeating when their bodies are actually craving water. By ensuring that hydration is a priority, individuals can avoid these cognitive pitfalls and keep their minds sharp.

In addition to drinking water, O'Neill highlights the importance of consuming water-rich foods, such as fruits and vegetables, to further support hydration. Foods like cucumbers, watermelons, and oranges not only provide hydration but also deliver essential vitamins and minerals that aid in cognitive function. This approach to hydration not only ensures that the brain stays properly hydrated but also provides the added benefit of delivering vital nutrients that support overall brain health.

Hydration also impacts the body's ability to manage stress. When the body is dehydrated, the production of stress hormones like cortisol increases. These elevated cortisol levels further exacerbate cognitive problems, as high stress levels are known to impair focus and mental clarity. By staying hydrated, individuals can help regulate cortisol levels, thus reducing the mental fatigue and fog associated with chronic stress.

Another key point to consider is how hydration impacts blood flow to the brain. Water helps to maintain proper blood viscosity, ensuring that oxygen and nutrients are efficiently transported to brain cells. When dehydration occurs, blood becomes thicker and less efficient at delivering these essential elements. This can lead to diminished mental performance and slower reaction times. Therefore, maintaining hydration supports not only cognitive function but also overall brain health by ensuring proper circulation.

3.3 Avoiding Processed Foods and Sugars

Processed foods and sugars are major contributors to cognitive decline, as they offer little nutritional value and often trigger inflammatory responses in the body. Inflammation, particularly in the brain, is a key factor in the development of cognitive disorders and mental fatigue. The consumption of highly processed foods, which are typically loaded with unhealthy fats, sugars, and artificial additives, can lead to a host of problems, including brain fog and impaired memory.

Processed foods often contain high levels of refined sugars, which cause rapid spikes and subsequent crashes in blood sugar levels. These fluctuations can result in a lack of sustained energy for the brain, leading to poor concentration and mood swings. The brain relies on a steady supply of glucose for energy, and when that supply is inconsistent due to sugar crashes, cognitive function suffers. Over time, the repeated consumption of sugary and processed foods can even contribute to insulin resistance, which has been linked to cognitive disorders like Alzheimer's disease.

Chapter 4: Natural Remedies for Brain Fog and Mental Fatigue

4.1 Reducing Mental Fatigue with Adaptogenic Herbs

Adaptogenic herbs are one of the most effective natural solutions for managing stress and combating mental fatigue. These herbs are unique in their ability to balance the body's response to stress, regulating hormones such as cortisol, which is often elevated during periods of prolonged stress. Two of the most widely recommended adaptogens for reducing mental fatigue are **ashwagandha** and **rhodiola**.

Ashwagandha is particularly valued for its ability to support the adrenal glands, which play a key role in the body's stress response. The adrenal glands release cortisol in response to stress, but when stress becomes chronic, the constant release of cortisol can lead to adrenal fatigue, a state in which the body is less able to cope with stress. Ashwagandha helps to regulate cortisol levels, reducing the negative impact of stress on both the body and the mind. As a result, it can significantly reduce symptoms of mental fatigue, improve cognitive function, and enhance overall mental resilience.

Rhodiola, another powerful adaptogen, works by boosting the brain's ability to handle stress. This herb has been shown to enhance the brain's resistance to physical and mental exhaustion, making it an ideal remedy for those experiencing burnout or cognitive decline due to stress. Rhodiola is also known to increase the production of neurotransmitters such as serotonin and dopamine, which are essential for maintaining mood balance and mental clarity. By supporting neurotransmitter function and balancing stress hormones, rhodiola helps to reduce mental fatigue and improve focus.

Both ashwagandha and rhodiola can be taken in supplement form, making them convenient for daily use. These adaptogens can also be brewed into teas, which offer a more traditional and soothing method of consumption. When brewed as a tea, the effects of these herbs can be felt more gradually, providing sustained support for mental clarity and resilience throughout the day. Barbara O'Neill recommends incorporating adaptogens into daily routines to enhance the body's ability to cope with stress, particularly in high-pressure environments.

Adaptogens are known for their gentle nature and long-term benefits. Unlike stimulants, which provide a temporary boost in energy but often result in a crash, adaptogenic herbs work to build the body's resilience over time. By regularly consuming ashwagandha, rhodiola, or other adaptogens, individuals can experience sustained improvements in mental performance and stress management. These herbs are especially beneficial for those who face ongoing mental challenges, such as demanding work schedules, caregiving responsibilities, or prolonged periods of emotional stress.

4.2 Enhancing Mental Clarity with Essential Oils

In addition to adaptogenic herbs, essential oils play an important role in improving mental clarity and focus. Essential oils have been used for centuries to support mental and physical health, and modern research has confirmed their efficacy in enhancing cognitive function. Two of the most popular essential oils for mental clarity are **peppermint** and **rosemary**.

Peppermint oil is widely recognized for its ability to stimulate the mind and improve concentration. The invigorating scent of peppermint helps to clear mental fog and sharpen focus, making it an ideal remedy for those who struggle with sluggishness or lack of clarity during the day. Peppermint oil works by increasing blood flow to the brain, which in turn enhances oxygen delivery and boosts cognitive performance. Inhaling peppermint oil through a diffuser or applying it to the temples can provide immediate mental stimulation, helping to overcome mental fatigue and improve alertness.

Another potent essential oil for improving mental clarity is rosemary oil. Known for its stimulating and memory-enhancing properties, rosemary has been used traditionally to improve focus and cognitive function. The compounds in rosemary oil, such as cineole, have been shown to increase mental clarity and promote sharper thinking. Rosemary is especially effective in improving memory recall and reducing cognitive decline, making it a valuable tool for individuals looking to boost productivity and mental performance.

Essential oils can be used in various ways to enhance focus and clarity. One of the most effective methods is to diffuse the oils in the air, creating an environment conducive to concentration. Diffusing peppermint or rosemary oil during work or study sessions can help maintain mental alertness and prevent distractions. Inhaling these oils directly from the bottle or applying them topically to pulse points, such as the wrists or neck, can also provide a quick boost in focus and mental energy.

Another method for using essential oils is to incorporate them into daily routines through the use of roll-on blends or sprays. These products allow individuals to carry the benefits of essential oils with them throughout the day, providing consistent support for mental clarity. For those who prefer a more immersive experience, essential oils can also be added to bathwater or used in a relaxing massage. This not only enhances mental focus but also promotes relaxation, helping to alleviate the physical and mental tension that often accompanies stress.

Essential oils are a versatile and natural way to support cognitive function. When used consistently, they help to create a more focused, productive environment, making them an excellent complement to other natural remedies such as adaptogenic herbs. By incorporating peppermint and rosemary oils into daily life, individuals can experience greater mental clarity, improved memory, and enhanced focus, all of which contribute to better overall cognitive health.

4.3 Physical Exercise for Cognitive Health

Physical activity plays a crucial role in maintaining and enhancing brain health. Regular exercise is known to increase blood flow to the brain, ensuring that essential nutrients and oxygen are delivered to support cognitive function. This improved circulation not only helps in maintaining clarity of thought but also enhances memory and concentration.

One of the key effects of regular physical exercise is the promotion of brain-derived neurotrophic factor (BDNF). BDNF is a protein that supports the survival of existing neurons and encourages the growth of new neurons and synapses, essential for neuroplasticity—the brain's ability to adapt and form new connections. Neuroplasticity is essential for memory, learning, and brain injury healing. Exercises that stimulate the release of BDNF, such as aerobic activities, walking, and yoga, provide essential support for mental clarity and overall cognitive health.

Walking, yoga, and aerobic exercises help the brain just as much as your body. In summary, engaging in regular physical exercise is essential for maintaining brain health. Activities such as walking, yoga, and aerobic exercises increase blood flow to the brain, promote the release of BDNF, and support neuroplasticity, all of which contribute to improved mental clarity and cognitive function.

Chapter 5: 12 Natural Remedies for Cognitive Health and Mental Clarity

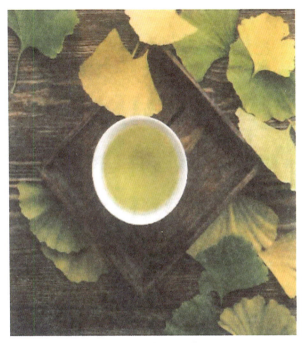

The appendix provides more details for each remedy.

1. Ginkgo Biloba Tea

2. Rosemary Oil Inhalation

3. Omega-3 Smoothie

4. Peppermint Essential Oil

5. Ashwagandha Tea

6. Bacopa Monnieri Supplement

7. Turmeric Golden Milk

8. Chamomile Tea

9. Ginseng Extract

10. Hydration Reminder

11. Lemon Balm Tea

12. B-Vitamin Complex

Part 18:
Weight Management and Metabolism Boosting

Chapter 1: Understanding Metabolism and Its Role in Weight Management

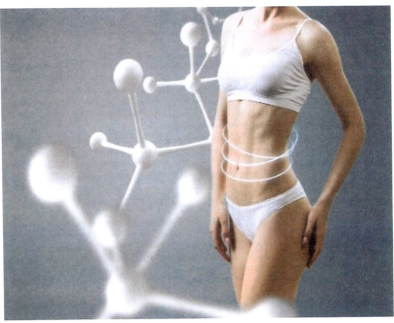

1.1 The Importance of a Healthy Metabolism

Metabolism is the process through which the body converts food into energy, an essential function for maintaining overall health and regulating body weight. Barbara O'Neill emphasizes that a healthy metabolism allows the body to efficiently use the nutrients from food, ensuring that energy is available for daily activities and vital bodily functions. This process involves not only the breakdown of food but also the conversion of it into usable energy or storage for future use.

Factors Affecting Metabolism

Several factors influence the body's metabolic rate, including age, diet, and lifestyle habits. As people age, their metabolism naturally slows down, leading to a decrease in the number of calories burned at rest. This is due to the gradual loss of muscle mass, which is more metabolically active than fat tissue. With less muscle mass, the body requires fewer calories to function, which can lead to weight gain if caloric intake is not adjusted accordingly. In contrast, younger individuals with more muscle tend to have faster metabolisms, allowing them to burn calories more efficiently.

Diet plays a significant role in metabolic health. Eating nutrient-dense foods that are high in vitamins and minerals supports the body's energy production processes. On the other hand, consuming processed foods high in sugars and unhealthy fats can slow down metabolism. Refined carbohydrates, for example, are quickly broken down into sugar, leading to spikes in blood glucose levels. These fluctuations can negatively impact metabolic function over time. A diet rich in whole foods, including fruits, vegetables, lean proteins, and healthy fats, supports a stable metabolic rate and prevents unnecessary weight gain.

Additionally, lifestyle habits such as physical activity and sleep quality have a direct impact on metabolism. Regular exercise increases the body's metabolic rate by building muscle mass and improving energy expenditure. Strength training, in particular, is effective at boosting metabolism, as muscle tissue burns more calories than fat, even at rest. Moreover, high-intensity workouts can increase calorie burn long after the activity is completed, a phenomenon known as the "afterburn effect."

Sleep is another crucial factor for metabolic health. Poor sleep patterns or lack of adequate rest can disrupt the body's natural rhythms and lead to hormonal imbalances that slow down metabolism. When the body does not receive enough sleep, the production of cortisol, a stress hormone, increases. Elevated cortisol levels can lead to increased appetite and cravings for high-calorie foods, which in turn contribute to weight gain.

Slow Metabolism and Weight Gain

A slow metabolism is often linked to difficulties in maintaining or losing weight. When the body's metabolic rate decreases, it becomes more challenging to burn calories efficiently, leading to the storage of excess energy as fat. This can create a cycle of weight gain, where the body stores more fat and burns fewer calories. Individuals with a slower metabolism may find it harder to shed excess weight, even with dietary changes and exercise. Factors like chronic stress, poor nutrition, and sedentary habits can further exacerbate this issue, making it even more difficult to achieve a healthy body weight.

One way to address a sluggish metabolism is by incorporating foods that naturally boost metabolic function. Certain foods, such as those high in protein, can temporarily increase the metabolic rate because they require more energy to digest compared to fats or carbohydrates. Spices like cayenne pepper and ginger are also known to stimulate metabolism due to their thermogenic properties, which raise the body's core temperature and increase calorie burn.

1.2 The Relationship Between Blood Sugar and Weight

The regulation of blood sugar levels plays a crucial role in managing body weight. Fluctuations in blood sugar, especially those caused by poor dietary choices, can lead to a cycle of cravings and overeating, making it difficult to maintain a healthy weight. The body responds to spikes and crashes in blood sugar by seeking quick energy sources, often leading individuals to consume processed foods and sugary drinks, which only exacerbate the problem.

Blood Sugar Spikes and Crashes

When someone consumes foods high in refined carbohydrates and sugars, such as white bread, sugary snacks, and soft drinks, it causes a rapid spike in blood glucose levels. This sudden increase triggers the pancreas to release insulin, a hormone responsible for lowering blood sugar by facilitating its storage in cells. However, this process can often result in a sharp drop in blood sugar, leading to what is commonly known as a "crash."

This crash leaves individuals feeling fatigued, irritable, and often craving more sugar or refined carbohydrates to quickly restore energy. As Barbara O'Neill points out, this creates a vicious cycle where the body continuously seeks high-sugar foods to counteract the drops in energy caused by insulin's action. Over time, this pattern can result in overeating and weight gain as the body stores excess glucose as fat, particularly when more sugar is consumed than is needed for immediate energy use.

Cravings and Overeating

One of the most common side effects of blood sugar imbalances is intense cravings for unhealthy foods. These cravings are not simply about hunger but are the body's response to low energy levels following a blood sugar crash. O'Neill explains that these imbalances can trigger overeating, particularly of foods that further disrupt blood sugar regulation, such as processed snacks, fast food, and sugary beverages. This leads to a cycle of consuming empty calories, which not only provide little nutritional value but also contribute to further weight gain.

When blood sugar levels are unstable, the body is unable to maintain consistent energy levels throughout the day. This fluctuation in energy can cause individuals to reach for quick fixes like sweets and junk food, which provide immediate but temporary boosts in energy, perpetuating unhealthy eating habits. Over time, this can lead to insulin resistance, where the body's cells become less responsive to insulin. This condition is often associated with weight gain, particularly around the abdominal area, and can increase the risk of developing type 2 diabetes.

The Role of Meal Timing and Portion Control

Along with food choices, meal timing and portion control are essential components in regulating blood sugar and managing weight. O'Neill highlights that eating smaller, balanced meals at regular intervals helps to prevent large fluctuations in blood sugar. Skipping meals or waiting too long between meals can lead to dips in energy, prompting cravings for high-sugar or high-carbohydrate foods. By maintaining consistent meal times and controlling portions, it becomes easier to manage appetite and avoid the overeating that often accompanies blood sugar crashes.

Furthermore, ensuring that meals contain a balance of macronutrients—proteins, fats, and carbohydrates—helps to keep blood sugar levels steady. By focusing on nutrient-dense foods, individuals can avoid the pitfalls of blood sugar spikes and crashes, ultimately supporting a healthier weight and reducing the likelihood of developing metabolic disorders.

Chapter 2: Supporting Healthy Metabolism with Natural Remedies

2.1 Green Tea for Boosting Metabolism

Green tea has long been recognized for its health benefits, particularly its ability to enhance metabolism. This popular beverage contains two key components—catechins and caffeine—that play a significant role in boosting thermogenesis, the process by which the body burns calories to produce heat. Catechins, a type of antioxidant, work by increasing fat oxidation, which allows the body to break down stored fat and convert it into energy. Caffeine, on the other hand, acts as a stimulant, increasing energy expenditure by raising the metabolic rate.

Barbara O'Neill highlights the value of incorporating green tea into daily routines, especially for individuals looking to manage their weight naturally. She emphasizes that drinking a few cups of green tea each day can support the body's ability to burn fat more efficiently. The combination of catechins and caffeine not only stimulates thermogenesis but also enhances the body's overall fat-burning capabilities. This makes green tea an ideal choice for those aiming to boost their metabolism without relying on synthetic supplements.

Green tea has many other health benefits in addition to its metabolic benefits. It is rich in antioxidants, which help protect the body from oxidative stress and inflammation, both of which can impair metabolic function. By reducing inflammation and oxidative damage, green tea contributes to maintaining a healthy, balanced metabolism. O'Neill recommends choosing high-quality green tea, preferably organic, to ensure maximum benefits without the potential exposure to pesticides or harmful additives.

For individuals who may not enjoy the taste of plain green tea, O'Neill suggests blending it with other herbs or flavors, such as lemon or ginger, to enhance its taste while maintaining its effectiveness. She also advises drinking green tea between meals, rather than with meals, to avoid interference with nutrient absorption. Green tea's inherent caffeine level gives you a steady, mild energy boost without the jitters or crashes that come with drinking other caffeinated drinks like coffee.

2.2 Cayenne Pepper: A Natural Metabolic Booster

Cayenne pepper is another powerful natural remedy known for its ability to stimulate metabolism. The active compound in cayenne, capsaicin, is responsible for its characteristic heat and fiery flavor. By raising the body's internal temperature—a process called thermogenesis—capsaicin enhances the body's ability to burn calories. This thermogenic effect makes cayenne pepper an excellent addition to a metabolism-boosting regimen.

Barbara O'Neill often points to the benefits of incorporating cayenne pepper into daily meals as a way to naturally enhance fat burning. By stimulating the body's heat production, capsaicin increases the amount of energy the body uses, even at rest. This not only helps in weight management but also improves overall metabolic function. Additionally, cayenne pepper can help suppress appetite, reducing the likelihood of overeating and supporting a balanced diet.

Beyond its metabolic effects, cayenne pepper offers a host of other health benefits. It has been shown to improve circulation, enhance digestion, and support cardiovascular health by reducing cholesterol levels and lowering blood pressure. For those looking to add cayenne pepper to their diet, O'Neill suggests starting with small amounts to gradually build tolerance, as the spice can be intense for some individuals.

One of the simplest ways to incorporate cayenne pepper is by adding a pinch to various dishes, such as soups, stews, and salads. It can also be sprinkled into smoothies or juices for a mild kick that boosts metabolism throughout the day. O'Neill cautions, however, that it is important to avoid overconsumption, as too much cayenne pepper can irritate the digestive system. A moderate amount, consumed consistently, is sufficient to provide the desired metabolic benefits.

For those who may be sensitive to the spice, O'Neill recommends combining cayenne pepper with cooling ingredients like yogurt or avocado to balance its heat while still reaping the benefits. The versatility of cayenne pepper makes it easy to incorporate into a variety of dishes, allowing individuals to enjoy its metabolic-boosting properties without drastically changing their eating habits.

2.3 Ginseng for Energy and Weight Loss

Ginseng is a well-known herbal remedy with a long history of use in traditional medicine, particularly for its energizing and adaptogenic properties. It plays a significant role in supporting energy levels and promoting weight loss, as it helps to combat fatigue and improve physical endurance, which are key factors in maintaining an active lifestyle and burning calories throughout the day.

One of the ways ginseng supports energy levels is by enhancing the body's resilience to physical and mental stress. When the body is better equipped to handle stress, energy reserves are conserved, and overall vitality is increased. This herb is particularly useful for individuals who experience fatigue, whether due to stress, a busy lifestyle, or other health concerns. Ginseng's adaptogenic properties help the body adapt to various stressors, balancing energy levels and allowing for more sustained physical activity, which in turn supports calorie expenditure and weight loss.

In addition to boosting energy, ginseng helps improve endurance during physical activity. Increased stamina allows for longer and more intense workouts, leading to higher calorie burn and enhanced weight management. Whether taken before exercise to boost performance or as part of a daily regimen to improve overall vitality, ginseng supports the body's ability to stay active, which is essential for anyone looking to lose weight or maintain a healthy weight.

Another benefit of ginseng is its ability to regulate blood sugar levels. Stabilizing blood sugar is crucial for preventing energy crashes and reducing cravings for sugary or high-calorie foods, both of which can hinder weight loss efforts. By helping to keep blood sugar levels balanced, ginseng supports sustained energy throughout the day and makes it easier to avoid overeating or snacking on unhealthy foods.

Ginseng can be consumed in a variety of forms to support energy and weight loss efforts. One popular method is to take it in capsule form, which provides a convenient way to incorporate the herb into a daily routine. Alternatively, ginseng can be brewed into a tea, allowing individuals to enjoy its benefits in a more traditional and soothing manner. Regardless of how it is consumed, ginseng remains an effective natural aid for enhancing energy levels and supporting weight management.

Chapter 3: Natural Appetite Suppressants and Fat-Burning Remedies

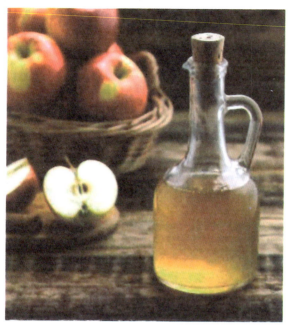

3.1 Natural Appetite Suppressants

Managing appetite is a critical aspect of weight loss and overall health. Certain foods and herbs can naturally suppress appetite, making it easier to control portion sizes and avoid overeating. One such food is flaxseeds, which are known for their high fiber content and rich supply of omega-3 fatty acids. These nutrients work together to help individuals feel fuller for longer periods of time, reducing the urge to snack between meals or consume large portions.

Flaxseeds are especially effective because they expand in the stomach, promoting a feeling of fullness. When consumed, the fiber in flaxseeds absorbs water and swells, which physically fills the stomach and signals to the brain that it's time to stop eating. This process not only curbs appetite but also supports digestive health by promoting regular bowel movements. The omega-3 fatty acids in flaxseeds further contribute to overall well-being by reducing inflammation and supporting metabolic processes, both of which are beneficial for weight management.

Another natural appetite suppressant that is highly recommended is apple cider vinegar. When consumed before meals, apple cider vinegar has been shown to slow the emptying of the stomach, which leads to a prolonged feeling of fullness and helps reduce overall calorie intake. This is particularly useful for those looking to manage portion sizes and avoid overeating during meals.

Apple cider vinegar works by enhancing the body's sensitivity to insulin and stabilizing blood sugar levels. Stable blood sugar levels are essential for controlling cravings, particularly for sugary and high-calorie foods. By preventing the rapid spikes and crashes in blood sugar that often lead to overeating, apple cider vinegar makes it easier to maintain a balanced diet and avoid unnecessary calorie consumption.

Incorporating apple cider vinegar into daily routines is simple and effective. It can be diluted in water and consumed before meals, or added to salad dressings and other dishes to provide a tangy flavor while simultaneously supporting appetite control. Over time, this natural remedy helps individuals develop healthier eating habits and better manage their calorie intake, which are crucial for long-term weight management.

Both flaxseeds and apple cider vinegar are powerful tools in the quest for natural appetite suppression. By incorporating these foods into a balanced diet, individuals can enjoy the benefits of reduced hunger, improved digestion, and better control over their eating habits.

3.2 Fat-Burning Foods

Certain foods are known for their ability to enhance the body's fat-burning processes. Grapefruit and chili peppers, in particular, are two powerful additions to a weight management plan. These foods not only help the body break down fat more efficiently, but they also support overall metabolism, making them valuable tools in any diet aimed at weight loss.

Grapefruit: Rich in Fat-Burning Enzymes

Grapefruit has long been recognized for its fat-burning properties. It is rich in enzymes that aid in the breakdown of fats, helping the body to metabolize them more effectively. These enzymes work by enhancing the body's ability to use stored fat as a source of energy, which can be particularly helpful for those looking to lose weight. Additionally, grapefruit is low in calories and high in fiber, making it a filling yet nutritious option for anyone trying to manage their weight.

The fruit's high vitamin C content is another benefit, as it supports overall metabolic health and helps to reduce inflammation in the body, which can often be a barrier to weight loss. Eating grapefruit before meals is believed to help reduce appetite, allowing for better portion control, which further aids in fat reduction.

Chili Peppers and Capsaicin: Boosting Fat Oxidation

Chili peppers, particularly those containing capsaicin, are another food known for their fat-burning effects. Capsaicin, the compound responsible for the heat in chili peppers, has been shown to increase fat oxidation in the body. This means that it helps to convert fat into energy, making it easier for the body to burn fat during physical activity or even at rest.

Capsaicin also has thermogenic properties, which means it raises the body's temperature and increases the metabolic rate. This increase in metabolism can lead to more calories being burned throughout the day, which is particularly beneficial for weight management. By incorporating chili peppers into meals, individuals can naturally stimulate their metabolism and support their body's fat-burning processes.

Incorporating Fat-Burning Foods into Regular Meals

Incorporating grapefruit and chili peppers into daily meals is a simple way to enhance the body's fat-burning potential. Grapefruit can be eaten as a snack, added to salads, or consumed as juice, while chili peppers can be used to spice up soups, stews, and stir-fries. By regularly including these foods in the diet, individuals can support their metabolism and promote fat loss more effectively.

Both grapefruit and chili peppers offer additional health benefits, such as providing essential nutrients like vitamins and antioxidants. These foods not only support weight management but also contribute to overall health and wellness, making them excellent choices for those looking to optimize their diet for fat burning.

Chapter 4: Sustainable Approaches to Weight Loss and Maintaining a Healthy Weight

4.1 Whole-Food, Plant-Based Diet for Weight Loss

A whole-food, plant-based diet is central to Barbara O'Neill's approach to achieving and maintaining a healthy weight. This type of diet prioritizes unprocessed or minimally processed foods, emphasizing fruits, vegetables, whole grains, nuts, and seeds. These foods are not only lower in calories compared to highly processed, calorie-dense options, but they are also packed with essential nutrients that support overall health.

The foundation of this diet is its focus on **nutrient density**, ensuring that individuals receive the vitamins, minerals, and antioxidants necessary for optimal bodily function without consuming excessive calories. Nutrient-dense foods, such as leafy greens, legumes, and whole grains, provide the body with energy while avoiding the empty calories often found in refined carbohydrates and processed snacks. This helps people lose weight while still feeling satisfied, which reduces the likelihood of overeating or experiencing cravings for unhealthy foods.

One of the main benefits of this plant-based approach is its ability to **balance blood sugar levels**. Consuming whole foods that are high in fiber—such as oats, brown rice, and quinoa—helps slow down the absorption of sugars into the bloodstream. This stabilizes insulin levels, preventing spikes and crashes that can trigger hunger and overeating. Maintaining stable blood sugar is crucial for weight loss, as it helps reduce cravings for sugary snacks and promotes more consistent energy levels throughout the day.

Additionally, the high fiber content in fruits, vegetables, and legumes is key to promoting **satiety**, which is the feeling of fullness after a meal. Fiber expands in the stomach and takes longer to digest, keeping hunger at bay for longer periods. This means that individuals following a whole-food, plant-based diet can naturally eat fewer calories without feeling deprived. High-fiber foods, such as lentils, chickpeas, and sweet potatoes, are ideal for this purpose, providing both nourishment and satisfaction.

Beyond managing hunger, this diet also helps in reducing the intake of **unhealthy fats** that are commonly found in processed foods and animal products. Whole, plant-based foods typically contain lower levels of saturated fats, which can contribute to weight gain and increase the risk of cardiovascular disease. By focusing on healthy fats from sources such as avocados, nuts, and seeds, individuals can improve their cholesterol levels and support heart health while managing their weight.

The **high water content** in many plant-based foods is another advantage. Foods like cucumbers, watermelon, and leafy greens are naturally hydrating and help with digestion, promoting a feeling of fullness without adding extra calories. These hydrating foods can also support detoxification processes, helping the body eliminate waste and function more efficiently.

To achieve sustainable weight loss, it is important to avoid **processed plant-based foods** that may be high in added sugars, unhealthy fats, and preservatives. While some packaged vegan foods may appear healthy, they can be just as detrimental to weight loss efforts as highly processed animal-based products. Instead, Barbara emphasizes whole, fresh ingredients that are minimally altered and free from artificial additives.

One of the most effective strategies she suggests for long-term success is **meal planning**. Preparing meals ahead of time using whole, plant-based ingredients helps individuals stay on track with their weight loss goals and avoid the temptation of reaching for quick, unhealthy options. Planning meals around vegetables, grains, and legumes ensures a balance of macronutrients, providing the necessary fuel for both physical activity and daily tasks without excessive caloric intake.

4.2 Incorporating Regular Exercise

Physical activity is a key component of Barbara O'Neill's weight loss philosophy, working in tandem with a whole-food, plant-based diet to support healthy weight management. Exercise not only burns calories but also plays a crucial role in **boosting metabolism**, which is essential for maintaining weight loss over time.

Cardiovascular exercises, such as walking and swimming, are particularly effective for burning calories and improving heart health. Walking, for example, is a low-impact activity that can be easily incorporated into daily routines. It helps improve circulation, supports heart function, and promotes fat burning without placing too much strain on the joints. Similarly, swimming offers a full-body workout that builds endurance and strengthens muscles while being gentle on the body.

Variety in exercise routines is essential for preventing boredom and ensuring that different muscle groups are engaged. In addition to walking, swimming, and yoga, incorporating activities like cycling, dancing, or hiking can help maintain motivation while providing a comprehensive workout for the entire body. Each form of exercise offers unique benefits, from improving endurance and cardiovascular health to building strength and enhancing mental clarity.

Chapter 5: 13 Natural Remedies for Boosting Metabolism and Managing Weight

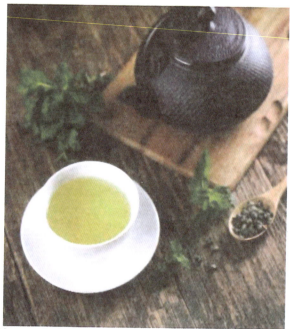

The appendix provides more details for each remedy.

1. Green Tea Infusion

2. Cayenne Pepper and Lemon Detox Drink

3. Apple Cider Vinegar Tonic

4. Ginger Tea

5. Ginseng Tea

6. Flaxseed Smoothie

7. Grapefruit Salad

8. Cinnamon Tea

9. Peppermint Tea

10. Cucumber and Mint Water

11. Turmeric Latte

12. Chili Pepper Infused Oil

13. Garlic and Lemon Detox Soup

Part 19:
Endocrine System Health and Hormonal Balance

Chapter 1: The Role of the Endocrine System in Overall Health

Understanding the Endocrine System

The endocrine system plays a critical role in regulating many of the body's essential functions, such as metabolism, growth, and reproduction, by secreting hormones into the bloodstream. This complex network of glands must work in harmony to ensure the body maintains balance and functions optimally. Among the key glands are the thyroid, adrenal glands, and reproductive organs, each with its specific role in producing hormones necessary for everyday processes.

The Role of the Thyroid

The thyroid gland is particularly significant in regulating metabolism. It produces hormones such as thyroxine (T4) and triiodothyronine (T3), which control the rate at which the body converts food into energy. When the thyroid functions optimally, it supports energy production and regulates body temperature. However, it can cause a variety of symptoms, such as anxiety, palpitations, and exhaustion, whether it becomes underactive (hypothyroidism) or hyperactive (hyperthyroidism).

An underactive thyroid often leads to a slowdown in metabolic processes, causing individuals to feel sluggish or experience weight gain despite maintaining regular eating habits. To support thyroid health, Barbara O'Neill advocates for a nutrient-dense diet that includes iodine, selenium, and zinc, which are essential for healthy thyroid function. Foods such as sea vegetables, brazil nuts, and seeds are particularly beneficial in promoting thyroid balance and ensuring the gland produces hormones efficiently.

Adrenal Glands and Stress Response

The adrenal glands, located above the kidneys, are responsible for producing hormones like cortisol, adrenaline, and aldosterone. These hormones are vital in managing the body's response to stress, regulating blood pressure, and maintaining fluid balance. When the adrenal glands are under constant pressure due to chronic stress, they may become overworked, leading to adrenal fatigue.

Adrenal fatigue is characterized by symptoms such as low energy, difficulty getting out of bed in the morning, and a feeling of being "burnt out." This condition arises when the adrenal glands can no longer produce sufficient amounts of cortisol to meet the body's demands. In this state, individuals may feel exhausted and overwhelmed, even when faced with minor stressors. To restore adrenal health, it is important to manage stress effectively through lifestyle adjustments, such as incorporating relaxation techniques like meditation, ensuring adequate sleep, and avoiding stimulants like caffeine.

Additionally, certain adaptogenic herbs, including ashwagandha and rhodiola, are known to support adrenal function and help the body adapt to stress more efficiently. These natural remedies help regulate cortisol production and promote a balanced stress response, enabling the adrenal glands to recover from exhaustion.

Supporting the Endocrine System Naturally

To maintain a healthy endocrine system, it is essential to adopt a holistic approach that includes dietary changes, lifestyle modifications, and the use of natural remedies. Reducing stress levels, getting adequate sleep, and engaging in regular physical activity are all key factors in promoting endocrine health. Additionally, incorporating specific nutrients, such as omega-3 fatty acids, iodine, and antioxidants, into the diet helps to nourish the glands and ensure optimal hormone production.

Chapter 2: Natural Support for Thyroid and Adrenal Health

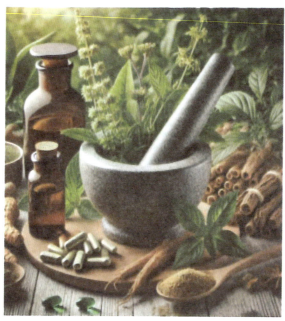

2.1 Supporting Thyroid Function Naturally

The thyroid gland plays a critical role in regulating metabolism, energy production, and overall bodily function. When the thyroid is not functioning optimally, specifically in the case of hypothyroidism (an underactive thyroid), various symptoms can arise, including fatigue, weight gain, depression, and even cognitive difficulties. Hypothyroidism occurs when the thyroid gland does not produce enough thyroid hormones, which are essential for energy regulation.

A key element in thyroid health is **iodine**, a mineral necessary for the production of thyroid hormones. Without sufficient iodine, the thyroid cannot produce enough hormones, leading to the aforementioned symptoms. Barbara O'Neill emphasizes the importance of incorporating iodine-rich foods into the diet to support the thyroid. Foods such as **seaweed** and **kelp** are excellent natural sources of iodine. She encourages the consumption of these foods in their natural forms, as they provide a concentrated dose of iodine, helping to ensure that the thyroid has enough of this essential mineral to function properly. Additionally, **iodized salt** can also be a convenient source of iodine for those who may not have access to seaweed or kelp in their regular diet.

In addition to iodine, other nutrients are equally important for optimal thyroid health. **Selenium** is one such nutrient, crucial for converting thyroid hormones into their active forms within the body. A selenium shortage can worsen hypothyroidism symptoms and affect thyroid function. Barbara recommends incorporating selenium-rich foods, particularly **Brazil nuts**, which are one of the most potent dietary sources of selenium. Consuming just a few Brazil nuts a day can provide a substantial portion of the recommended daily intake of selenium, supporting the thyroid in its hormone production and conversion processes.

Another essential mineral for thyroid function is **zinc**, which plays a role in both the synthesis of thyroid hormones and the regulation of the immune system. Zinc deficiency is associated with impaired thyroid function, so ensuring adequate zinc intake is critical for those looking to maintain thyroid health. Barbara suggests eating foods such as **pumpkin seeds**, which are high in zinc, or taking a zinc supplement if needed.

Finally, **vitamin D** is another vital nutrient for thyroid health, particularly in supporting the immune system and reducing the risk of autoimmune thyroid conditions. Low levels of vitamin D are common in individuals with thyroid disorders, and supplementing with vitamin D or consuming vitamin D-rich foods like fatty fish or fortified dairy products can help to restore balance and promote overall thyroid function.

2.2 Restoring Adrenal Balance

The adrenal glands are responsible for producing hormones such as cortisol and adrenaline, which help the body manage stress. In times of acute stress, these hormones are essential for survival, as they trigger the body's "fight or flight" response. However, when stress becomes chronic, the adrenal glands can become fatigued, leading to what is commonly known as **adrenal fatigue**. Symptoms of adrenal fatigue include persistent exhaustion, difficulty concentrating, low energy, and cravings for sugar or salty foods.

Chapter 3: Herbs and Lifestyle Changes for Managing Hormonal Imbalances

3.1 Adaptogens for Hormonal Balance

Adaptogenic herbs play a crucial role in helping the body regulate its hormonal balance. These herbs are particularly beneficial for managing the stress hormone cortisol, supporting the thyroid and adrenal glands, and improving overall endocrine function. Among the most potent adaptogens are **ashwagandha** and **rhodiola**, which Barbara O'Neill frequently highlights for their ability to regulate the body's response to stress.

Ashwagandha, a key adaptogen, is well-known for its ability to lower cortisol levels. Cortisol, often referred to as the "stress hormone," plays a significant role in the body's response to stress. While short-term spikes in cortisol can be beneficial for managing immediate threats, chronic high levels of cortisol can disrupt the body's hormonal balance. Ashwagandha helps modulate cortisol production, reducing the damaging effects of prolonged stress on the body. By promoting relaxation and improving the body's stress response, ashwagandha not only balances cortisol but also supports overall hormonal health.

In addition to its effects on cortisol, ashwagandha is known for its positive impact on **thyroid function**. It can stimulate thyroid hormone production, which is particularly beneficial for individuals experiencing hypothyroidism or an underactive thyroid. The thyroid plays a central role in regulating metabolism, energy levels, and overall hormonal balance, making ashwagandha a valuable tool in supporting endocrine function.

Rhodiola is another powerful adaptogen that Barbara recommends for stress management and hormonal regulation. Like ashwagandha, rhodiola helps to balance cortisol levels, but it is also particularly effective in combating mental fatigue and improving cognitive function. This adaptogen enhances the body's ability to cope with stress by promoting resilience and endurance, which in turn supports adrenal health. The **adrenal glands** are responsible for producing several key hormones, including cortisol, adrenaline, and aldosterone, which help the body manage stress, maintain blood pressure, and regulate fluid balance.

Rhodiola is also known to improve **mood and emotional well-being,** making it a useful remedy for those experiencing anxiety or depression, which can often result from hormonal imbalances. By enhancing mental clarity and reducing stress-induced fatigue, rhodiola indirectly supports the body's hormonal equilibrium, making it a key component in any strategy aimed at restoring balance to the endocrine system.

Maca root is another adaptogen Barbara recommends, particularly for its ability to balance reproductive hormones. Maca is particularly helpful for ladies who are having irregular periods or menopausal symptoms. It works by supporting the endocrine system, helping to regulate the production of hormones such as estrogen and progesterone. For women in menopause, maca can help alleviate common symptoms like hot flashes, mood swings, and night sweats by modulating estrogen levels.

Maca is also effective in promoting **fertility** and **sexual health,** as it enhances libido and supports healthy hormone production in both men and women. Additionally, it helps stabilize energy levels and reduce the mood fluctuations that can accompany hormonal changes, making it a valuable tool for maintaining hormonal balance throughout different stages of life.

3.2 Diet for Hormonal Health

A key principle emphasized in Barbara O'Neill's teachings is the importance of a whole-food, plant-based diet to support hormonal health. She highlights the role of nutrition in regulating and balancing hormones, particularly in how certain foods can either support or disrupt the body's delicate hormonal system.

One of the cornerstones of maintaining hormonal balance is the inclusion of **healthy fats** in the diet. These fats are essential for the production of hormones, which are made from cholesterol and fatty acids. Foods such as **avocados, nuts,** and **seeds** are excellent sources of these beneficial fats. Avocados, for instance, are rich in monounsaturated fats, which are crucial for the synthesis of hormones like estrogen, progesterone, and testosterone. Similarly, nuts and seeds, particularly **flaxseeds** and **chia seeds,** contain omega-3 fatty acids that help reduce inflammation in the body, supporting overall hormonal function.

In addition to healthy fats, O'Neill underscores the importance of avoiding **refined sugars** and **processed foods**. These foods can cause significant disruptions in hormonal balance by spiking blood sugar levels, which in turn leads to insulin resistance. Insulin, a hormone that regulates blood sugar, plays a vital role in how the body stores fat and processes energy. When insulin is constantly elevated due to high sugar intake, it can lead to imbalances in other hormones, such as cortisol and estrogen. O'Neill advises steering clear of sugary snacks, sodas, and refined carbohydrates to prevent these hormonal disruptions.

Another important aspect of hormonal health is the detoxification of excess hormones, particularly **estrogen**, which can accumulate in the body and lead to conditions such as estrogen dominance. To support this detoxification process, O'Neill recommends incorporating **cruciferous vegetables** into the diet. Vegetables like **broccoli**, **kale**, **cauliflower**, and **Brussels sprouts** contain a compound called **indole-3-carbinol**, which helps the liver break down excess estrogen and remove it from the body. This process is vital for maintaining the balance of estrogen with other hormones, such as progesterone and testosterone.

Cruciferous vegetables are also high in **fiber**, which plays a crucial role in hormonal health by binding to excess hormones and toxins in the digestive tract and promoting their elimination. This reduces the likelihood of reabsorbing these hormones into the bloodstream. Fiber-rich foods, such as **leafy greens**, **whole grains**, and **legumes**, should therefore be a staple in any diet aimed at balancing hormones.

Additionally, O'Neill points out the benefits of **herbs and spices** that can support hormonal health. For example, **turmeric** has powerful anti-inflammatory properties that can help alleviate symptoms of hormonal imbalance, such as bloating and mood swings, by reducing inflammation in the body. Incorporating these herbs into daily meals can further support the body's natural ability to regulate hormones.

Chapter 4: 14 Natural Remedies for Endocrine System Health and Hormonal Balance

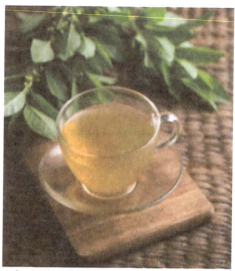

The appendix provides more details for each remedy.

1. Ashwagandha Tea
2. Rhodiola Supplement
3. Licorice Root Tea
4. Maca Root Powder
5. Seaweed Salad
6. Brazil Nuts
7. Pumpkin Seed Snack
8. Broccoli Stir-Fry
9. Coconut Oil Supplement
10. Flaxseed Pudding
11. Chia Seed Smoothie
12. Holy Basil Tea
13. Evening Primrose Oil
14. Thyme and Honey Elixir

Part 20:
Eye Health and Natural Vision Support

Chapter 1: Protecting Your Vision with the Right Nutrients

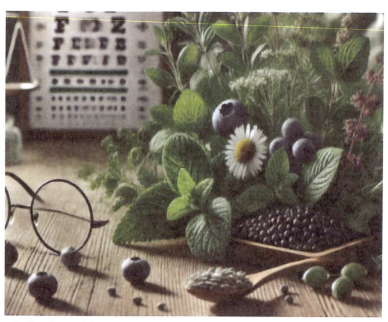

1.1 The Role of Nutrition in Eye Health

Nutrients play a vital role in maintaining eye health and preventing vision deterioration. Specific vitamins and minerals are essential to support the structure and function of the eyes, and without them, the risk of developing degenerative conditions like macular degeneration and cataracts increases significantly.

Protection Against Oxidative Stress

Oxidative stress is one of the primary contributors to vision deterioration as we age. The eyes are particularly vulnerable to this type of stress due to their constant exposure to light and oxygen. When the body's levels of antioxidants and free radicals are out of balance, oxidative stress results in cellular damage. This damage can affect various parts of the eyes, including the lens and the retina, and is a significant factor in the development of cataracts and macular degeneration.

To combat oxidative stress, consuming foods rich in **antioxidants** is essential. Antioxidants help neutralize free radicals, preventing them from causing damage to the cells in the eyes. **Lutein** and **zeaxanthin**, two carotenoids found in high concentrations in the macula, are particularly important for eye health. These antioxidants act as natural filters for harmful blue light and help protect the retina from damage. Foods like kale, spinach, and egg yolks are excellent sources of lutein and zeaxanthin.

Additionally, incorporating **zinc** into the diet is beneficial for eye health. Zinc plays a critical role in transporting vitamin A from the liver to the retina, where it is used to produce melanin, a protective pigment in the eyes. Zinc is also involved in maintaining the structural integrity of the retina and may help reduce the risk of macular degeneration. Foods rich in zinc include oysters, beef, and pumpkin seeds.

1.2 Lutein and Zeaxanthin: Antioxidants for Vision Protection

Lutein and zeaxanthin are carotenoids that play a crucial role in protecting eye health. Naturally concentrated in the retina, particularly in the macula, these powerful antioxidants help filter harmful blue light from digital screens and sunlight, which can cause oxidative damage over time. Blue light is known to contribute to the risk of developing age-related eye conditions such as cataracts and macular degeneration. Protecting the eyes from these damaging effects is essential, particularly as one ages, since the natural levels of lutein and zeaxanthin in the retina tend to decline.

Both lutein and zeaxanthin serve as internal sunglasses, shielding the sensitive structures of the eye. By absorbing blue light, they prevent it from penetrating deeply into the eye tissues where it can generate free radicals that damage cells. When consumed in sufficient amounts through the diet, these carotenoids help maintain optimal eye function and reduce the risk of progressive vision loss associated with aging.

Lutein and Zeaxanthin in Foods

These carotenoids cannot be synthesized by the body, so they must be obtained through dietary sources. Among the best sources of lutein and zeaxanthin are dark, leafy greens such as spinach, kale, and Swiss chard. These vegetables are not only rich in these antioxidants but are also packed with other nutrients like vitamins A, C, and K, which further support eye health and overall wellness.

Spinach, in particular, is a standout source of lutein. Just one cup of cooked spinach provides a significant portion of the daily recommended intake of lutein and zeaxanthin. Kale is another excellent option, offering high concentrations of both carotenoids. The rich, vibrant green color of these vegetables is a visual indicator of their antioxidant content, and regular consumption of them can make a noticeable difference in long-term eye health.

In addition to leafy greens, Barbara highlights the benefits of including corn in the diet. Yellow corn is a good source of zeaxanthin, which is particularly effective in protecting the central vision by absorbing excess light energy that could damage the retina. Regularly consuming corn, either fresh or as part of a balanced meal, can help boost the levels of zeaxanthin in the eye, offering an additional layer of protection against oxidative stress.

Egg yolks also contain both lutein and zeaxanthin, and although their levels are lower compared to leafy greens, they are highly bioavailable, meaning that the body can absorb and utilize these antioxidants more efficiently from eggs. Including a variety of these foods in the diet ensures that the body receives a steady supply of these vision-protecting carotenoids.

Daily Consumption for Eye Health

Barbara advocates for the daily consumption of lutein- and zeaxanthin-rich foods as part of a balanced diet to support long-term eye health. She emphasizes that while supplements are available, the most effective and natural way to increase these antioxidants in the body is through whole foods. Regular intake of these nutrients helps maintain the density of the macular pigment, which in turn preserves sharp, central vision and reduces the risk of developing age-related conditions such as macular degeneration and cataracts.

Chapter 2: Herbal Remedies for Common Eye Conditions

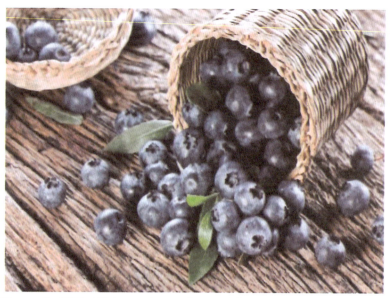

2.1 Bilberry for Night Vision and Macular Health

Bilberry is highly regarded for its potent effects on improving vision, especially when it comes to night vision. The herb is rich in anthocyanins, a group of powerful antioxidants that play a critical role in enhancing circulation to the eyes and strengthening the delicate capillaries in the retina. This improved circulation ensures that the eyes receive the necessary oxygen and nutrients to function optimally, particularly in low-light conditions. Barbara O'Neill emphasizes that bilberry is particularly beneficial for individuals who struggle with vision at night, helping to sharpen eyesight and reduce strain when visibility is compromised.

The anthocyanins found in bilberry are known to protect the retina by reinforcing the structure of the capillaries, making them less susceptible to damage or leakage. This protective effect is especially important for maintaining the health of the macula, the central part of the retina responsible for clear, sharp vision. Macular degeneration, a common concern as people age, can lead to significant vision impairment if not addressed. By improving capillary strength and enhancing blood flow to this vital area, bilberry serves as a natural defense against this degenerative condition.

One of the most convenient ways to incorporate bilberry into a daily routine is through supplements, which provide a concentrated dose of anthocyanins for sustained eye health. However, bilberry can also be consumed as a tea, which offers a gentler yet effective way to reap its benefits. Drinking bilberry tea regularly helps to support overall eye function, providing ongoing protection to the retina and macula. For those looking for natural solutions to maintain or improve their night vision, bilberry serves as an accessible and effective remedy.

Bilberry's ability to enhance circulation in the eyes is not limited to just night vision. Individuals who suffer from eye strain due to prolonged exposure to screens or other demanding visual tasks can also benefit from this herb. By improving blood flow to the eyes, bilberry helps alleviate fatigue and ensures that the eyes remain nourished and oxygenated throughout the day. This makes it an ideal herb for those who experience frequent eye discomfort or who want to preserve their visual acuity as they age.

2.2 Eyebright for Eye Irritations

Eyebright is another powerful herb frequently recommended for soothing various eye irritations. It has a long history of use in traditional herbal medicine for relieving symptoms such as redness, dryness, and discomfort in the eyes. Whether caused by environmental factors like dust and pollution, or conditions such as conjunctivitis and allergies, eyebright offers a gentle yet effective way to reduce irritation and restore comfort to the eyes.

The herb works primarily by reducing inflammation in the eye tissues. Its anti-inflammatory properties help to calm the irritated surfaces of the eyes, making it a popular remedy for conditions like allergic conjunctivitis, where the eyes become red, itchy, and swollen due to an allergic reaction. By reducing the inflammation and soothing the affected areas, eyebright helps to alleviate the discomfort and restore clarity to the eyes.

Eyebright can be prepared as a tea and used as an eye wash or compress to directly apply its healing properties to the eyes. This method is particularly useful for treating external irritations, where the herb can immediately reduce redness and swelling. When used as an eye wash, the cooling effect of the tea helps to flush out any irritants or debris that may be exacerbating the problem, offering relief for conditions like dry eyes or irritation caused by excessive screen time.

For those suffering from seasonal allergies that affect the eyes, eyebright is a natural alternative to over-the-counter allergy medications. By addressing the inflammation and calming the irritated tissues, eyebright helps to reduce the need for stronger pharmaceutical interventions. In cases of mild to moderate eye irritations, it can be an effective first line of defense.

Moreover, eyebright is not only limited to external applications. Consuming eyebright tea can also help to support eye health from within. The herb's anti-inflammatory and antioxidant properties work systemically to reduce inflammation in the body, including the eyes. This internal support complements the topical applications, making eyebright a versatile herb for comprehensive eye care.

In addition to its benefits for eye irritations, eyebright has been noted for its astringent properties, which help to tighten and tone the tissues of the eyes. This is particularly beneficial for individuals who experience watery eyes or excessive tearing, as it helps to regulate moisture levels and maintain the integrity of the eye tissues.

Eyebright's effectiveness as an herbal remedy is enhanced when used in combination with other eye-supporting herbs. It pairs well with bilberry, as both herbs work to strengthen and protect the eyes in different ways.

2.3 Ginkgo Biloba for Improved Circulation

Ginkgo biloba is a well-known herb that has been praised for its cognitive benefits, particularly its ability to improve memory and focus by increasing blood flow to the brain. However, it is also highly beneficial for eye health, especially in cases where circulation to the optic nerve and retina needs support. Poor circulation to these areas can result in various eye conditions, including glaucoma, which is caused by increased pressure within the eye that can damage the optic nerve. By enhancing blood flow, Ginkgo biloba may help protect against such conditions and promote overall ocular health.

Ginkgo biloba works by increasing blood circulation throughout the body, including to the smallest capillaries in the eyes. This is especially important for maintaining a healthy optic nerve, which plays a vital role in vision. The herb helps to dilate blood vessels, thereby reducing pressure and allowing for improved oxygen and nutrient delivery to the retina and other critical parts of the eye. This process is essential in preventing degeneration, which can lead to conditions like glaucoma or age-related macular degeneration.

Another benefit of Ginkgo biloba for eye health is its ability to protect the eyes from oxidative stress. The herb is rich in antioxidants, which help to neutralize free radicals that can cause damage to the delicate tissues in the eyes. By reducing oxidative damage, Ginkgo biloba helps maintain the health of the retina, which is responsible for converting light into neural signals that are processed by the brain. Regular use of Ginkgo biloba can, therefore, support long-term eye health by protecting these vital structures.

Ginkgo biloba is also beneficial for individuals who experience eye strain or fatigue due to prolonged screen time or exposure to harsh lighting. Enhanced circulation can alleviate the discomfort associated with tired eyes by ensuring that the optic nerve receives an adequate supply of blood. This increased circulation not only improves overall visual acuity but also aids in the healing and recovery of eye tissues after extended use.

Ginkgo biloba's protective properties extend beyond just improving circulation. The herb also has anti-inflammatory effects, which can help reduce swelling and pressure within the eyes. This is particularly relevant for individuals who are at risk of developing glaucoma or other eye conditions related to increased intraocular pressure. By supporting circulation and reducing inflammation, Ginkgo biloba serves as a natural remedy to maintain eye health and prevent future complications.

Chapter 3: Simple Exercises and Dietary Tips for Maintaining Good Eyesight

3.1 Eye Exercises for Vision Support

Maintaining vision strength and flexibility is essential for overall eye health, especially in a world where prolonged screen time and other visual strains have become the norm. Regular eye exercises can help to reduce strain and support long-term vision health. Barbara O'Neill recommends incorporating simple practices into daily routines to strengthen the eyes and enhance their resilience.

One of the most effective exercises she suggests is **palming**. Palming involves covering the eyes with the palms of the hands, ensuring no light reaches the eyes. This simple action helps relax the eye muscles and gives them a break from focusing. By allowing the eyes to rest in complete darkness, palming can relieve tension and strain that builds up from prolonged use, such as staring at a computer screen or reading for extended periods.

Another useful exercise is **focusing on distant and close objects alternately**. This practice helps to improve the flexibility of the eye muscles, which are responsible for adjusting focus between near and far distances. To perform this exercise, one should start by focusing on an object up close, then shift their gaze to an object far away. Alternating between the two distances several times helps the eyes adapt to different focal lengths, which can improve overall focus and reduce eye fatigue.

Eye rotations are another recommended exercise. To perform eye rotations, gently move the eyes in a circular motion, first clockwise and then counterclockwise. This helps to strengthen the eye muscles and increase their range of motion. By regularly performing eye rotations, individuals can prevent stiffness in the eye muscles and maintain their ability to move freely, which is important for overall vision health.

These exercises not only help to reduce immediate eye strain but also serve as preventive measures to maintain long-term vision. They are particularly helpful for individuals who spend a significant amount of time engaged in visually demanding tasks, such as working on a computer, reading, or driving. By incorporating these simple exercises into daily routines, it's possible to support the strength and flexibility of the eyes, promoting better vision and reducing the risk of eye fatigue.

3.2 Hydration and Eye Health

Dry eyes occur when the eyes are not able to produce enough tears or when the tears evaporate too quickly. The tear film, which covers the surface of the eye, is essential for protecting and lubricating the eyes, and water is a key component of this tear film.

Adequate water intake helps ensure that the body's mucous membranes, including those in the eyes, remain hydrated. When the body is dehydrated, it prioritizes water for essential organs, which means that non-essential functions, like tear production, may be compromised. Drinking water regularly throughout the day helps to support this natural process, ensuring that the eyes remain lubricated and protected from environmental irritants such as dust and pollutants.

3.3 Omega-3 Fatty Acids for Dry Eye Relief

Omega-3 fatty acids are another critical component in maintaining eye health, particularly in preventing and treating dry eyes. These essential fatty acids are known for their anti-inflammatory properties and their ability to support healthy cell membranes throughout the body, including the eyes. A deficiency in omega-3 fatty acids can result in increased inflammation and dryness in the eyes, as well as impaired tear production.

Fish oil, derived from fatty fish such as salmon, mackerel, and sardines, is another excellent source of EPA and DHA. Consuming fish oil supplements or regularly eating fatty fish can help improve the lipid layer of the tear film, reducing evaporation and promoting longer-lasting eye lubrication. This is especially beneficial for individuals who suffer from dry eye syndrome, as omega-3 fatty acids can enhance tear production and improve tear quality, resulting in more comfortable, well-moisturized eyes.

For individuals who experience frequent dry eyes, increasing omega-3 intake through both food and supplements can help alleviate symptoms and support overall eye health. In addition to flaxseed and fish oil, other plant-based sources of omega-3s, such as chia seeds and walnuts, can be beneficial.

Chapter 4: Reducing Eye Strain Naturally

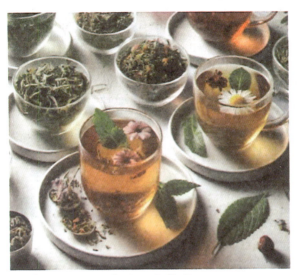

4.1 Herbal Teas and Compresses for Eye Relief

Chamomile and fennel are two powerful herbs known for their anti-inflammatory and soothing properties, which make them particularly useful for relieving eye strain and discomfort. Chamomile, a mild sedative and anti-inflammatory herb, has been used for centuries to calm irritated skin and reduce inflammation. Fennel, on the other hand, contains antioxidants and anti-inflammatory agents that can help reduce swelling and soothe strained eyes.

To prepare a chamomile or fennel tea compress, start by brewing the tea as you normally would. Once the tea has steeped and cooled, the tea bags can be placed directly over the eyes for 10-15 minutes. This simple technique helps to calm irritated eyes and reduce inflammation. The cooling effect of the tea compress also provides a soothing sensation, which can alleviate discomfort caused by prolonged screen use or general eye strain. Chamomile, in particular, is known for its ability to reduce puffiness and redness around the eyes, offering relief to those who spend long hours staring at digital devices or reading.

Fennel tea, with its additional antioxidant properties, supports eye health by reducing oxidative stress in the delicate tissues around the eyes. Regular use of fennel or chamomile tea compresses can help maintain overall eye health and prevent the strain that often leads to more severe discomfort. For those experiencing persistent eye strain, these natural remedies offer a gentle yet effective approach to eye care, supporting the body's natural healing mechanisms.

Using herbal teas like chamomile and fennel as both a drink and a compress provides a dual benefit: the tea, when consumed, nourishes the body with anti-inflammatory and antioxidant compounds, while the external application of the tea bags on the eyes provides targeted relief from strain and discomfort.

4.2 Limiting Screen Time and Blue Light Exposure

In today's digital age, eye strain from prolonged screen use is a common complaint. Blue light emitted by phones, computers, and other digital devices can contribute to digital eye strain, leading to symptoms such as dry eyes, headaches, and blurred vision. One of the most effective ways to manage this strain is to limit exposure to screens and take regular breaks throughout the day.

The 20-20-20 rule, as recommended by Barbara O'Neill, calls for taking a 20-second break every 20 minutes to stare at anything 20 feet away. This simple practice helps to reduce the continuous focus on a close-up screen, giving the eyes a chance to rest and recalibrate. Additionally, taking frequent breaks from digital devices can prevent the accumulation of eye strain over the course of the day.

Positioning screens correctly is another critical aspect of reducing eye strain. O'Neill recommends that screens be kept at eye level to avoid unnecessary strain on the eyes and neck. When screens are too high or too low, the eyes must work harder to focus, exacerbating strain and discomfort. Ensuring that the lighting in your environment is adequate also helps reduce glare from the screen, which can worsen digital eye strain.

For those who spend extended periods in front of screens, blue light-blocking glasses can be an effective solution. These glasses filter out the harmful blue light that can interfere with sleep patterns and cause additional strain on the eyes. Blue light exposure, especially in the evening, can disrupt the body's natural circadian rhythm by suppressing the production of melatonin, a hormone that regulates sleep. By wearing blue light-blocking glasses, particularly in the hours leading up to bedtime, individuals can protect their eyes from the negative effects of blue light while also improving their sleep quality.

Another practical step is to reduce screen brightness or switch to "night mode" on devices, which minimizes blue light emission and helps ease the strain on the eyes. This feature is especially useful for those who work in low-light environments or use screens extensively during evening hours.

Chapter 5: 12 Natural Remedies and Recipes for Eye Health

The appendix provides more details for each remedy.

1. Bilberry Tea

2. Eyebright Eye Wash

3. Ginkgo Biloba Supplement

4. Carrot and Spinach Juice

5. Chamomile Eye Compress

6. Flaxseed Oil Supplement

7. Blueberry Smoothie

8. Palming Exercise

9. Lutein Salad

10. Fennel Tea Eye Compress

11. Golden Milk with Turmeric

12. Warm Water Hydration

Part 21:
Dental Health –
Herbal Remedies for
Strong Teeth and
Gums

Chapter 1: Natural Oral Care for Strong Teeth and Healthy Gums

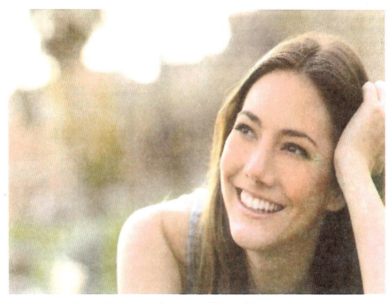

The Importance of Oral Hygiene for Overall Health

Maintaining good oral hygiene is essential not only for healthy teeth and gums but also for overall health. Strong oral health can help prevent systemic infections and support the immune system's ability to defend against disease.

Oral Health as a Reflection of Overall Well-Being

The condition of the mouth is often a reflection of what is happening in the body as a whole. Issues like gum disease and tooth decay can be indicators of underlying health problems, such as nutritional deficiencies, chronic inflammation, or even systemic infections. When oral health is neglected, it can create an environment where harmful bacteria thrive. These bacteria can enter the bloodstream through the gums and spread throughout the body, contributing to conditions such as heart disease and respiratory infections.

The immune system is closely linked to oral health. The mouth serves as one of the primary entry points for pathogens, and a healthy oral environment helps prevent harmful microbes from gaining a foothold in the body. Conversely, poor oral hygiene can overwhelm the immune system, leaving it vulnerable to infections. Daily practices that support strong oral health, such as brushing and flossing, are therefore critical for maintaining the body's natural defenses.

Gum Disease and Its Impact on Systemic Health

Gum disease, also known as periodontal disease, is one of the most common consequences of poor oral hygiene. It begins as gingivitis, characterized by swollen and bleeding gums, and can progress into more serious forms that affect the bone and tissue supporting the teeth. If left untreated, gum disease can lead to tooth loss and may have far-reaching effects beyond the mouth.

There is growing evidence that chronic gum disease can contribute to systemic inflammation, which is a factor in many chronic diseases, including heart disease, diabetes, and rheumatoid arthritis. The bacteria associated with gum disease can enter the bloodstream through damaged gums, triggering an inflammatory response that affects the entire body. This systemic inflammation is thought to contribute to the buildup of plaque in the arteries, which increases the risk of cardiovascular problems.

Addressing gum disease early and maintaining good oral hygiene practices can prevent these complications and reduce the burden on the immune system.

The Role of Daily Oral Hygiene Practices

Good oral hygiene is built on simple, consistent daily practices. It is essential to brush your teeth twice a day to help get rid of food particles and plaque, which can cause gum disease and cavities. Barbara O'Neill stresses the importance of using natural toothpaste without harsh chemicals or additives that could irritate the gums or disrupt the balance of good bacteria in the mouth. Natural ingredients such as baking soda and essential oils can effectively clean the teeth while promoting a healthy oral environment.

Chapter 2: Herbal Remedies for Common Oral Health Issues

2.1 Herbal Mouthwashes and Toothpastes

Barbara O'Neill advocates for the use of natural ingredients in oral care, emphasizing the benefits of avoiding chemicals commonly found in commercial toothpaste and mouthwash. She recommends simple, homemade solutions using ingredients that are both effective and gentle on the body, while promoting overall oral health.

Baking Soda for Alkalizing the Mouth

Baking soda, or sodium bicarbonate, is one of the key ingredients O'Neill suggests for maintaining a healthy oral environment. Baking soda is a natural alkalizer, helping to neutralize acids in the mouth that can lead to tooth decay and gum disease. By maintaining a more alkaline environment, harmful bacteria are less likely to thrive, reducing the risk of cavities and infections. Additionally, baking soda is mildly abrasive, making it an effective agent for removing surface stains and plaque without damaging tooth enamel.

When incorporated into toothpaste or mouthwash, baking soda helps to cleanse the mouth and refresh breath. O'Neill often points out that its natural alkalizing properties are superior to many commercial products, which may contain artificial additives and harsh chemicals that disrupt the mouth's natural balance.

Essential Oils for Antibacterial Benefits

Essential oils are another important component in O'Neill's natural oral care recommendations. Tea tree oil and peppermint oil, in particular, are noted for their antibacterial and antimicrobial properties. Tea tree oil is known to fight off bacteria and fungi that contribute to gum disease and bad breath, while peppermint oil provides a refreshing flavor and helps kill harmful bacteria that can accumulate in the mouth.

O'Neill encourages the use of these essential oils in both mouthwash and toothpaste formulations to enhance oral hygiene naturally. Peppermint oil, with its cooling and soothing properties, also helps to relieve minor oral discomfort while leaving the mouth feeling clean and invigorated. Tea tree oil's potent antimicrobial properties make it ideal for combating the bacteria responsible for plaque buildup and gum infections.

A Simple Homemade Toothpaste Recipe

One of the simple recipes shared by O'Neill for homemade toothpaste includes coconut oil, baking soda, and peppermint essential oil. Coconut oil is a natural antibacterial and antifungal agent, which helps reduce the bacterial load in the mouth while also moisturizing the gums. When combined with baking soda, it creates a paste that can effectively clean the teeth and neutralize acids, making it a powerful yet gentle option for everyday oral care.

The recipe calls for mixing equal parts of coconut oil and baking soda, with a few drops of peppermint essential oil for flavor and added antibacterial benefits. This combination forms a smooth, gentle toothpaste that not only cleans the teeth but also supports overall gum health. Coconut oil's natural properties make it an excellent carrier for the other ingredients, ensuring that the mixture remains easy to use and provides thorough coverage when applied to the teeth.

2.2 Garlic and Clove for Toothaches

Garlic is renowned for its potent antibacterial properties and has been used for centuries as a natural remedy for a variety of ailments, including toothaches. This powerful herb contains allicin, a compound that acts as a natural antibiotic, helping to fight bacterial infections that can cause tooth pain. To use garlic for toothaches, the recommended method is to crush a clove of garlic and apply it directly to the affected area. The crushed garlic releases allicin, which penetrates the site of infection, reducing inflammation and killing harmful bacteria. While it may cause a temporary burning sensation, garlic's ability to reduce pain and prevent the spread of infection makes it an effective remedy for toothaches.

Clove oil is another natural remedy often recommended for tooth pain due to its analgesic and anti-inflammatory properties. Cloves contain eugenol, a compound known for its numbing effects and ability to reduce inflammation. When applied directly to the sore tooth or gum area, clove oil can provide fast pain relief.

A small amount of clove oil can be placed on a cotton ball or swab and gently dabbed onto the affected area. The eugenol in clove oil works by numbing the nerve endings, offering relief from the sharp, throbbing pain associated with toothaches. Additionally, its anti-inflammatory properties help reduce swelling and irritation in the surrounding gum tissue.

Both garlic and clove oil not only address the symptoms of a toothache but also tackle the underlying causes, such as bacterial infections or inflammation. These remedies can be used together or individually, depending on the severity of the pain and the specific needs of the individual. However, it's important to use them cautiously, especially with clove oil, as it can be quite strong and should not be applied in excessive amounts.

How to Use Garlic and Clove Oil for Toothaches

For immediate relief from a toothache, the following steps can be followed:

Garlic: Take a fresh clove of garlic, crush it to release the allicin, and apply it directly to the painful tooth or gum area. After a few minutes, remove it with some warm water and rinse your mouth. This can be repeated a few times a day until the pain subsides.

Clove Oil: Dip a cotton swab or cotton ball in clove oil and apply it to the affected tooth or gum. Leave it in place for a few minutes, then remove the cotton ball. Avoid swallowing the oil. This method can provide fast relief from pain and should be repeated as needed throughout the day.

In addition to its pain-relieving qualities, clove oil can also be diluted in a carrier oil, such as coconut or olive oil, and massaged into the gums to prevent future infections or reduce inflammation in the gum tissue. Combining these two natural remedies can create a synergistic effect, providing both immediate relief and long-term protection against oral health issues.

2.3 Aloe Vera for Gum Inflammation

Aloe vera, a well-known plant for its soothing and healing properties, has been traditionally used to treat a variety of skin and oral conditions. It is particularly effective in addressing gum inflammation and bleeding, conditions that are often caused by poor oral hygiene, bacterial infections, or chronic irritation. The gel from the aloe vera plant can be applied directly to the gums to reduce inflammation, ease discomfort, and promote tissue regeneration.

Soothing Gum Inflammation

Aloe vera gel is rich in anti-inflammatory compounds that help calm irritated tissues. When applied to inflamed gums, it works to reduce swelling and discomfort. The natural enzymes and antioxidants present in the gel, such as vitamins C and E, also assist in neutralizing harmful bacteria that may be contributing to the inflammation. In cases of gingivitis or early-stage periodontal disease, aloe vera can be a helpful addition to regular oral care routines by addressing the root causes of gum irritation.

The cooling sensation provided by the gel not only soothes the gums but also accelerates the healing process. As the inflammation subsides, the gums can begin to heal, and the tissue can regenerate. Regular application of aloe vera to the gums ensures that the inflammation remains under control and prevents further damage to the gum tissue.

Promoting Healing of Bleeding Gums

In addition to reducing inflammation, aloe vera is effective in treating bleeding gums. Bleeding often occurs when the gum tissue becomes fragile or damaged due to infection or irritation. Aloe vera's antimicrobial properties help fight off bacterial infections that may be causing the bleeding, while its healing properties strengthen the gums.

Aloe vera contains compounds such as glucomannan and gibberellins, which are known to promote collagen production. Collagen is essential for the repair and regeneration of damaged gum tissue. By enhancing collagen synthesis, aloe vera supports the rebuilding of healthy gum tissue, reducing the likelihood of further bleeding or irritation.

For individuals experiencing chronic gum bleeding, incorporating aloe vera into their oral care regimen can be an effective natural remedy. Whether used as a gel applied directly to the gums or as part of a mouth rinse, aloe vera's healing properties help restore the gums to their natural, healthy state.

Application of Aloe Vera Gel

To use aloe vera for gum inflammation, it is essential to apply the gel directly to the affected areas. The pure gel from the aloe vera leaf is the most effective form, free from additives or preservatives. A small amount of the gel can be gently massaged into the gums, focusing on areas where the inflammation or bleeding is most severe. For best results, this should be done after brushing and flossing, allowing the gel to penetrate the gum tissue without interference from food particles or plaque.

Regular use of aloe vera gel can prevent the recurrence of gum issues and promote overall oral health. While it is important to maintain proper dental hygiene practices, such as brushing twice a day and regular flossing, aloe vera provides an additional natural method to support gum health.

Chapter 3: Preventing Cavities and Gum Disease with Natural Remedies

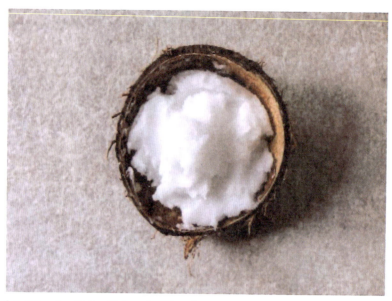

3.1 Oil Pulling for Detoxifying the Mouth

Oil pulling is a traditional Ayurvedic practice that has gained popularity for its ability to support oral health and detoxify the mouth. Barbara O'Neill emphasizes the importance of this technique as a natural method to cleanse the mouth of harmful bacteria, reduce plaque buildup, and prevent cavities. The practice involves swishing oil in the mouth for 15 to 20 minutes, which helps to "pull" out toxins and impurities that contribute to oral health issues such as gum disease and tooth decay.

One of the primary oils recommended for oil pulling is **cold-pressed coconut oil**. This oil is favored for its antibacterial, antiviral, and antifungal properties, which make it particularly effective at targeting the harmful microorganisms in the mouth. The lauric acid found in coconut oil is especially potent in killing off bacteria like *Streptococcus mutans*, a significant contributor to tooth decay and plaque formation. By swishing the oil around the mouth, these bacteria are trapped and expelled when the oil is spit out, preventing them from causing further damage to the teeth and gums.

Barbara advocates for making oil pulling a part of the daily routine, especially in the morning before eating or drinking anything. The process of oil pulling helps to clean the mouth and prepare it for the day by reducing the bacterial load and promoting a cleaner environment for the teeth and gums. Regular practice of oil pulling can lead to noticeable improvements in oral hygiene, including fresher breath, whiter teeth, and healthier gums. It is particularly beneficial for those dealing with early stages of gum disease or chronic bad breath, as it helps remove the bacteria that can cause these conditions.

The correct technique for oil pulling is to take about one tablespoon of cold-pressed coconut oil and swish it gently in the mouth for the recommended 15-20 minutes. It is essential not to swallow the oil, as it becomes laden with toxins and bacteria during the process. After swishing, the oil should be spit out, ideally into a trash bin rather than a sink, as the oil can solidify and clog pipes. Following the oil pulling session, rinsing the mouth with warm water and brushing the teeth as usual helps to ensure that any remaining residue is fully cleared away.

3.2 Green Tea for Reducing Gum Inflammation

Another natural remedy endorsed for oral health is **green tea**, known for its powerful antioxidant and anti-inflammatory properties. Green tea contains catechins, which are potent antioxidants that help reduce inflammation and fight bacterial growth in the mouth. This makes it an effective tool for preventing gum disease and promoting overall oral health.

The anti-inflammatory properties of green tea are particularly beneficial for those suffering from gum inflammation, a common precursor to more severe conditions such as gingivitis and periodontitis. Gum inflammation occurs when bacteria in the mouth accumulate around the gum line, leading to redness, swelling, and irritation. Over time, if left untreated, this inflammation can cause gums to recede and lead to tooth loss. Green tea helps to counteract this process by reducing bacterial activity and soothing the gums.

Drinking **green tea** daily is a simple yet effective way to incorporate its benefits into a regular oral care routine. It not only helps in maintaining healthy gums but also contributes to fresher breath and overall improved oral hygiene. The catechins in green tea, particularly epigallocatechin gallate (EGCG), are known to inhibit the growth of harmful oral bacteria, such as *Porphyromonas gingivalis*, which is associated with gum disease. Additionally, green tea's natural fluoride content helps to strengthen tooth enamel, further protecting against decay.

Green tea also promotes a healthy balance in the oral microbiome by supporting the growth of beneficial bacteria while reducing the harmful varieties. This balance is crucial for maintaining a healthy environment in the mouth, as an imbalance in the oral microbiome can lead to various dental issues, including cavities and gum disease. Regular consumption of green tea, either as a beverage or as an ingredient in oral care products, can significantly contribute to the health of teeth and gums over time.

For best results, it is recommended to drink at least one to two cups of unsweetened green tea daily. It is important to avoid adding sugar or sweeteners, as these can negate the beneficial effects and contribute to bacterial growth. In addition to drinking green tea, some may find benefit in using it as a mouth rinse. Steeping green tea and allowing it to cool can create a natural, antioxidant-rich mouthwash that can be used to rinse the mouth after meals or as part of a daily oral care routine.

Incorporating green tea into daily life can complement other oral hygiene practices, such as brushing, flossing, and oil pulling, to create a comprehensive approach to maintaining oral health.

Chapter 4: 14 Natural Remedies and Recipes for Dental Health

Baking Soda Toothpaste

Baking soda is a powerful yet gentle abrasive that helps whiten teeth and neutralize acids in the mouth, which can prevent cavities. To create a natural toothpaste, mix one teaspoon of baking soda with a few drops of peppermint essential oil and coconut oil. This combination not only cleans the teeth but also helps reduce harmful bacteria that can cause tooth decay and gum disease. Use this paste two to three times a week to avoid over-abrasion of the enamel.

Oil Pulling with Coconut Oil

Oil pulling is an ancient practice that helps detoxify the mouth and reduce plaque buildup. Coconut oil, in particular, has antimicrobial properties that help kill harmful bacteria in the mouth. To perform oil pulling, swish one tablespoon of coconut oil in your mouth for 15-20 minutes daily, preferably in the morning before eating or drinking anything. Spit out the oil (never swallow it) and rinse your mouth with warm water afterward. This practice can be done daily to support overall oral hygiene and reduce plaque buildup over time.

Garlic Poultice for Toothache

Garlic contains allicin, a compound with potent antibacterial and anti-inflammatory properties. To alleviate a toothache, crush one garlic clove and apply it directly to the sore tooth or gum area. The garlic may sting initially, but it can help reduce pain and fight off infection. This remedy can be used as needed when tooth pain arises, though it is important to seek dental care for persistent or severe toothaches.

Clove Oil for Toothache

Clove oil is known for its numbing and anti-inflammatory effects, making it an excellent remedy for toothaches and gum inflammation. To use, apply one or two drops of clove oil directly to the affected tooth or gums using a cotton swab. Be sure to dilute the oil with a carrier oil, such as coconut or olive oil, to avoid irritation. This remedy can be applied up to three times a day to relieve pain and inflammation.

Aloe Vera Gel for Gum Health

Aloe vera is well known for its soothing properties, particularly when it comes to reducing inflammation and healing wounds. For gum health, apply fresh aloe vera gel directly to inflamed or bleeding gums. Gently massage the gel into the gums and leave it on for 10-15 minutes before rinsing with water. Use this remedy two to three times a week to help soothe gum irritation and reduce bleeding.

Herbal Mouthwash with Tea Tree Oil

Tea tree oil is a powerful antimicrobial agent that can help reduce bacteria in the mouth and freshen breath. To create an herbal mouthwash, mix one cup of water with a pinch of salt and 2-3 drops of tea tree oil. Swish the mixture in your mouth for 30 seconds to one minute before spitting it out. Use this mouthwash once a day for a natural way to combat bad breath and kill harmful bacteria in the mouth.

Green Tea Rinse

Green tea is rich in antioxidants and has natural anti-inflammatory properties, making it an effective rinse for reducing gum inflammation and fighting bacteria. Brew a cup of green tea and let it cool. Once cool, use the tea as a mouth rinse by swishing it in your mouth for 30 seconds to one minute. This can be done daily to support gum health and reduce the risk of gum disease.

Calcium-Rich Smoothie

Calcium is essential for maintaining strong teeth and supporting overall dental health. To ensure you're getting enough calcium, blend spinach, kale, and almond milk into a smoothie. Both spinach and kale are high in calcium, and almond milk is often fortified with calcium, making this smoothie a great addition to your daily routine. Drink this smoothie regularly, ideally once a day, to help maintain strong teeth and bones.

Turmeric Paste for Gum Inflammation

Turmeric is well known for its anti-inflammatory properties, making it an excellent remedy for inflamed gums. To create a turmeric paste, mix one teaspoon of turmeric powder with a few drops of water until a paste forms. Apply this paste directly to the gums and let it sit for 10-15 minutes before rinsing with water. This can be used two to three times a week to help reduce inflammation and promote gum healing.

Neem Powder Toothpaste

Neem is traditionally used for its antibacterial properties, making it an effective ingredient for preventing cavities and maintaining oral health. To create a natural toothpaste, mix one teaspoon of neem powder with water to form a paste. Use this paste to brush your teeth once a day, as neem can help fight bacteria and prevent plaque buildup.

Clove and Cinnamon Mouth Rinse

Clove and cinnamon are both antimicrobial spices that can help freshen breath and fight bacteria. To make a mouth rinse, simmer **five whole cloves** and **one cinnamon stick** in **two cups of water** for 10-15 minutes. Let the mixture cool, strain it, and use it as a mouth rinse. Swish the rinse in your mouth for **30 seconds**, then spit it out. Use this rinse **once daily** to promote oral health and reduce bad breath.

Sesame Oil for Oil Pulling

Similar to coconut oil, sesame oil can also be used for oil pulling. Swish **one tablespoon of sesame oil** in your mouth for **10-15 minutes** to reduce bacteria and support healthy teeth and gums. Spit the oil into a trash can and rinse your mouth with warm water. Sesame oil has been used in Ayurvedic practices for centuries and helps to strengthen the teeth and gums while reducing plaque buildup.

Sea Salt Rinse

Sea salt is a natural disinfectant that can help cleanse the mouth and promote healing of sore gums. Dissolve **one teaspoon of sea salt** in **a glass of warm water** and use it as a rinse. Swish the solution in your mouth for **30 seconds to one minute**, then spit it out. Use this rinse **two to three times a day** to soothe inflamed gums and cleanse the mouth. Sea salt helps reduce swelling and aids in healing minor infections or irritations in the gums.

Peppermint Tea Mouthwash

Peppermint tea is a soothing, refreshing option for a natural mouthwash. Brew **a cup of peppermint tea**, let it cool, and use it as a mouth rinse. Swish the tea in your mouth for **30 seconds to one minute**, then spit it out. Use this mouthwash **once or twice a day** to freshen breath and soothe gum inflammation. The menthol in peppermint provides a cooling sensation that helps reduce irritation in the gums while freshening breath.

Part 22:
Hair and Nail Health – Boosting Growth Naturally

Chapter 1: Nutrition and Hair Growth

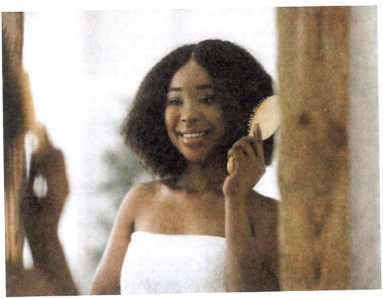

1.1 The Role of Nutrition in Healthy Hair and Nails

Hair and nail health is deeply connected to overall nutrition. Deficiencies in key vitamins and minerals can lead to visible issues, such as brittle nails or thinning hair. Ensuring the body receives the proper nutrients is essential for maintaining strength and promoting healthy growth in both hair and nails.

Nutrient-Dense Foods for Strong Hair and Nails

Incorporating a variety of nutrient-dense foods into the diet is essential for preventing deficiencies that can negatively impact hair and nails. **Almonds** are particularly beneficial, as they are rich in both biotin and vitamin E, which helps to protect hair and nails from oxidative damage. **Sunflower seeds** are another excellent source of vitamin E, along with zinc and other vital nutrients that contribute to the health of hair and nails.

Leafy greens, such as spinach and kale, are packed with vitamins A and C, as well as iron, which are essential for maintaining hair and nail health. Vitamin A helps in the production of sebum, a natural oil that keeps the scalp hydrated and hair nourished, while vitamin C aids in collagen production and protects hair and nails from damage. Iron supports the transport of oxygen to cells, which is crucial for hair growth and nail strength.

In addition, **whole grains** like oats and quinoa provide a steady supply of silica, zinc, and B vitamins, all of which are vital for the growth and maintenance of healthy hair and nails. These grains also offer a good source of energy, ensuring the body has the resources needed to support cellular repair and regeneration.

1.2 Omega-3 Fatty Acids for Hair and Scalp Health

For the purpose of encouraging hair development and preserving a healthy scalp, omega-3 fatty acids are essential. Found abundantly in flaxseeds and walnuts, these essential fats provide the nourishment necessary for both the hair and scalp to thrive. They are known for their anti-inflammatory properties, which help to reduce scalp inflammation—a condition that can contribute to hair thinning and loss.

Inflammation of the scalp can often be a precursor to hair thinning or more serious hair loss conditions. The presence of omega-3s in the diet helps to combat this by addressing the underlying inflammation. Omega-3s work to hydrate the scalp from within, ensuring that the hair follicles are adequately nourished and supported in their natural growth cycle. Without proper nourishment, hair can become dry, brittle, and prone to breakage, but incorporating sources of omega-3 into daily meals can alleviate these issues and contribute to stronger, healthier hair.

Flaxseeds are a particularly rich source of omega-3 fatty acids, especially in the form of alpha-linolenic acid (ALA), which is converted by the body into more active forms like EPA and DHA. These fats are essential for maintaining the lipid layer of the scalp, which helps to keep moisture locked in and the scalp well-hydrated. A well-hydrated scalp is less likely to suffer from common issues like dandruff, itchiness, or excessive oil production, all of which can negatively affect hair health.

Similarly, walnuts are another excellent source of omega-3 fatty acids, as well as other beneficial nutrients like biotin and vitamin E. These nutrients work in tandem with omega-3s to enhance the strength and shine of the hair, while also promoting a healthy scalp environment that supports sustained hair growth. By regularly consuming these foods, individuals can ensure that their hair remains nourished from the inside out, reducing the likelihood of breakage or thinning.

Brittle, cracked, or peeling nails are often a sign of nutrient deficiency, and omega-3s can help to address this issue. These essential fats work by improving the moisture content of the nails, which prevents them from becoming dry and prone to splitting. Omega-3s also reduce inflammation around the nail bed, promoting better nail growth and strength.

In the same way that omega-3s nourish the scalp, they also support the health of the cuticles and the skin around the nails. This can prevent conditions like hangnails and promote smoother, stronger nails that are less likely to break or crack. Regular consumption of foods rich in omega-3s ensures that the nails are fortified from within, making them more resilient and healthy over time.

In summary, omega-3 fatty acids found in foods like flaxseeds and walnuts offer a multitude of benefits for both hair and nail health. These essential fats work to reduce inflammation, nourish the hair and scalp, and promote stronger, healthier nails, making them a key component of a balanced diet aimed at enhancing overall beauty and wellness.

Chapter 2: Herbal Remedies for Strengthening Hair and Nails

2.1 Horsetail for Silica Support

Horsetail is a powerful herb known for its high silica content, which plays a crucial role in promoting the health of hair and nails. Silica is a vital mineral responsible for the formation of collagen, a structural protein that is essential for maintaining the strength and elasticity of various tissues in the body, including hair, skin, and nails. Collagen provides the support needed for healthy hair and nail growth, ensuring that these structures remain strong and resilient against damage.

Regular consumption of horsetail can help replenish the body's silica levels, which may become depleted due to poor diet, aging, or other factors. Silica supports the natural repair and regeneration processes within the body, helping to improve the texture and strength of hair and nails. This mineral also aids in the formation of keratin, the protein that makes up the outer layer of hair and nails, further contributing to their robustness.

Horsetail can be used in several forms to boost silica intake. One of the most common ways is by consuming horsetail as a tea. The tea is made by steeping dried horsetail leaves in hot water, allowing the beneficial compounds to infuse into the liquid. Drinking horsetail tea regularly provides a steady supply of silica, supporting the body's natural processes of strengthening and rejuvenating hair and nails.

For those seeking a more concentrated source of silica, horsetail is also available in supplement form. These supplements contain extracts of the herb that are rich in silica, making it easier to achieve higher doses of the mineral for individuals looking to accelerate the improvement of hair and nail health. Barbara O'Neill advises integrating horsetail into one's routine, whether through tea or supplements, to ensure consistent support for hair and nail growth.

Apart from its role in hair and nail health, silica has additional benefits for the skin and bones. By supporting collagen production, silica contributes to maintaining skin elasticity and preventing the formation of wrinkles. In the case of bones, silica works alongside other minerals like calcium to strengthen bone density, making horsetail a well-rounded herb that benefits multiple systems within the body.

The effects of regular silica intake through horsetail can be observed in improved hair texture, increased elasticity, and reduced brittleness in nails. Hair may become less prone to breakage and split ends, while nails grow stronger, resisting common issues like chipping or cracking. This is particularly beneficial for individuals who have weak or thinning hair and nails, as silica directly addresses the structural weaknesses in these areas.

2.2 Rosemary for Hair Stimulation

Rosemary is a well-known herb in the realm of natural hair care, praised for its ability to stimulate hair growth and improve scalp health. The herb is widely used for its capacity to increase circulation to the scalp, which is crucial for delivering essential nutrients and oxygen to hair follicles. This enhanced blood flow stimulates hair follicles, encouraging the growth of stronger, healthier hair.

One of the primary ways to use rosemary for hair stimulation is through the application of rosemary oil. By massaging the oil into the scalp, the stimulating properties of rosemary enhance blood flow to the hair follicles, promoting hair growth and helping to prevent hair thinning. The oil can be left on the scalp for a period of time before rinsing, allowing the active compounds to penetrate deeply into the scalp and nourish the hair roots.

In addition to oil treatments, rosemary can also be used as a hair rinse. Rosemary tea, made by steeping rosemary leaves in hot water, can be used as a final rinse after shampooing and conditioning the hair. This practice not only promotes hair growth but also improves the overall health of the scalp, preventing issues such as dandruff and dryness. Rosemary's antifungal and antibacterial properties help to maintain a clean and healthy scalp environment, reducing the likelihood of scalp infections that can inhibit hair growth.

Rosemary's ability to prevent hair thinning makes it a versatile remedy for those experiencing hair loss or reduced hair density. The herb strengthens the hair shaft and reduces breakage, making it particularly beneficial for individuals dealing with fragile or brittle hair. Regular use of rosemary treatments can result in thicker, fuller hair, as the herb's properties support both the growth and maintenance of strong, healthy strands.

Additionally, rosemary helps to combat dandruff by reducing scalp flakiness and irritation. The herb's soothing properties calm the scalp and reduce inflammation, which is often a contributing factor to dandruff and other scalp conditions. This makes rosemary a valuable ingredient for maintaining overall scalp health, ensuring that the hair grows in an optimal environment.

For those looking to incorporate rosemary into their hair care routine, it can be used in combination with other natural ingredients to maximize its effects. Mixing rosemary oil with carrier oils such as coconut or jojoba oil can provide additional moisture to the scalp and hair, enhancing the overall health and appearance of the hair. Likewise, combining rosemary tea with other herbs like nettle or sage can create a more comprehensive hair rinse that addresses multiple aspects of hair and scalp health.

Overall, the regular use of rosemary as part of a hair care regimen can lead to noticeable improvements in hair growth, thickness, and scalp condition. Its ability to stimulate circulation and nourish hair follicles makes it an excellent natural remedy for individuals seeking to improve the health and vitality of their hair.

2.3 Nettle for Hair and Nail Strength

Nettle is a powerful herb recommended for its high mineral content, particularly iron, calcium, and silica. These nutrients are crucial for the health of hair and nails, as they play a significant role in strengthening the keratin structure of both. Keratin is the protein that forms the foundation of hair and nails, and its integrity is directly impacted by the availability of key minerals in the body.

Iron is essential for proper oxygen transport in the blood, and when the body has adequate iron levels, it ensures that hair follicles receive the necessary oxygen to support hair growth. Low iron levels, often seen in individuals with anemia or poor diet, can lead to hair thinning or even hair loss. Incorporating nettle into the diet can help prevent these issues, as nettle is known for its high iron content, making it a natural remedy for promoting strong, healthy hair.

In addition to iron, **calcium** is another critical mineral found in nettle. Calcium is not only important for bone health, but it also supports the structural integrity of nails. Brittle nails are often a sign of calcium deficiency, and regular consumption of nettle tea or supplements can help address this deficiency, making the nails more resilient and less prone to breakage.

Silica, a trace mineral found in abundance in nettle, is also essential for strengthening both hair and nails. It promotes collagen production, which helps maintain the elasticity and strength of hair strands and nail beds. Silica also supports the growth of new hair and nails, ensuring that they remain healthy and strong over time.

Incorporating **nettle tea** into the daily routine is an excellent way to absorb these essential minerals. Drinking a cup or two of nettle tea each day can help boost the body's mineral levels, supporting overall hair and nail health. Nettle can also be used topically. Applying nettle-infused oil directly to the scalp nourishes the hair follicles, while massaging the oil into the nails strengthens them from the outside.

Chapter 3: External Care and Treatment for Hair and Nail Health

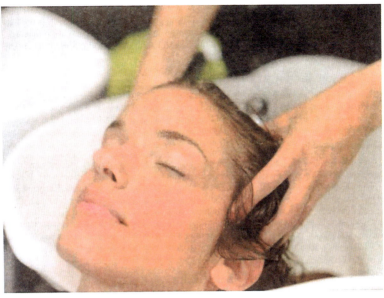

3.1 Scalp Massage and Oil Treatments

For hair health, it is essential to encourage blood flow to the scalp. Massaging the scalp regularly is one of the most effective ways to stimulate circulation, which in turn delivers essential nutrients and oxygen to the hair follicles. Healthy follicles are crucial for the growth and strength of hair.

Barbara O'Neill emphasizes the importance of daily or weekly scalp massages to ensure that the hair follicles remain nourished and active. Scalp massage not only stimulates blood flow but also helps remove dead skin cells and excess oil, creating a cleaner environment for hair growth.

Natural oils like **coconut oil** and **olive oil** are excellent bases for scalp massage. Both oils are rich in nutrients that hydrate and nourish the scalp. Because it can deeply condition hair by into the shaft, coconut oil is especially advantageous. This helps to reduce protein loss from hair strands, making them stronger and less prone to breakage.

Olive oil is another highly recommended oil for scalp treatments. Rich in antioxidants, olive oil helps to fight free radical damage on the scalp and hair follicles. It also contains vitamin E, which supports hair growth by promoting healthy blood circulation. Regular use of olive oil on the scalp helps prevent dryness, which can often lead to itching and dandruff—conditions that can inhibit hair growth if left untreated.

For an enhanced effect, adding **essential oils** to the base oil can further boost the benefits of scalp massage. **Lavender essential oil** is known for its calming properties, but it is also highly effective in promoting hair growth. Studies suggest that lavender oil can increase the number of hair follicles, thus enhancing hair density. It is also effective in soothing the scalp, reducing inflammation, and providing relief from itchiness or irritation.

Peppermint essential oil is another powerful addition to scalp treatments. Its cooling sensation stimulates the scalp and improves blood flow, which is crucial for delivering nutrients to hair follicles. Peppermint oil also has antimicrobial properties, which help keep the scalp clean and free from infections that could otherwise impede hair growth.

When massaging the scalp, it is recommended to gently warm the oil mixture before application. Warming the oil allows it to penetrate the skin more effectively, providing deeper nourishment to the hair follicles. Using gentle, circular motions during the massage encourages blood flow and helps distribute the oils evenly across the scalp.

By incorporating scalp massages with nutrient-rich oils and essential oils, one can significantly improve the condition of the scalp and hair. The combined effect of stimulating circulation and providing the hair follicles with essential nutrients ensures that the hair grows stronger and healthier. Regular scalp massage not only promotes hair growth but also helps to maintain the overall health of the scalp, preventing conditions like dandruff and dryness.

3.2 Natural Remedies for Brittle Nails

Brittle nails are often an indication of underlying issues such as mineral deficiencies or dehydration. They can become weak, prone to splitting, and lack flexibility, especially when the body is not receiving the necessary nutrients for optimal nail health. Environmental factors, such as cold or dry weather, can also exacerbate the problem, making it essential to take preventive measures.

Mineral Deficiencies and Hydration

When it comes to brittle nails, one of the primary causes is a deficiency in key minerals such as calcium, magnesium, and silica. These minerals are crucial for maintaining strong and flexible nails. When the body lacks sufficient levels of these nutrients, nails can become dry and prone to breakage. Ensuring an adequate intake of mineral-rich foods is essential for reversing this condition. Foods such as leafy greens, almonds, and seeds are excellent sources of magnesium and calcium, which contribute to overall nail health.

Hydration is another important factor in maintaining healthy nails. When the body is dehydrated, nails can become brittle and lose their natural flexibility. Drinking plenty of water throughout the day helps to hydrate the body from within, which in turn supports nail strength. For individuals who struggle with dry nails, ensuring proper hydration is a simple yet effective remedy.

The Benefits of Oils for Nail and Cuticle Health

Applying oils directly to the nails and cuticles is a natural and effective way to improve nail strength and flexibility. Oils such as castor oil and almond oil are particularly beneficial due to their nourishing and moisturizing properties. Castor oil, which is rich in fatty acids, helps to promote healthy nail growth while improving flexibility, reducing the likelihood of nails splitting or breaking. Applying a small amount of castor oil to the nails and cuticles regularly can also help protect them from environmental damage.

Almond oil is another excellent choice for nail and cuticle care. It is rich in vitamins, including vitamin E, which is known for its ability to hydrate and repair damaged skin and nails. Regularly massaging almond oil into the nails and cuticles can help to lock in moisture and prevent dryness, especially during colder months when the air tends to be drier. This practice not only strengthens the nails but also promotes healthier cuticle tissue, which is important for overall nail integrity.

Moisturizing and Protecting the Nails

In addition to using oils, regularly moisturizing the nails and cuticles is essential for preventing splitting and breakage. Exposure to cold or dry weather can cause nails to lose moisture, leading to brittleness. Applying a moisturizer or oil to the nails and cuticles on a daily basis creates a protective barrier that helps retain moisture and prevent further damage. This is particularly important for individuals who live in climates with harsh winters, where the cold air can quickly dry out the skin and nails.

Wearing gloves during outdoor activities in cold weather can also help protect the nails from environmental damage. For those who frequently work with water or chemicals, such as cleaning agents, wearing protective gloves is advisable to prevent further dehydration and weakening of the nails.

Chapter 4: 11 Natural Remedies and Recipes for Hair and Nail Health

The appendix provides more details for each remedy.

1. Horsetail Tea
2. Rosemary Oil Scalp Massage
3. Nettle Tea
4. Flaxseed Smoothie
5. Castor Oil Nail Treatment
6. Lavender Oil Hair Treatment
7. Biotin Supplement
8. Aloe Vera Hair Mask
9. Peppermint Oil Scalp Treatment
10. Silica-Rich Hair Rinse
11. Almond Oil Cuticle Massage

Part 23:
Managing Allergies Naturally

Chapter 1: Understanding Allergies and Their Triggers

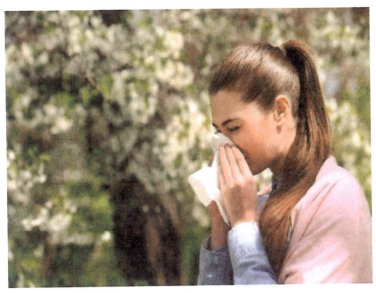

1.1 The Body's Immune Response to Allergens

Barbara O'Neill explains that allergies are a result of an overactive immune system. When the body encounters certain substances like pollen, dust, pet dander, or specific foods, it can mistakenly identify these as harmful invaders, triggering an immune response. This reaction involves the release of histamines and other chemicals in the body that cause symptoms such as itching, swelling, sneezing, and difficulty breathing. The immune system's hyper-reactivity in these situations is at the core of allergic reactions, and managing this overactive response is critical to alleviating symptoms.

Inflammation and Allergic Reactions

At the root of allergic reactions lies inflammation. When the body senses an allergen, it responds by creating inflammation to protect itself, even though the perceived threat is not inherently harmful. This inflammation leads to many of the uncomfortable symptoms associated with allergies, such as runny nose, skin rashes, and respiratory issues. O'Neill stresses that controlling inflammation is the key to reducing allergic responses. When inflammation is well-managed, the immune system is less likely to overreact to harmless substances.

Environmental Factors and Allergies

Environmental factors play a significant role in exacerbating allergic reactions. Exposure to pollutants, chemicals, and toxins can burden the immune system, making it more susceptible to overreacting when exposed to allergens. Pollen from trees and flowers, dust mites, mold, and household cleaning chemicals are common environmental triggers that can increase the likelihood of an allergic response. These irritants cause the body's immune system to be constantly on alert, weakening its ability to distinguish between true threats and harmless substances.

Barbara emphasizes the importance of reducing exposure to environmental toxins to manage allergies. This can involve using natural, non-toxic cleaning products, avoiding areas with heavy air pollution, and ensuring good ventilation in the home to prevent mold growth. Additionally, purifying the air in living spaces and maintaining a clean, dust-free environment can help reduce exposure to allergens like dust mites and pet dander. By limiting these external triggers, the immune system is less likely to become overwhelmed, helping to reduce allergic reactions.

Toxin Exposure and Allergies

Toxins from both the environment and food sources can weaken the immune system and contribute to allergic reactions. Exposure to heavy metals, pesticides, and pollutants places a significant burden on the body, as it must work harder to detoxify itself. This constant effort to eliminate toxins can deplete the immune system, making it more likely to overreact to allergens. The liver, which is responsible for detoxification, plays a critical role in filtering out harmful substances, but when it is overloaded, it cannot perform its functions effectively, leading to a buildup of toxins in the body.

To alleviate the strain on the immune system and manage allergies, it is important to reduce toxin exposure. This includes choosing organic foods to avoid pesticides, drinking filtered water, and avoiding plastic containers that may leach chemicals. Additionally, supporting liver function through detoxifying herbs such as dandelion and milk thistle can help the body process toxins more efficiently. By reducing the overall toxic burden on the body, the immune system can function more effectively, reducing the frequency and severity of allergic reactions.

1.2 Common Allergy Symptoms and Their Impact on Health

Allergies manifest in a variety of symptoms that can significantly affect daily life. Sneezing, itchy eyes, nasal congestion, and skin irritations are common reactions that occur when the immune system encounters an allergen. These symptoms are primarily the result of the body's release of histamines, a chemical that triggers inflammation and other immune responses aimed at neutralizing perceived threats. Histamines cause the blood vessels to dilate, leading to swelling and irritation in the affected areas, which is why allergic reactions often involve redness, itchiness, and congestion.

Prolonged exposure to allergens without addressing the underlying causes can lead to chronic inflammation, which, over time, may damage respiratory health. When histamine levels remain elevated for extended periods, it not only worsens symptoms but can also place additional strain on the immune system. The body, constantly fighting off what it perceives as a threat, can become exhausted, leading to reduced immune resilience. In more severe cases, chronic exposure to allergens can exacerbate respiratory conditions like asthma or bronchitis, making it essential to address allergies before they evolve into more serious health concerns.

Allergic reactions are not limited to environmental triggers like pollen, dust, or pet dander. Food allergies can also produce a range of symptoms, from mild digestive discomfort to more severe reactions such as hives or difficulty breathing. Barbara O'Neill emphasizes the importance of recognizing how food sensitivities can lead to systemic inflammation, which affects the digestive tract and overall health. Certain common foods, including dairy, gluten, and nuts, are frequent culprits that trigger immune responses in sensitive individuals.

Addressing these allergies naturally is key to reducing the body's sensitivity to allergens and preventing the escalation of symptoms. One of the most effective ways to do this is by strengthening the immune system. A well-functioning immune system is better equipped to distinguish between harmful pathogens and benign substances, reducing the likelihood of overreacting to allergens. Strengthening the immune system involves adopting a diet rich in nutrient-dense foods, particularly those that contain vitamins and minerals known to support immune health. Foods high in vitamin C, such as citrus fruits, berries, and leafy greens, act as natural antihistamines by lowering the production of histamine in the body. Zinc-rich foods, including seeds, nuts, and legumes, help to bolster the immune response, allowing the body to better manage allergenic substances without triggering excessive inflammation.

In addition to dietary changes, herbs like stinging nettle and butterbur are well-known natural remedies that can reduce the severity of allergy symptoms. Stinging nettle contains compounds that help block histamine receptors, preventing the typical inflammatory response that accompanies allergic reactions. Butterbur has been used traditionally to treat hay fever and seasonal allergies due to its anti-inflammatory properties, which reduce swelling in the nasal passages and alleviate symptoms of congestion.

Managing allergies also involves reducing exposure to allergens in the environment. Simple practices like using air purifiers to filter out dust and pollen, regularly washing bedding, and keeping windows closed during high pollen seasons can greatly minimize exposure and, consequently, the frequency and severity of allergic reactions. Additionally, staying hydrated helps to thin mucus, making it easier for the body to expel allergens trapped in the nasal passages and airways. Drinking plenty of water and consuming hydrating foods such as cucumbers, melons, and other water-rich fruits and vegetables can support the body's natural detoxification processes, helping to flush out irritants.

Lifestyle factors also play an important role in managing allergies. Stress, for instance, can exacerbate allergic reactions by weakening the immune system. High-stress levels increase the body's production of cortisol, a hormone that, when elevated for prolonged periods, suppresses immune function and makes it harder for the body to manage allergic responses. Techniques such as meditation, deep breathing exercises, and yoga can help to lower stress levels, thus indirectly improving the body's ability to cope with allergens. Regular physical activity is also beneficial, as it promotes healthy circulation and helps to regulate immune function.

Lastly, probiotics are another key component in supporting immune health and managing allergies. The balance of gut flora plays a significant role in the body's immune response, and maintaining a healthy gut can help reduce the likelihood of allergic reactions. Probiotic-rich foods like yogurt, kefir, and fermented vegetables introduce beneficial bacteria into the gut, which can modulate the immune system and help reduce inflammation.

Chapter 2: Strengthening the Immune System to Combat Allergies

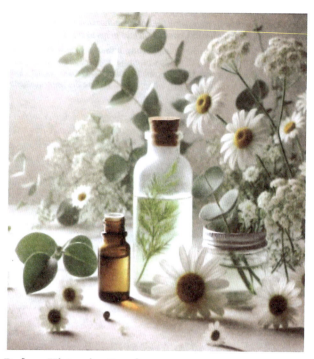

2.1 Herbs to Reduce Histamine Levels

Histamine reactions in the body, such as those experienced during allergy season, can cause discomfort, including sneezing, itching, and inflammation. To manage these reactions, Barbara O'Neill suggests turning to natural antihistamines, particularly nettle and quercetin. These natural remedies help reduce the body's histamine response and minimize the symptoms associated with allergic reactions.

Nettle (Urtica dioica) is a powerful herb known for its ability to reduce hay fever symptoms and other allergic reactions. It works by inhibiting the production of histamines, which are chemicals produced by the immune system in response to allergens. When histamine levels are too high, they cause inflammation and other allergy symptoms. Nettle helps to block this overproduction, making it an effective remedy for conditions like hay fever and allergic rhinitis. The best results come when nettle is used consistently, particularly during high-pollen seasons or other times when allergy symptoms are at their peak. Barbara suggests that incorporating nettle into one's daily routine during allergy season can help prevent the onset of severe symptoms.

Another natural antihistamine Barbara advocates is quercetin, a flavonoid found in common foods such as apples, onions, and tea. Quercetin has strong anti-inflammatory properties that make it highly effective in reducing allergic reactions. It works by stabilizing mast cells, which release histamines when exposed to allergens. By preventing the release of these histamines, quercetin helps to mitigate the severity of allergic responses, including sneezing, itching, and swelling. Quercetin is especially helpful for individuals who suffer from seasonal allergies, as it targets the immune system's response to pollen and other airborne allergens. It can be taken in supplement form or consumed through a diet rich in quercetin-containing foods.

Barbara emphasizes the importance of integrating these herbs into a daily regimen, especially during allergy season, to reduce the immune system's heightened response to allergens. Nettle can be consumed as a tea or taken in capsule form, while quercetin can be increased through the diet or with supplements. Using these natural antihistamines consistently allows the body to better cope with exposure to allergens without the harsh side effects that often accompany pharmaceutical antihistamines.

2.2 Vitamin C and Allergies

In addition to herbs like nettle and quercetin, vitamin C plays a crucial role in managing allergies. Vitamin C acts as both an antioxidant and a natural antihistamine, reducing the production of histamine in the body. By lowering histamine levels, vitamin C helps to prevent the inflammatory responses that are common during allergic reactions, making it an essential tool in managing seasonal and environmental allergies.

Vitamin C is well-known for its immune-boosting properties. It enhances the body's ability to fight off infections and respond to allergens by supporting the function of white blood cells, which play a key role in immune defense. For individuals dealing with allergies, maintaining adequate levels of vitamin C can help reduce the frequency and intensity of allergy symptoms. This is particularly important during allergy season, when the immune system is constantly challenged by airborne allergens like pollen, dust, and mold.

Foods rich in vitamin C include citrus fruits, such as oranges, lemons, and grapefruits, as well as vegetables like broccoli, bell peppers, and kale. Barbara recommends incorporating these foods into the diet regularly, especially during times of high allergen exposure. Not only do these foods provide vitamin C, but they also supply other nutrients that support overall immune health and reduce inflammation.

By combining the power of vitamin C with natural antihistamines like nettle and quercetin, individuals can create a robust defense against seasonal allergies. These natural remedies work synergistically to reduce histamine levels, support the immune system, and prevent the body from overreacting to allergens.

Chapter 3: Detoxifying the Body to Alleviate Allergies

The Connection Between Allergies and Toxins

Allergies are often a reflection of the body's internal environment, with a high toxin load being a significant contributing factor. Toxins from processed foods, chemicals, and environmental pollutants accumulate in the body, placing additional strain on the immune system. This toxin burden can exacerbate allergic reactions, making the body more sensitive to allergens that it might otherwise tolerate.

When the body is overwhelmed by toxins, the immune system becomes hyperactive, overreacting to otherwise harmless substances like pollen, dust, or certain foods. Barbara O'Neill explains that this heightened reactivity occurs because the immune system is already working overtime to deal with the internal toxin load, leaving it less capable of distinguishing between real threats and benign particles. As a result, the body mounts an inflammatory response, leading to the typical symptoms of allergies, such as sneezing, itching, and respiratory issues.

One of the key organs involved in managing this toxin load is the liver, which plays a central role in detoxification. The liver processes and eliminates harmful substances from the body, but when it becomes overloaded with toxins from processed foods, alcohol, chemicals, and environmental pollutants, its function is compromised. This can lead to the accumulation of toxins in the bloodstream, further aggravating the immune system and making the body more reactive to allergens.

To address this, O'Neill advocates for the detoxification of the liver and kidneys, the organs primarily responsible for filtering and eliminating toxins. By supporting these organs, the body can more effectively process and expel harmful substances, thereby reducing the overall inflammatory response to allergens. One of the most effective ways to detoxify the liver is through the use of specific herbs known for their detoxifying properties. **Dandelion** and **milk thistle** are two herbs O'Neill recommends for this purpose. Dandelion is a potent liver tonic that helps stimulate bile production, aiding in the digestion and removal of fats and toxins from the body. Milk thistle, on the other hand, is renowned for its protective effects on liver cells, helping to regenerate damaged tissue and promote overall liver health.

By incorporating these herbs into a detoxification regimen, the liver is better able to perform its role in cleansing the body, which in turn reduces the burden on the immune system. When the liver and kidneys are functioning optimally, the body becomes less reactive to allergens, as it is no longer constantly on high alert due to toxin overload.

Chapter 4: Natural Remedies for Managing Seasonal Allergies

4.1 Herbal Teas and Tinctures for Relief

Herbal remedies are an integral part of natural approaches to alleviating respiratory discomfort, especially during allergy season. Certain herbs have long been used to soothe symptoms such as sneezing, nasal congestion, and irritation. Barbara O'Neill emphasizes the use of **chamomile, peppermint**, and **elderflower** in the form of teas for their ability to relieve the respiratory system and ease symptoms caused by allergens.

4.2 Essential Oils for Allergy Relief

Essential oils offer another natural approach to managing allergic reactions, particularly when it comes to relieving nasal congestion and reducing inflammation. Barbara recommends several essential oils, including **eucalyptus, lavender**, and **peppermint**, for their ability to open the airways and ease respiratory discomfort.

Eucalyptus oil is one of the most powerful natural decongestants available. When used in steam inhalation or a diffuser, eucalyptus oil works by opening the nasal passages and facilitating clearer breathing. The active compound in eucalyptus, cineole, helps to reduce inflammation in the sinuses, making it easier to expel mucus and breathe more comfortably. Eucalyptus is especially effective during high-pollen seasons when nasal congestion is at its worst. By adding a few drops of eucalyptus oil to hot water and inhaling the steam, individuals can experience immediate relief from sinus congestion.

Lavender oil is another essential oil with potent anti-inflammatory and calming effects. Lavender is known for its ability to relax both the mind and body, and when used for allergy relief, it can help soothe irritated respiratory tissues. Lavender oil can be diffused in the air to create a calming environment that reduces stress and inflammation caused by allergens. This oil is especially helpful for individuals who experience anxiety or restlessness due to their allergic symptoms, as it provides both respiratory and emotional relief.

Peppermint oil also plays a significant role in managing allergies naturally. Like eucalyptus, peppermint oil contains menthol, which has a cooling and soothing effect on the respiratory system. When used as a natural decongestant, peppermint oil helps to clear the nasal passages and reduce the discomfort associated with blocked sinuses. Peppermint oil can be diffused or used in a steam inhalation to provide fast relief from congestion during allergy season. It is particularly effective when combined with steam therapy, as the warm steam helps to open the airways, allowing the essential oils to penetrate more deeply into the respiratory system.

For a more targeted approach to sinus relief, Barbara suggests combining these essential oils with **steam therapy**. This method involves adding a few drops of the chosen essential oil, such as eucalyptus, lavender, or peppermint, to a bowl of hot water and then inhaling the steam. Steam therapy helps to open the sinuses, relieve nasal congestion, and reduce inflammation. This combination of essential oils and steam not only provides immediate relief from sinus pressure but also supports long-term respiratory health by reducing the buildup of allergens and mucus in the nasal passages.

Chapter 5: Managing Allergies with Natural Remedies and Recipes

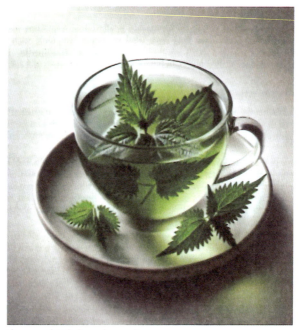

The appendix provides more details for each remedy.

1. Nettle Tea

2. Quercetin Supplement

3. Vitamin C Smoothie

4. Butterbur Tincture

5. Chamomile Tea Compress

6. Elderflower Tea

7. Eucalyptus Steam Inhalation

8. Peppermint Oil Inhalation

9. Apple Cider Vinegar Drink

10. Dandelion Root Tea

11. Milk Thistle Supplement

Part 24: Natural Pain Management and Reducing Inflammation

Chapter 1: Understanding Pain from a Holistic Perspective

1.1 The Body's Natural Pain Responses

Pain is a fundamental signal from the body, serving as a protective mechanism that alerts us when something is wrong. It is the body's way of drawing attention to an area that requires care and healing. Barbara O'Neill highlights the importance of understanding that pain, while uncomfortable, is not the enemy. Rather, it is a symptom that signals deeper underlying issues that need to be addressed.

Pain as a Protective Mechanism

The body's natural response to injury or dysfunction is often pain, which plays a crucial role in preventing further damage. Acute pain, for example, prompts us to remove ourselves from harmful stimuli, such as when touching something hot or sharp. This immediate response allows the body to protect itself from further harm. Pain also forces rest, giving the body the time it needs to heal. In many cases, when the source of the pain is addressed, the body is able to repair itself, and the pain subsides.

However, chronic pain is a different matter. Unlike acute pain, chronic pain persists long after the initial cause has been resolved. This type of pain can become a cycle of ongoing discomfort, often linked to unresolved inflammation or circulation problems in the affected area. It is this chronic pain that requires deeper exploration to identify its root causes, rather than just focusing on the symptoms.

Poor Circulation and Pain

Poor circulation is another common factor contributing to chronic pain. When blood flow to an area is restricted, the delivery of oxygen and nutrients to the cells is impaired, slowing down the healing process. This can result in ongoing pain, particularly in areas like the joints, muscles, and extremities. Inadequate circulation often leads to a buildup of metabolic waste in the tissues, which can cause pain and discomfort.

Focusing on the Underlying Causes

Rather than merely addressing pain symptoms with medication or temporary solutions, it is essential to identify and treat the underlying causes of pain. Inflammation and poor circulation are two major contributors to chronic pain, and they often stem from lifestyle factors that can be modified. By focusing on these root causes, it is possible to alleviate pain more effectively and support the body's natural ability to heal.

This approach aligns with the broader holistic view of health, which emphasizes prevention and long-term healing over symptom suppression.

1.2 Inflammation and Its Role in Chronic Pain

Chronic inflammation is widely recognized as a key factor in the development and persistence of many pain conditions, including arthritis, fibromyalgia, and autoimmune disorders. Inflammation is the body's natural response to injury or infection, but when it becomes chronic, it can lead to lasting damage to tissues, joints, and organs, contributing to prolonged pain and discomfort.

Chronic Inflammation and Tissue Damage

Inflammation plays a protective role in the body by helping to repair damaged tissues and fight infections. However, when inflammation becomes chronic, it ceases to be helpful and instead begins to harm the body. In the case of arthritis, for example, inflammation targets the joints, causing swelling, stiffness, and pain. Over time, this constant state of inflammation can erode cartilage, the protective tissue that cushions the ends of bones, resulting in more severe joint pain and reduced mobility.

In conditions like fibromyalgia and autoimmune disorders, chronic inflammation disrupts the body's ability to regulate its immune response. Instead of protecting the body, the immune system begins attacking healthy tissues, leading to widespread pain, fatigue, and other symptoms. As a result, individuals with these conditions experience ongoing pain, often without a clear external cause.

According to Barbara O'Neill, one of the most important steps in managing chronic pain is reducing the inflammation that underlies it. She explains that chronic inflammation is often fueled by poor lifestyle choices, particularly in diet. Certain foods can exacerbate inflammation, while others help to reduce it, making dietary adjustments essential for anyone suffering from chronic pain conditions.

Supporting a Pain-Free Lifestyle

In addition to incorporating anti-inflammatory herbs and dietary changes, lifestyle modifications can play a critical role in reducing chronic pain. Regular physical activity, especially gentle exercises like yoga and swimming, helps to improve circulation, reduce stiffness, and promote joint health. Managing stress is also essential, as stress hormones like cortisol can exacerbate inflammation and increase pain sensitivity.

Chapter 2: Herbal and Natural Remedies for Pain Relief

2.1 Turmeric for Inflammation

Turmeric has long been recognized for its potent anti-inflammatory properties, and it plays a crucial role in managing inflammation naturally. The active compound in turmeric, **curcumin**, is the primary element responsible for its therapeutic effects. Curcumin has been studied extensively for its ability to reduce inflammation in the body, making it an essential remedy for individuals suffering from conditions like arthritis, where chronic inflammation leads to joint pain and stiffness.

Curcumin works by targeting specific pathways in the body that regulate the inflammatory response. It inhibits enzymes like **cyclooxygenase-2 (COX-2)**, which are responsible for promoting inflammation. This is similar to the action of many non-steroidal anti-inflammatory drugs (NSAIDs), but without the side effects that are often associated with long-term medication use. Curcumin also reduces levels of **tumor necrosis factor-alpha (TNF-α)**, a pro-inflammatory molecule that plays a role in many autoimmune and inflammatory conditions.

For individuals dealing with **arthritis**, curcumin can be especially beneficial. Arthritis, whether rheumatoid or osteoarthritis, is characterized by persistent inflammation in the joints, leading to pain, swelling, and reduced mobility. Research shows that curcumin helps alleviate these symptoms by reducing inflammation at the source, allowing for better joint function and less discomfort. Incorporating turmeric into meals, such as adding it to soups, stews, or smoothies, is a practical way to reap its benefits. Additionally, curcumin supplements offer a more concentrated form of this powerful compound for those needing higher doses to manage chronic conditions.

2.2 Ginger as a Natural Anti-Inflammatory

Another natural remedy for inflammation that Barbara frequently mentions is **ginger**. Ginger has been used for centuries in traditional medicine for its ability to reduce pain and inflammation. The active compounds in ginger, particularly **gingerols** and **shogaols**, are known to block certain inflammatory markers in the body, much like curcumin in turmeric.

Ginger's effectiveness lies in its ability to inhibit pro-inflammatory cytokines, which are molecules that signal the immune system to promote inflammation. By reducing the production of these cytokines, ginger helps to lower the inflammatory response in the body. This makes ginger particularly effective for **joint pain** and **muscle soreness**, two common complaints associated with chronic inflammation.

To incorporate ginger into the diet, fresh ginger root can be added to teas, smoothies, or stir-fries. For those who prefer a more concentrated form, ginger supplements are widely available and provide a convenient way to ensure regular intake. Like turmeric, ginger can be easily integrated into daily routines for ongoing support in managing inflammation.

Both turmeric and ginger offer powerful, natural solutions for reducing inflammation and managing chronic pain. By incorporating these herbs into daily life, either through food or supplements, individuals can experience relief from inflammation-related symptoms and support their body's natural healing processes.

2.3 White Willow Bark for Headaches and Muscle Pain

White willow bark has been used for centuries as a natural remedy for pain relief. Often referred to as "nature's aspirin," its effectiveness stems from its high content of **salicin**, a compound that the body converts into salicylic acid, which is closely related to the active ingredient in aspirin. Unlike synthetic aspirin, however, white willow bark is gentler on the stomach, making it a preferred choice for those seeking natural pain management without the harsh side effects of pharmaceutical alternatives.

For headaches, white willow bark works by reducing inflammation and easing the pressure that can cause pain. It is especially useful for tension headaches, which often result from stress or muscle tightness in the neck and shoulders. By addressing both the inflammation and muscle soreness, white willow bark provides a comprehensive approach to headache relief. Barbara O'Neill advises using **white willow bark tea** or

tincture as an effective method for managing these symptoms. When consumed as a tea, the body absorbs the salicin gradually, offering a steady and prolonged relief from pain.

In cases of **muscle soreness**, such as those following strenuous physical activity or injury, white willow bark serves as an anti-inflammatory agent, helping to reduce the swelling that contributes to pain. Muscle pain is often caused by tiny tears in the muscle fibers, which leads to inflammation. White willow bark, by reducing this inflammation, accelerates the healing process, allowing the body to recover faster from the injury or strain. Barbara recommends using a tincture for more targeted relief, especially when muscle pain is persistent or widespread.

Another area where white willow bark is highly beneficial is in the treatment of **menstrual cramps**. Menstrual cramps are caused by the contraction of the uterus, which is often accompanied by inflammation. The anti-inflammatory properties of white willow bark help alleviate this discomfort by targeting the root cause. Additionally, its pain-relieving qualities help reduce the overall sensation of cramping, making it a natural alternative to over-the-counter pain medications commonly used for menstrual pain. The tea is a gentle option, offering soothing relief without the GI irritation that often accompanies conventional medicines.

Chapter 3: Natural Techniques for Pain Management

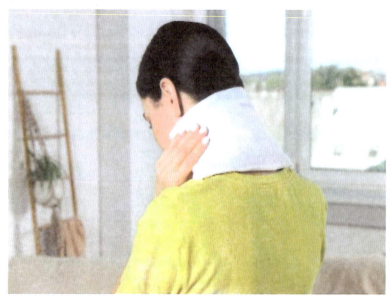

3.1 Heat and Cold Therapy

When it comes to managing pain from injuries or chronic conditions, the use of **heat and cold therapy** has long been recognized as an effective, non-invasive treatment. Barbara highlights the importance of alternating between these two forms of therapy to maximize pain relief and promote healing. By understanding the specific benefits of heat and cold therapy, individuals can tailor their approach to pain management based on their symptoms and the type of pain they are experiencing.

Heat therapy is particularly useful for relaxing muscles, improving circulation, and reducing stiffness in areas of the body that may be tense or tight. Applying heat to sore or stiff muscles increases blood flow to the area, bringing oxygen and nutrients that aid in the repair of damaged tissues. For those suffering from **chronic pain** conditions such as arthritis, where joint stiffness and muscle tightness are common, heat therapy provides a soothing effect that allows for greater mobility and comfort. Barbara suggests using **heat packs**, **warm towels**, or even soaking in a warm bath to target specific areas of discomfort. The key to effective heat therapy is to ensure that the warmth is applied at a comfortable level—too much heat can lead to burns or irritation, while mild warmth can offer deep relaxation and relief.

For **acute pain**, especially in the case of injury, **cold therapy** is an essential tool in reducing inflammation and numbing sharp pain. Cold works by constricting blood vessels, which helps reduce swelling and inflammation at the site of injury. It also has a numbing effect on the nerves, which can provide immediate relief from intense pain. Cold therapy is most effective when applied shortly after an injury occurs, as it helps to prevent further swelling and promotes faster recovery. Barbara recommends using **ice packs** or **cold compresses** for injuries such as sprains, strains, or acute muscle tears. However, cold therapy should not be applied directly to the skin to avoid frostbite—wrapping ice in a towel is an effective way to protect the skin while delivering the cooling effect.

Alternating between heat and cold therapy, known as **contrast therapy**, combines the benefits of both treatments and is particularly useful for **injury recovery**. By alternating heat and cold, the body experiences increased circulation during the heat phase, followed by reduced inflammation during the cold phase. This method helps to flush out toxins and waste products from the injured area, promoting faster healing and reducing pain more effectively than using heat or cold alone. Barbara advocates for this approach in cases of **muscle sprains**, **strains**, and **joint injuries**, where both stiffness and inflammation need to be addressed.

In addition to injuries, **heat and cold therapy** can also be beneficial for managing **chronic conditions** like **back pain** or **fibromyalgia**, where inflammation and muscle tightness are common complaints. By applying heat to relax muscles and cold to reduce inflammation, individuals can experience a greater range of motion and less discomfort in their daily activities.

3.2 Massage and Essential Oils

Massage therapy, when combined with essential oils, is an integral part of Barbara O'Neill's recommendations for pain relief and relaxation. Essential oils like lavender, peppermint, and eucalyptus play a key role in enhancing the therapeutic effects of massage by alleviating muscle tension, reducing inflammation, and calming the mind. These natural oils, when applied through gentle massage, can penetrate the skin and deliver their active compounds directly to the area of discomfort.

Lavender essential oil is widely known for its soothing and calming properties. When used in massage, it can help relax tense muscles and promote a sense of overall relaxation. Lavender is especially useful for individuals dealing with stress-induced pain, as its scent and active components help to reduce anxiety and induce calm, which in turn can lower the body's pain response. By encouraging the relaxation of both body and mind, lavender is particularly effective in easing chronic muscle tension that often accompanies stress or overexertion.

Peppermint oil is another key component of pain relief, particularly for headaches and sore muscles. It contains menthol, which has a cooling effect that helps to numb pain and soothe discomfort. O'Neill highlights the effectiveness of peppermint oil in treating tension headaches, especially when massaged onto the temples or neck. The oil's analgesic properties make it highly effective in reducing inflammation and relieving muscle pain. When applied during a massage, peppermint oil provides both immediate relief and long-term benefits by helping to reduce swelling in the muscles.

Eucalyptus oil, with its anti-inflammatory and analgesic properties, is ideal for easing muscle aches and joint pain. The oil's active compounds, such as cineole, help to reduce inflammation and improve circulation to the affected areas. When eucalyptus oil is combined with massage, it helps to relax the muscles and promote healing by enhancing blood flow. This makes it particularly useful for individuals suffering from conditions like arthritis or chronic muscle stiffness. Regular massages with eucalyptus oil can support the body's natural healing processes by reducing swelling and promoting mobility in affected joints.

Essential oils can also be mixed into carrier oils like almond or coconut oil to make them more suitable for massage. These carrier oils allow for smoother application and help prevent irritation, ensuring the essential oils are absorbed effectively into the skin. The combination of essential oils and massage not only targets pain at its source but also helps to activate the body's relaxation response, lowering stress levels and reducing the overall perception of pain.

3.3 Physical Activity and Movement

Maintaining an active lifestyle is one of the most effective ways to manage chronic pain, according to Barbara O'Neill. Physical activity helps to improve circulation, strengthen muscles, and promote flexibility, all of which are essential for preventing injury and reducing pain. Movement, even in the form of gentle exercises, encourages the release of endorphins, which are the body's natural pain relievers. For individuals dealing with chronic pain, regular physical activity helps to break the cycle of immobility and discomfort.

Overall, physical activity plays a crucial role in pain management by improving circulation, promoting flexibility, and reducing muscle tension. Incorporating exercises like walking, swimming, stretching, and yoga into a daily routine can greatly enhance one's ability to cope with chronic pain.

Chapter 4: Natural Remedies and Recipes for Pain Relief

Turmeric-Ginger Tea

Turmeric and ginger are two powerful anti-inflammatory herbs that work synergistically to relieve chronic pain. To prepare **Turmeric-Ginger Tea**, take 1 teaspoon of ground turmeric and 1 teaspoon of freshly grated ginger. Brew these in hot water for 10 minutes, then strain the mixture. This tea can be consumed once daily, particularly in the morning, to help reduce inflammation in the body. The active compound in turmeric, curcumin, has been shown to inhibit inflammatory markers, while ginger enhances the absorption of turmeric and provides its own anti-inflammatory benefits. Drinking this tea regularly can be especially helpful for conditions such as arthritis and joint pain.

White Willow Bark Tea

White willow bark has long been used as a natural remedy for pain due to its salicin content, which acts similarly to aspirin. To prepare **White Willow Bark Tea**, steep 1 to 2 teaspoons of dried white willow bark in boiling water for 10 minutes, then strain. This tea can be taken up to twice a day to alleviate headaches, muscle pain, and menstrual cramps. White willow bark is known for its effectiveness in reducing inflammation, making it an excellent option for those suffering from chronic pain conditions. However, it is important to avoid exceeding recommended doses as it can irritate the stomach in sensitive individuals.

Peppermint Oil Massage

Peppermint essential oil is widely recognized for its cooling, analgesic properties, making it effective for relieving muscle pain and headaches. For a **Peppermint Oil Massage**, mix 5 drops of peppermint essential oil with a tablespoon of carrier oil, such as coconut or olive oil. Gently massage the mixture onto sore muscles or apply it to the temples to reduce headache tension. This method can be used once or twice a day as needed. The menthol in peppermint oil increases blood flow and helps relax muscles, making it especially useful for tension headaches or muscle stiffness.

Lavender Oil Bath

Lavender essential oil has calming properties that make it ideal for reducing stress-related pain and tension. To prepare a **Lavender Oil Bath**, add 10-15 drops of lavender essential oil to a warm bath and soak for 20-30 minutes. This practice can be done 2-3 times a week, particularly after a long day or when experiencing muscle tension. Lavender helps soothe both the mind and body, reducing pain caused by stress and anxiety, and promoting relaxation. For individuals dealing with sleep-related muscle tension or migraines, this bath can provide significant relief.

Ginger Compress

Ginger is well known for its warming and anti-inflammatory properties. A **Ginger Compress** can be made by grating fresh ginger and placing it in a cloth or cheesecloth. The compress is then placed on sore joints or muscles for 20 minutes. This should be applied once or twice daily, particularly after physical activity or during flare-ups of joint pain. The heat from the ginger helps stimulate circulation and reduce inflammation, making it a natural remedy for arthritis, muscle pain, or other inflammatory conditions.

Turmeric Golden Milk

Another effective use of turmeric for pain relief is in the form of **Turmeric Golden Milk**. To make this drink, mix 1 teaspoon of turmeric powder with 1 cup of almond milk. Add a pinch of black pepper to increase the bioavailability of curcumin, turmeric's active compound, and sweeten with honey if desired. Drink this soothing beverage before bed to help with inflammation, particularly for those with arthritis pain. This can be consumed daily, as it is a gentle and nourishing way to incorporate turmeric into the diet while benefiting from its anti-inflammatory properties.

Arnica Salve

Arnica is a traditional remedy used to reduce swelling and promote the healing of bruises and sprains. **Arnica Salve** can be applied directly to the affected area 2-3 times a day to help relieve pain and reduce inflammation. Its anti-inflammatory and circulation-boosting properties make it ideal for sore muscles, sprains, and even joint pain. Arnica works by stimulating the body's own healing response, making it a preferred natural remedy for those recovering from minor injuries or dealing with persistent muscle soreness.

Epsom Salt Bath

Epsom salts, rich in magnesium, are a well-known remedy for relieving muscle tension and reducing inflammation. For an **Epsom Salt Bath**, dissolve 2 cups of Epsom salts in a warm bath and soak for 20-30 minutes. This can be done up to three times a week, especially after strenuous physical activity or during periods of heightened muscle tension. Magnesium helps relax muscles and can be particularly beneficial for individuals dealing with chronic pain, fibromyalgia, or muscle cramps. The warm water also helps to increase circulation, promoting overall relaxation and pain relief.

Heat and Cold Therapy Packs

Heat and cold therapy is a simple yet effective way to manage both acute and chronic pain. **Heat Packs** can be applied to areas of tension or soreness to increase blood flow and relax muscles. Heat should be applied for 15-20 minutes, up to three times a day. **Cold Compresses** help reduce inflammation and numb acute pain, particularly after an injury. Apply cold for 10-15 minutes, then alternate with heat if needed. This combination therapy can be highly effective for managing joint pain, muscle strains, or back pain.

Chamomile Tea

Chamomile is well known for its muscle-relaxing properties, making it a gentle remedy for pain caused by stress and tension. Steep 1-2 tablespoons of dried chamomile flowers in boiling water for 5-10 minutes to prepare chamomile tea. Drink the tea up to twice daily, particularly in the evening, to help relax muscles and reduce stress-induced pain. Chamomile is particularly useful for relieving tension headaches, menstrual cramps, and digestive discomfort caused by stress.

Cayenne Pepper Salve

Cayenne pepper contains capsaicin, a compound known for its pain-relieving properties by blocking pain signals to the brain. To make a **Cayenne Pepper Salve**, mix 1 teaspoon of cayenne pepper powder with 1/4 cup of olive oil and 2 tablespoons of melted beeswax. Allow the mixture to cool before applying it to the skin. This salve can be used once or twice daily on areas of joint or muscle pain. The heat from the capsaicin stimulates circulation, helping to relieve pain, especially in cases of arthritis or muscle stiffness. It is important to avoid using the salve on broken skin, as the capsaicin can cause irritation.

Part 25:
Seasonal Health and
Herbal Support

Chapter 1: Adapting Health Routines to the Seasons

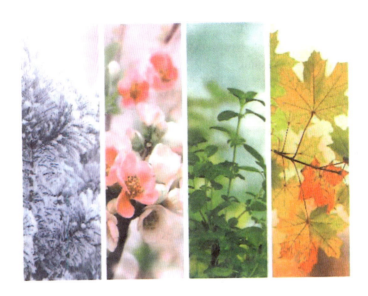

1.1 The Impact of Seasonal Changes on Health

Seasonal changes significantly impact the body's overall health, affecting everything from immune system function to energy levels and mood. Adjusting health practices in response to these changes can help maintain balance and vitality throughout the year. The body responds differently to each season, making it essential to modify dietary, physical, and lifestyle habits according to the time of year.

Winter: Cold Weather and Immune System Support

In colder months, the body is more susceptible to respiratory infections, as cold, dry air tends to dry out mucous membranes, weakening the immune system's ability to fend off pathogens. Warming foods and practices that boost immunity are particularly important during this season. This can include focusing on nutrient-dense, warming foods like soups and stews, which help maintain body temperature and provide essential vitamins and minerals that support immune function.

Warming herbs and spices such as ginger, garlic, and turmeric are also invaluable. They not only aid digestion but have natural anti-inflammatory properties, making them effective in reducing the risk of infection. Along with these, incorporating foods rich in vitamin C, such as citrus fruits and bell peppers, strengthens the immune system by enhancing the body's ability to fight off pathogens.

Barbara O'Neill emphasizes the importance of staying physically active, even in cold weather. Physical movement remains essential during winter to improve circulation and stimulate the lymphatic system, both of which are vital for detoxification. Despite the cold weather, light exercises such as stretching, indoor yoga, or brisk walks can support the body's ability to stay resilient against seasonal illnesses.

Spring: Detoxification and Renewal

Spring is a time of renewal, both for nature and the body. It's an ideal period for detoxification, as the body naturally begins to shed the excesses accumulated during the colder months. During this season, it's beneficial to incorporate lighter, cleansing foods into the diet, particularly those that support liver function. Leafy greens, dandelion, and artichokes are excellent for promoting detoxification and improving liver health. The liver is the primary organ responsible for filtering toxins, and supporting it during this time helps prepare the body for the warmer months ahead.

Engaging in physical activities that promote circulation and eliminate toxins through sweat, such as jogging or more vigorous forms of exercise, is beneficial in the spring. Additionally, maintaining hydration is crucial, as it aids in flushing toxins from the body and supports kidney function.

Summer: Hydration and Cooling

As the temperature rises during the summer, the body's need for hydration increases. The risk of dehydration is higher due to increased sweating, making it essential to focus on water intake and hydrating foods. Water-rich foods like cucumbers, watermelon, and leafy greens provide hydration while also helping to regulate body temperature.

Cooling herbs and teas, such as peppermint and hibiscus, help to reduce internal heat and maintain electrolyte balance. These herbs not only aid in digestion but also calm the nervous system, which can become overstimulated in hot weather. It's also recommended to avoid heavy, oily foods and instead focus on lighter meals that are easier to digest.

Physical activities such as swimming or light outdoor activities are excellent during summer, as they allow the body to stay active without overheating. Swimming, in particular, provides full-body exercise while keeping the body cool.

Fall: Preparation for the Colder Months

Autumn is a time of preparation, when the body naturally starts to build up its defenses for the colder months ahead. This is a good time to introduce more grounding and nutrient-dense foods, such as root vegetables and whole grains. These foods provide the body with the necessary nutrients to strengthen the immune system in anticipation of winter.

Herbs like astragalus and elderberry, known for their immune-boosting properties, can be incorporated into the diet during this season. These herbs help fortify the body against seasonal illnesses such as colds and flu, which often become more prevalent as the weather cools.

Moderate physical activity is also beneficial during fall. Activities like walking or hiking in cooler, crisp air can improve circulation and support the immune system without straining the body.

Adapting to Circadian Rhythms and Energy Levels

In addition to dietary and lifestyle changes, it is essential to pay attention to the body's circadian rhythms, which are influenced by seasonal changes in daylight. During winter, shorter days and longer nights can lead to decreased energy and mood fluctuations. It's natural for the body to require more rest during this time, making it important to prioritize sleep and create a calm evening routine that supports relaxation.

In contrast, the longer days of summer often increase energy levels, allowing for more outdoor activities and social engagements. However, it's important to balance this increased activity with adequate rest to avoid burnout.

1.2 Strengthening Immunity During the Cold and Flu Season

During the colder months, the immune system is particularly vulnerable to seasonal challenges, such as colds and the flu. To strengthen the body's natural defenses, it is essential to support the immune system through diet, lifestyle choices, and natural remedies. By increasing the intake of specific vitamins, avoiding foods that weaken the immune response, and incorporating herbs known for their immune-boosting properties, individuals can significantly enhance their body's ability to ward off infections.

The Role of Vitamin C in Immune Health

Vitamin C plays a crucial role in supporting the immune system, particularly during cold and flu season. It is known for its antioxidant properties, which help neutralize free radicals and protect cells from oxidative stress. This nutrient also enhances the production of white blood cells, which are essential for fighting infections.

During winter months, when the immune system faces heightened risks, increasing the intake of vitamin C-rich foods can help protect the body from illness.

Citrus fruits such as oranges, lemons, and grapefruits are some of the most well-known sources of vitamin C. Other excellent sources include bell peppers, strawberries, and broccoli. Incorporating these foods into the daily diet provides the body with the tools it needs to mount a strong defense against viruses and bacteria.

In addition to fresh fruits and vegetables, vitamin C supplementation may also be beneficial, especially for those with limited access to fresh produce during the winter. Ensuring adequate levels of this vital nutrient helps the body maintain a robust immune response during the months when colds and flu are most prevalent.

Echinacea and Elderberry: Herbal Immune Boosters

Herbs such as echinacea and elderberry have long been recognized for their immune-boosting properties. Echinacea is particularly well-known for its ability to stimulate the immune system, helping to increase the activity of white blood cells and reduce the duration of colds and flu symptoms. It is commonly used at the onset of a cold to reduce the severity of symptoms and support faster recovery.

Elderberry, another powerful herb, is rich in antioxidants and has been shown to enhance the immune system's ability to fight infections. It is often used as a preventative measure during the winter months and can also help alleviate symptoms if an infection occurs. Elderberry's antiviral properties are especially beneficial in protecting against influenza viruses.

You can take these two herbs in a variety of forms, including teas, tinctures, and capsules. Incorporating them into a daily health regimen during cold and flu season provides natural support for the body's defenses and helps prevent illness before it takes hold.

Avoiding Foods That Weaken Immunity

During flu season, it is essential to avoid foods that can weaken the immune system and increase susceptibility to infections. Processed foods, refined sugars, and unhealthy fats are some of the main culprits that compromise immune function. These foods contribute to inflammation in the body and place additional stress on the immune system, making it less capable of fighting off infections.

Refined sugar, in particular, has been shown to suppress the activity of white blood cells, which are essential for immune defense. Consuming high amounts of sugar can reduce the body's ability to respond effectively to pathogens, leaving it more vulnerable to infections such as colds and the flu. Replacing sugary snacks and processed foods with whole, nutrient-dense options supports immune health and reduces the risk of illness during the winter months.

A diet rich in fresh fruits, vegetables, whole grains, and healthy fats from sources such as nuts and seeds provides the body with the nutrients it needs to maintain a strong immune system. In addition to avoiding harmful foods, incorporating immune-boosting herbs and supplements further enhances the body's natural defenses.

Hydration and Immune Function

Staying hydrated is another key component of supporting the immune system during cold and flu season. Proper hydration helps the body flush out toxins and maintain healthy mucous membranes, which act as the first line of defense against pathogens entering the respiratory system. Drinking sufficient water throughout the day is essential for keeping the body's defenses strong.

Herbal teas, especially those made from immune-boosting herbs like ginger and turmeric, provide additional benefits while keeping the body hydrated. Ginger has natural anti-inflammatory properties, and turmeric is rich in antioxidants that help support the immune system. Sipping on these warming teas not only hydrates but also provides additional immune support during the colder months.

Chapter 2: Seasonal Superfoods for Health

21 Winter Superfoods

During the winter months, it is essential to focus on nutrient-dense foods that provide warmth and support the body in maintaining energy levels and immunity. Root vegetables such as sweet potatoes, carrots, and other seasonal produce play a significant role in nourishing the body during colder weather. These vegetables are rich in antioxidants, vitamins, and minerals, which help the body stay energized and fight off illness.

Sweet Potatoes

Sweet potatoes are a winter staple, offering a variety of health benefits. They are rich in beta-carotene, a powerful antioxidant that the body converts into vitamin A. Vitamin A plays a crucial role in supporting the immune system by enhancing the production and function of white blood cells, which fight infection. The high fiber content in sweet potatoes also aids digestion, which is particularly important during winter when the body's metabolism may slow down due to lower activity levels.

Sweet potatoes are also a good source of complex carbohydrates, providing sustained energy without spiking blood sugar levels. Their naturally sweet flavor makes them a versatile ingredient that can be used in both savory and sweet dishes, from soups and stews to baked goods.

Carrots and Other Root Vegetables

Carrots, like sweet potatoes, are rich in beta-carotene and provide similar immune-boosting properties. In addition to being an excellent source of vitamins A and C, carrots contain a variety of phytochemicals that help protect the body from oxidative stress. Winter weather can be harsh on the body, and consuming antioxidants helps mitigate the damage caused by free radicals, which are more prevalent during times of physical stress or illness.

Other root vegetables such as parsnips, beets, and turnips offer a range of nutrients that support overall health during the winter. Beets, for example, are known for their ability to improve circulation and support heart health, which can be particularly beneficial when colder temperatures may cause circulation to slow down.

Warming Spices

Along with root vegetables, spices play a significant role in winter nutrition. Warming spices such as cinnamon, ginger, and cloves are not only flavorful but also have medicinal properties that enhance circulation and immune function.

Cinnamon is a powerful antioxidant and has anti-inflammatory properties that can help reduce the risk of illness. It also helps regulate blood sugar levels, making it a useful spice for those trying to maintain energy levels during the winter months.

Ginger is well-known for its warming and digestive properties. It stimulates circulation, which is often sluggish in cold weather, and helps the body fight off infections by boosting the immune system. Additionally, ginger can alleviate digestive issues that may arise from heavier winter meals.

Cloves contain compounds that are highly effective in reducing inflammation and fighting infections. They also have antioxidant properties, helping the body detoxify and maintain health through the colder months.

Barbara O'Neill emphasizes the importance of incorporating these warming spices into meals, particularly in soups, teas, and baked goods, as they help the body maintain warmth and circulation, which are critical during cold weather.

2.2 Spring Superfoods

As winter gives way to spring, the body's nutritional needs shift. Spring is a time of renewal and detoxification, and incorporating fresh greens into the diet can help cleanse the body of toxins accumulated over the winter. Barbara O'Neill advises focusing on greens like spinach, kale, and dandelion leaves to support liver health and aid in the detoxification process.

Spinach

Spinach is a versatile green that is particularly beneficial during spring. It has high concentrations of important minerals like iron and magnesium, as well as vitamins A, C, and K. These nutrients are crucial for maintaining healthy blood and supporting the liver's detoxification processes. The high chlorophyll content in spinach helps remove heavy metals and toxins from the bloodstream, making it an ideal food for spring cleansing.

Spinach also supports digestive health due to its high fiber content, which promotes regular bowel movements and aids in the elimination of waste. As the body transitions from the heavier foods of winter, spinach helps to lighten the digestive load and prepare the body for the increased activity of spring.

Kale

Kale is another green that plays a significant role in spring detoxification. Like spinach, it is high in vitamins A, C, and K, but it also contains compounds called glucosinolates, which have been shown to help detoxify the liver. These compounds assist in neutralizing harmful substances that accumulate in the body, allowing the liver to process and eliminate them more efficiently.

Kale is also a rich source of calcium, which is essential for maintaining strong bones and teeth, especially as the body becomes more active during the spring months. Its high fiber content supports digestion, and its anti-inflammatory properties make it a valuable addition to a spring detox diet.

Dandelion Leaves

Dandelion leaves have long been used in traditional medicine for their powerful detoxifying properties. They are a natural diuretic, helping to flush excess water and toxins from the body. Dandelion leaves are particularly effective in supporting liver health, as they stimulate bile production, which is essential for breaking down fats and eliminating waste.

Rich in vitamins A, C, and K, as well as potassium, dandelion leaves help to replenish nutrients lost during the detoxification process. Incorporating dandelion leaves into salads, teas, or smoothies during the spring can provide the body with the necessary support to cleanse and rejuvenate itself after the winter months.

Supporting Liver Detoxification

The liver is the primary organ responsible for detoxifying the body, and supporting its function is key during the spring. In addition to consuming greens like spinach, kale, and dandelion leaves, it is beneficial to reduce the intake of processed foods and increase the consumption of whole, plant-based foods. This helps the liver focus on eliminating toxins rather than processing harmful substances found in processed foods.

Drinking plenty of water and herbal teas, such as dandelion or ginger tea, further supports the liver's detoxification processes by helping to flush out toxins. Staying hydrated is crucial, as it allows the liver and kidneys to work efficiently in eliminating waste from the body.

2.3 Summer Superfoods

In summer, it is crucial to focus on foods that help the body stay hydrated and cool. High temperatures can lead to dehydration, heat exhaustion, and sluggishness, making hydration a top priority. Barbara O'Neill suggests incorporating water-rich foods such as cucumbers, watermelon, and leafy greens into the diet to support overall hydration and maintain energy levels.

Cucumbers

Cucumbers are a quintessential summer food, containing over 90% water, which makes them highly effective at hydrating the body. They are also rich in essential vitamins such as vitamin K and various B vitamins, which support energy metabolism and help combat fatigue often experienced in hot weather. Cucumbers are known for their cooling properties, helping to lower body temperature naturally. In addition to hydration, cucumbers also contain anti-inflammatory compounds that support skin health, particularly during summer when the skin is more exposed to heat and sun.

Adding cucumbers to salads or smoothies is an easy way to ensure you are staying hydrated throughout the day. They are also excellent in infused water, which adds a refreshing twist to regular hydration routines.

Watermelon

Watermelon, another staple of summer, is not only a delicious and refreshing fruit but also an excellent source of hydration. Comprising around 92% water, watermelon is particularly effective at keeping the body cool and hydrated. Watermelon also contains electrolytes such as potassium, which help maintain fluid balance in the body. This is essential during hot weather when the body loses more fluids through sweat.

In addition to hydration, watermelon is rich in antioxidants like lycopene, which supports heart health and protects the skin from sun damage. Lycopene helps reduce oxidative stress, making watermelon an ideal food for combatting the effects of prolonged sun exposure.

Eating watermelon on its own as a snack or incorporating it into salads and juices can significantly boost hydration and provide essential nutrients during the summer.

Leafy Greens

Leafy greens such as spinach, lettuce, and arugula are excellent for keeping the body cool and energized. These greens are not only water-dense but also packed with vital nutrients like vitamins A, C, and K, which support immune function, skin health, and overall vitality. Leafy greens are light, making them easy to digest, which is especially important during the summer when the body's digestive capacity can be reduced due to heat.

Incorporating leafy greens into salads or smoothies helps maintain hydration and provides essential vitamins and minerals without burdening the digestive system. Their cooling effect also helps to regulate body temperature, making them ideal for hot summer days.

Peppermint and Hibiscus for Cooling

In addition to hydrating foods, certain herbs can help cool the body and refresh the mind during hot weather. **Peppermint** is particularly effective in reducing body heat due to its natural cooling properties. Peppermint contains menthol, which has a soothing effect on the body and helps reduce the perception of heat. Peppermint tea or infused water is an excellent way to stay hydrated while also benefiting from its cooling effects.

Hibiscus, another powerful cooling herb, is rich in antioxidants and helps reduce body temperature. Hibiscus tea, known for its tart and refreshing flavor, is often consumed cold in the summer to provide relief from the heat. It also supports hydration and is known for its ability to help regulate blood pressure, which can be affected by high temperatures. Drinking hibiscus tea throughout the day not only cools the body but also provides essential antioxidants that support overall health during the summer months.

2.4 Fall Superfoods

As the weather begins to cool and the body prepares for the upcoming winter, it is important to focus on foods that support digestion, immunity, and overall strength. Barbara recommends fiber-rich foods such as apples, pumpkins, and squashes, which help prepare the body for the colder months by boosting digestion and providing essential nutrients.

Apples

Apples are a quintessential fall food that offers numerous health benefits. They include a lot of dietary fiber, especially pectin, which promotes healthy blood sugar regulation and digestion. This is particularly important as the body transitions from lighter summer foods to the heartier meals typical of colder months.

In addition to their fiber content, apples are rich in antioxidants such as quercetin and vitamin C. These antioxidants help fortify the immune system, protecting the body from seasonal illnesses that often arise in the fall. Apples are also hydrating and can be eaten raw, cooked, or added to salads and desserts, making them a versatile food to include in the fall diet.

Pumpkins

Pumpkins are another nutrient-dense food that plays a vital role in fall nutrition. They are rich in beta-carotene, which the body converts into vitamin A, an essential nutrient for maintaining healthy skin, vision, and immune function. As the body faces colder weather, vitamin A becomes crucial in supporting the immune system and keeping the skin healthy, which can become dry and irritated in colder temperatures.

Pumpkins are also high in fiber, which supports digestive health. The fiber content helps to regulate bowel movements and promote a healthy gut microbiome, both of which are important as the body prepares for the rich, heavier foods consumed during winter. Pumpkin seeds, in particular, are an excellent source of magnesium, which supports muscle function and helps reduce stress, making them a valuable addition to fall meals.

Pumpkins can be roasted, pureed, or added to soups and stews, providing both nutrition and comfort as the temperatures begin to drop.

Squashes

Like pumpkins, squashes are rich in fiber and beta-carotene, providing many of the same health benefits. They help to keep the digestive system functioning smoothly, which is essential as the body adjusts to more substantial fall meals. Squashes are also packed with vitamins A and C, which support immune function and help the body fight off infections that are more common in the colder months.

Squashes are versatile and can be roasted, baked, or pureed into soups. Their sweet, earthy flavor pairs well with warming spices like cinnamon and nutmeg, making them a comforting and nutritious addition to fall dishes. Incorporating squashes into meals helps the body prepare for winter by boosting immunity and ensuring a healthy digestive system.

Part 26:
Sleep and
Restorative Health
with Herbal Support

Chapter 1: The Importance of Restorative Sleep for Overall Health

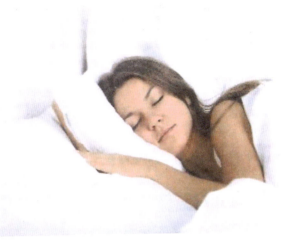

1.1 The Role of Sleep in Healing and Recovery

Sleep is a crucial aspect of the body's natural healing processes. The cells of the body regenerate at twice the rate during sleep, making restful and consistent sleep essential for tissue repair, immune function, and overall recovery. Adequate sleep allows the body to repair damage done throughout the day, whether from physical strain, exposure to pathogens, or emotional stress.

The Role of the Circadian Rhythm

Barbara O'Neill emphasizes the importance of maintaining a regular sleep routine to support the body's internal clock, also known as the circadian rhythm. This rhythm regulates various bodily functions, including the sleep-wake cycle, hormone production, and digestion. When this natural rhythm is disrupted by irregular sleep patterns or insufficient sleep, the body struggles to maintain its normal functions.

The pineal gland, located in the brain, releases melatonin during the night to promote restful sleep. This hormone plays a critical role in signaling the body that it is time to rest. When the circadian rhythm is disrupted, melatonin production can be suppressed, leading to difficulties falling asleep or staying asleep. Regular exposure to natural sunlight during the day and reduced exposure to artificial light in the evening can help regulate melatonin production, making it easier to maintain a healthy sleep-wake cycle.

The Impact of Sleep Deprivation

Chronic sleep deprivation can have a range of negative effects on the body and mind. Fatigue, reduced concentration, and a weakened immune system are among the most immediate consequences. Over time, insufficient sleep can contribute to the development of chronic conditions such as hypertension, diabetes, and cardiovascular diseases. These conditions are closely linked to prolonged periods of stress and inflammation, both of which are exacerbated by a lack of restorative sleep.

In terms of mental health, sleep deprivation is associated with increased anxiety, depression, and mood swings. The brain's inability to properly regulate emotions without sufficient sleep can lead to heightened stress levels, which in turn disrupt the body's ability to heal and recover. Thus, a regular and restorative sleep routine is essential not only for physical health but also for mental and emotional well-being.

Establishing Healthy Sleep Habits

Establishing a consistent sleep routine is essential for maintaining optimal health. This includes going to bed and waking up at the same time each day, even on weekends. Better sleep is encouraged and the circadian cycle is regulated with the support of consistency. Creating a relaxing bedtime routine, such as dimming lights, avoiding screens, and engaging in calming activities like reading or meditation, can signal to the body that it is time to wind down and prepare for sleep.

In addition, the timing and quality of meals can also affect sleep. Barbara O'Neill recommends having lighter meals in the evening to prevent digestive discomfort that can interfere with sleep. Heavier meals should be consumed earlier in the day, while the evening meal should focus on easily digestible foods. This allows the digestive system to rest and the body to focus on healing and recovery during sleep.

1.2 How Lack of Sleep Affects Hormones

Sleep is essential for maintaining hormonal balance, particularly regarding two critical hormones: cortisol and melatonin. A lack of sufficient sleep can disrupt these hormones, leading to significant negative effects on overall health, including weight gain, stress, and immune dysfunction. Barbara O'Neill explains how sleep deprivation can disturb the natural regulation of these hormones, particularly under chronic stress conditions.

Cortisol: The Stress Hormone

As covered in previous chapters, cortisol is referred to as the "stress hormone" and is released by the adrenal glands in response to physical or emotional stress. Cortisol levels are naturally higher in the morning and decrease throughout the day. However, when sleep is disrupted, this natural rhythm can be thrown off, causing cortisol levels to remain elevated. High cortisol levels can trigger the storage of fat, particularly around the abdominal area, as the body perceives a state of ongoing stress. This can lead to weight gain, particularly in people already prone to stress-related eating patterns.

Melatonin: The Sleep Hormone

Melatonin is another crucial hormone that directly impacts sleep. It is produced by the pineal gland in response to darkness, signaling the body that it is time to rest. Melatonin is not only essential for regulating the sleep-wake cycle, but it also plays a role in protecting the body from oxidative stress and supporting the immune system.

When sleep is disrupted, melatonin production is also affected, making it harder to fall asleep and stay asleep. Reduced melatonin levels can lead to insomnia or poor-quality sleep, perpetuating the cycle of hormonal imbalance. Melatonin is also linked to the regulation of other hormones, such as those that control reproductive functions and circadian rhythms.

Barbara O'Neill emphasizes the importance of creating an environment conducive to melatonin production by ensuring exposure to natural light during the day and limiting exposure to artificial light at night. The suppression of melatonin caused by exposure to bright screens or artificial lighting at night can further exacerbate sleep issues. Poor melatonin production leads to a lack of deep, restorative sleep, which is critical for hormonal balance and overall health.

Chapter 2: Herbs for Improving Sleep Quality

2.1 Valerian for Deep Sleep

Valerian is widely recognized for its potent sedative properties, making it one of the most effective natural remedies for improving sleep quality. This herb has been used for centuries to promote relaxation and calm the nervous system, which is particularly beneficial for those suffering from insomnia or frequent night waking. Valerian works by increasing levels of gamma-aminobutyric acid (GABA) in the brain, a neurotransmitter responsible for regulating nerve activity and inducing a calming effect on the mind and body.

Valerian can be consumed in different forms, including teas, tinctures, or capsules, and is an excellent alternative to pharmaceutical sleeping pills, which often come with side effects such as grogginess and dependency. Valerian's ability to enhance sleep without the harsh side effects of synthetic drugs makes it a preferred choice for those looking to treat sleep issues naturally.

For those who experience difficulty falling asleep or staying asleep throughout the night, valerian offers a natural and gentle solution. The herb's calming effect on the nervous system helps reduce the mental overactivity that often prevents people from relaxing enough to fall asleep. By soothing the brain and body, valerian makes it easier to enter a state of deep sleep and maintain it for longer periods. Additionally, valerian's natural sedative properties support the body's ability to achieve the kind of deep, restorative sleep necessary for proper recovery and rejuvenation.

Valerian is most effective when taken consistently over a period of time. Drinking valerian tea or taking valerian tincture in the evening, about 30 minutes to an hour before bed, can help prepare the body for sleep. By creating a relaxing pre-sleep routine that includes valerian, individuals can improve both the duration and quality of their sleep over time.

While valerian is generally considered safe, it is important to note that its effectiveness can vary from person to person. Some individuals may experience drowsiness or mild digestive upset after using valerian, so it is recommended to start with a lower dose and gradually increase it if necessary. Furthermore, valerian should not be used in combination with alcohol or other sedative medications without consulting a healthcare provider.

2.2 Passionflower for Calming the Mind

Passionflower is another herb highly recommended for its calming properties, particularly for individuals who struggle with anxiety or racing thoughts at bedtime. Like valerian, passionflower works by increasing the levels of GABA in the brain, which helps reduce overactivity and induces a state of relaxation. This makes passionflower especially effective for those whose insomnia is linked to mental or emotional stress.

Passionflower is a mild sedative that can be consumed in the form of tea, tinctures, or capsules. For people who experience difficulty falling asleep due to anxiety, passionflower provides a natural way to calm the mind and ease the transition into sleep. Its calming effects are gentle yet powerful enough to reduce the mental tension that can lead to restless nights.

For individuals who tend to overthink or experience racing thoughts before bed, passionflower can help quiet the mind and promote mental clarity. By reducing the overactivity in the brain, passionflower helps individuals enter a more peaceful state, which is conducive to falling asleep faster and enjoying uninterrupted sleep.

Passionflower also offers additional benefits beyond promoting sleep. It is known for its ability to ease symptoms of generalized anxiety and nervous tension, making it a useful herb not only for insomnia but also for managing daily stress. By addressing the underlying issues of anxiety and mental overactivity, passionflower helps create a more relaxed mental and emotional state, which directly supports better sleep hygiene.

To incorporate passionflower into a nighttime routine, it can be consumed as a tea or taken as a tincture about an hour before bed. Passionflower tea, made by steeping dried passionflower leaves in hot water, can be a soothing way to unwind in the evening. Alternatively, passionflower tincture can be added to a small amount of water and taken before bed to promote relaxation.

Barbara O'Neill emphasizes that, like valerian, passionflower is a natural and effective alternative to conventional sedatives, offering a way to improve sleep without the risk of side effects associated with prescription medications. While passionflower is generally safe for most people, it should be used cautiously in combination with other sedative substances. For those with preexisting health conditions or those who are pregnant, it is advisable to consult with a healthcare professional before using passionflower as part of a sleep regimen.

Supporting Sleep with Natural Remedies

In addition to valerian and passionflower, there are several other lifestyle practices and natural remedies that can further support sleep quality. Creating a consistent sleep routine, minimizing screen time before bed, and using essential oils like lavender can all help create an optimal sleep environment. Both valerian and passionflower can be complemented with these practices to maximize their benefits for sleep.

A holistic approach to sleep, incorporating these herbs along with relaxation techniques, not only improves sleep but also promotes overall mental and physical well-being. Regular use of these herbs, combined with healthy sleep hygiene, can help individuals develop better long-term sleep patterns, making it easier to achieve the deep, restorative rest that is vital for health.

2.3 Chamomile for Relaxation

Chamomile has been widely recognized for its calming and anti-inflammatory properties. It has been used for centuries as a remedy for promoting relaxation and aiding digestion. Barbara O'Neill emphasizes the value of chamomile tea as a natural way to soothe both the body and mind, particularly before bedtime. Chamomile can reduce mild digestive discomforts that often disrupt sleep, such as indigestion or bloating, and it promotes a sense of calm that helps the body transition into a state of rest.

The Calming Effects of Chamomile

Chamomile contains compounds such as apigenin, an antioxidant that binds to specific receptors in the brain, potentially promoting relaxation and reducing feelings of anxiety. For individuals who struggle with restlessness or mild anxiety, chamomile tea is an excellent evening drink to help prepare the body for sleep. By calming the nervous system, chamomile encourages a peaceful state of mind, which is essential for deep and restorative sleep.

Chamomile is especially beneficial for individuals who experience stress-related sleep disturbances. The soothing aroma, combined with its physical effects, helps alleviate tension and promotes a smoother transition into a relaxed state. This herb not only enhances sleep but also plays a role in reducing the mental clutter that can often keep one awake at night.

Incorporating Chamomile Into a Bedtime Routine

Drinking a warm cup of chamomile tea in the evening signals to the body that it is time to relax. Over time, the body begins to associate this ritual with relaxation, creating a mental and physical connection to restfulness.

Chamomile can be consumed in various forms, but tea is one of the most accessible and beneficial methods. The warm liquid not only aids in the absorption of the calming compounds but also helps to relax the digestive system and provide a comforting prelude to sleep. For those who prefer a stronger concentration, chamomile extract can be added to tea or taken as a tincture.

Chapter 3: Creating Routines and Habits for Restorative Sleep

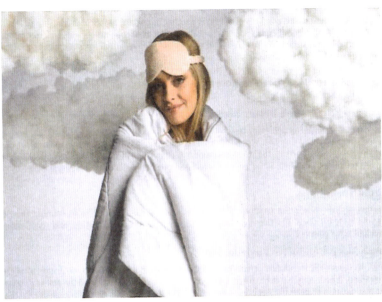

3.1 Establishing a Sleep Routine

Establishing a consistent sleep routine is essential for promoting regular sleep patterns and improving overall sleep quality. Barbara O'Neill emphasizes that going to bed and waking up at the same time each day helps to regulate the body's circadian rhythm, which governs the natural sleep-wake cycle. A well-maintained circadian rhythm makes it easier to fall asleep and wake up feeling refreshed.

The Importance of Consistency

Maintaining a regular sleep schedule helps synchronize the body's internal clock, ensuring that it functions optimally. The body thrives on routine, and when it receives consistent signals about when to rest and wake, it becomes easier to maintain energy levels throughout the day. This consistency also aids in improving the quality of sleep, as the body knows when it should enter its most restorative phases of the sleep cycle.

O'Neill highlights that a stable sleep schedule helps prevent sleep disorders, such as insomnia, that are often caused by erratic sleep patterns. By committing to a regular bedtime and wake-up time, the body can enter a predictable rhythm that supports deeper and more effective rest.

Creating a Bedtime Ritual

In addition to maintaining consistent sleep times, establishing a bedtime ritual can further enhance the quality of sleep. Barbara O'Neill suggests practices such as dimming the lights, drinking a cup of herbal tea, and avoiding screen time before bed. These habits help signal to the body that it is time to wind down and prepare for rest.

Dimming the lights in the evening mimics the natural decline of sunlight and encourages the production of melatonin, the hormone responsible for sleep regulation. Exposure to bright lights or screens, particularly blue light from phones and computers, can suppress melatonin production and interfere with the body's ability to fall asleep. Reducing screen time and using dim lighting in the hours leading up to bedtime supports the body's natural rhythm and facilitates a smoother transition into sleep.

Drinking herbal tea, such as chamomile, as part of this evening routine, further enhances relaxation by calming the nervous system and aiding digestion. Incorporating a relaxing activity, like reading or meditation, can also be beneficial in creating a sense of calm before bed.

The Role of Environment in Sleep Quality

Creating an environment that is conducive to sleep is another important aspect of establishing a healthy sleep routine. Barbara O'Neill recommends ensuring that the bedroom is cool, quiet, and dark to promote better sleep. A comfortable and supportive mattress and pillows are also essential for maintaining proper posture and reducing discomfort during sleep.

Reducing noise and light disturbances, such as from outside traffic or electronic devices, is key to maintaining uninterrupted sleep. For those who are sensitive to noise, the use of earplugs or a white noise machine can be helpful in creating a peaceful environment.

3.2 Managing Stress for Better Sleep

Managing stress is essential for achieving restorative sleep, as stress can significantly disrupt the body's natural rhythms and prevent restful slumber. When the mind remains active with concerns or worries, the body tends to produce higher levels of cortisol, the stress hormone, which inhibits the ability to relax and fall asleep. Stress management techniques can help lower cortisol levels and promote relaxation, making it easier to fall into a deep, restful sleep.

Relaxation Techniques

Incorporating specific relaxation techniques before bed can be highly effective in calming the mind and preparing the body for sleep. Practice deep breating, progressive muscle relaxation, and meditation to calm your mind and relax your body.

Creating a Sleep-Conducive Environment

In addition to relaxation techniques, creating a calm and comfortable bedroom environment is crucial for promoting sleep. A bedroom that is too bright, noisy, or cluttered can interfere with the ability to relax and fall asleep. It is important to keep the sleeping environment **cool**, as lower temperatures encourage the body to produce melatonin, which signals that it is time to sleep. A cooler room also supports the body's natural drop in core temperature, which occurs as part of the sleep cycle.

Minimizing exposure to **bright lights** before bed is another important step. Bright artificial lighting, especially from screens and devices, can suppress melatonin production and make it harder to fall asleep. To avoid this, it is helpful to dim the lights in the evening and refrain from using electronic devices at least an hour before bedtime. **Blackout curtains** or sleep masks can also be used to block out light and create a darker sleeping environment, further promoting melatonin production.

Lastly, reducing **noise** is critical for uninterrupted sleep. Whether it's outside traffic or household noise, creating a quiet space can significantly improve sleep quality. Earplugs or white noise machines can help mask disruptive sounds and create a peaceful sleeping environment.

3.3 Nutritional Support for Sleep

Diet plays a crucial role in supporting healthy sleep cycles. Certain foods and nutrients can either enhance or disrupt sleep, and it is important to be mindful of eating habits, particularly in the evening. Barbara O'Neill emphasizes the importance of avoiding stimulants like caffeine and sugar, which can interfere with sleep, and incorporating foods rich in magnesium and other calming nutrients that promote relaxation and restorative sleep.

Avoiding Stimulants

Caffeine is a well-known stimulant that can disrupt sleep by blocking adenosine receptors in the brain, which normally promote relaxation and drowsiness. Consuming caffeine in the afternoon or evening can lead to difficulty falling asleep and reduce the overall quality of sleep. To prevent this, it is best to avoid coffee, tea, chocolate, and other sources of caffeine several hours before bed. Even **decaffeinated beverages** can contain small amounts of caffeine, so it is important to be aware of these hidden sources.

Similarly, **sugar** can cause spikes and crashes in blood sugar levels, leading to restlessness and wakefulness during the night. Eating sugary snacks in the evening can create fluctuations in energy levels that make it harder to fall and stay asleep. It is recommended to opt for complex carbohydrates and low-sugar options, especially before bedtime, to maintain stable blood sugar levels.

Magnesium-Rich Foods

Magnesium is a vital mineral that supports muscle relaxation and nervous system function, both of which are important for promoting restful sleep. Foods rich in magnesium, such as **leafy greens**, **nuts**, and **seeds**, can help calm the body and prepare it for sleep. Magnesium deficiency has been linked to insomnia and other sleep disturbances, so including magnesium-rich foods in the diet is a natural way to improve sleep quality.

Spinach, kale, and **almonds** are particularly high in magnesium and are easy to incorporate into evening meals. Additionally, **pumpkin seeds** and **sunflower seeds** provide a good source of magnesium and can be consumed as a snack before bed. These foods not only promote muscle relaxation but also support overall nervous system function, which is critical for reducing stress and anxiety.

Sleep-Friendly Foods

In addition to magnesium, there are several sleep-friendly foods that can naturally improve sleep quality. **Bananas**, for example, are rich in potassium and magnesium, both of which help relax muscles. Additionally, they contain tryptophan, an amino acid that the body uses to produce melatonin and serotonin, which induce feelings of calm and sleepiness.

Almonds are another excellent option for promoting sleep, as they contain both magnesium and healthy fats that support relaxation. Consuming a small handful of almonds before bed can help stabilize blood sugar levels and reduce the chances of waking up during the night.

Herbal teas, such as **chamomile** and **passionflower**, are also beneficial for promoting sleep. Chamomile tea has long been used for its calming properties and ability to reduce anxiety. Passionflower tea can also promote relaxation by increasing levels of gamma-aminobutyric acid (GABA) in the brain, which helps reduce brain activity and promotes restful sleep.

Chapter 4: Natural Remedies for Sleep and Restorative Health

Achieving deep and restorative sleep is crucial for maintaining overall health and well-being. Sleep allows the body to repair and regenerate, ensuring that physical and mental processes function optimally. Natural remedies can play a vital role in supporting better sleep quality by addressing common sleep disturbances such as stress, anxiety, and hormonal imbalances. Below are 20 effective natural remedies that can be used to improve sleep and enhance the body's restorative health processes.

The appendix provides more details for each remedy.

1. Valerian Root

2. Chamomile

3. Lavender

4. Passionflower

5. Magnesium

6. Melatonin

7. Ashwagandha

8. Tart Cherry Juice

9. Lemon Balm

10. Glycine

11. Hops

12. Skullcap

13. Kava

14. L-Theanine

15. Holy Basil

16. 5-HTP (5-Hydroxytryptophan)

17. California Poppy

18. Reishi Mushroom

19. GABA

20. St. John's Wort

Part 27:
Healing Recipes

Barbara O'Neill's Approach to Healing through Nutrition

Barbara O'Neill emphasizes that the foundation of health lies in the foods we consume daily. Her philosophy centers on a plant-based, nutrient-dense diet, which supports the body's natural healing processes. According to her approach, whole foods provide the necessary nutrients for preventing disease, promoting detoxification, and strengthening the immune system. O'Neill underscores the importance of returning to a simpler diet, one that excludes processed foods and focuses on natural ingredients.

Whole-Food Diet for Disease Prevention

A central aspect of Barbara O'Neill's approach is the prevention of disease through a whole-food diet. She advocates for meals rich in vegetables, fruits, nuts, seeds, and legumes, which are naturally packed with vitamins, minerals, and antioxidants. These nutrients play a critical role in supporting the immune system, reducing inflammation, and protecting the body from chronic conditions. By consuming a variety of plant-based foods, the body receives the necessary tools to repair itself and maintain optimal health.

Processed foods, on the other hand, are seen as a major contributor to disease. O'Neill encourages individuals to avoid refined sugars, unhealthy fats, and artificial additives, which burden the body's detoxification systems and contribute to the development of illnesses. Instead, she promotes natural, whole foods that provide clean energy and support the body's healing mechanisms.

Boosting Digestion and Vitality

A well-functioning digestive system is crucial for overall health, and Barbara O'Neill believes that the right foods can improve digestion and enhance vitality. She advocates for meals that are easy to digest, such as soups, smoothies, and salads rich in raw vegetables and herbs. Fermented foods, like sauerkraut and kefir, are also recommended for promoting a healthy gut microbiome, which is essential for digestion and immune function.

Chapter 1: Healing Soups

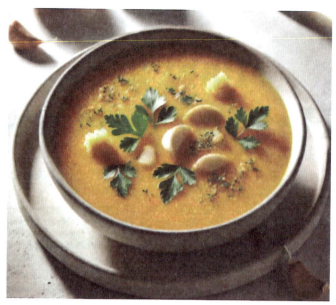

Immune-Boosting Garlic and Ginger Soup

Ingredients: Garlic (4 cloves), ginger (2-inch piece), onion (1), vegetable broth (4 cups), olive oil (2 tbsp), lemon juice (1 tbsp), salt, and pepper to taste.

Instructions: Sauté garlic, ginger, and onion in olive oil until fragrant. Add vegetable broth, bring to a boil, and simmer for 20 minutes. Blend until smooth, season with lemon juice, salt, and pepper.

Detoxifying Green Broccoli Soup

Ingredients: Broccoli (2 heads), spinach (1 cup), onion (1), garlic (2 cloves), vegetable broth (4 cups), olive oil (2 tbsp), lemon juice (1 tbsp), salt, and pepper to taste.

Instructions: Sauté onion and garlic in olive oil, add broccoli and spinach, and cook for 5 minutes. Pour in the broth, simmer for 15 minutes, then blend until smooth. Add lemon juice, salt, and pepper to taste.

Carrot and Turmeric Healing Soup

Ingredients: Carrots (4), turmeric powder (1 tsp), ginger (1-inch piece), onion (1), vegetable broth (4 cups), coconut milk (1/2 cup), olive oil (2 tbsp), salt, and pepper.

Instructions: Sauté onion, ginger, and turmeric in olive oil. Add carrots and broth, simmer for 20 minutes, then blend. Stir in coconut milk, season with salt and pepper.

Sweet Potato and Lentil Nourishing Soup

Ingredients: Sweet potatoes (2), red lentils (1 cup), onion (1), garlic (2 cloves), vegetable broth (4 cups), cumin (1 tsp), olive oil (2 tbsp), salt, and pepper.

Instructions: Sauté onion and garlic in olive oil. Add sweet potatoes, lentils, and broth. Simmer for 25 minutes until lentils are soft. Blend for a smoother texture, and season with cumin, salt, and pepper.

Gut-Soothing Miso and Seaweed Broth

Ingredients: Miso paste (2 tbsp), wakame seaweed (1 tbsp), tofu (1/2 cup, cubed), green onions (2), water (4 cups).

Instructions: Boil water, add miso paste, stir well. Add wakame and tofu, simmer for 5 minutes. Top with green onions before serving.

Immune-Supporting Mushroom and Garlic Soup

Ingredients: Mushrooms (2 cups), garlic (4 cloves), onion (1), vegetable broth (4 cups), olive oil (2 tbsp), thyme (1 tsp), salt, and pepper.

Instructions: Sauté garlic, onion, and mushrooms in olive oil. Add broth and thyme, simmer for 20 minutes. Blend if desired and season with salt and pepper.

Anti-Inflammatory Pumpkin and Ginger Soup

Ingredients: Pumpkin (2 cups, cubed), ginger (2-inch piece), coconut milk (1/2 cup), vegetable broth (4 cups), onion (1), olive oil (2 tbsp), salt, and pepper.

Instructions: Sauté onion and ginger in olive oil. Add pumpkin and broth, simmer for 20 minutes. Blend, stir in coconut milk, and season with salt and pepper.

Liver-Cleansing Beet and Carrot Soup

Ingredients: Beets (2), carrots (3), ginger (1-inch piece), onion (1), vegetable broth (4 cups), olive oil (2 tbsp), lemon juice (1 tbsp), salt, and pepper.

Instructions: Sauté onion and ginger in olive oil. Add beets, carrots, and broth, simmer for 30 minutes. Blend, season with lemon juice, salt, and pepper.

Warming Butternut Squash and Cinnamon Soup

Ingredients: Butternut squash (1, cubed), cinnamon (1 tsp), vegetable broth (4 cups), onion (1), olive oil (2 tbsp), coconut milk (1/2 cup), salt, and pepper.

Instructions: Sauté onion and cinnamon in olive oil. Add squash and broth, simmer for 25 minutes. Blend, stir in coconut milk, and season with salt and pepper.

Bone Broth with Healing Herbs and Vegetables

Ingredients: Beef or chicken bones (1 lb), carrots (2), celery (2 stalks), onion (1), garlic (4 cloves), bay leaves (2), thyme (1 tsp), water (8 cups).

Instructions: Simmer bones, vegetables, and herbs in water for 8-12 hours. Strain broth, season with salt and pepper before serving.

Cabbage and Fennel Digestive Soup

Ingredients: Cabbage (1/2 head, shredded), fennel bulb (1, sliced), onion (1), garlic (2 cloves), vegetable broth (4 cups), olive oil (2 tbsp), salt, and pepper.

Instructions: Sauté garlic, onion, and fennel in olive oil. Add cabbage and broth, simmer for 25 minutes. Season with salt and pepper. This soup helps support digestion due to the digestive properties of fennel and cabbage.

Green Detox Zucchini Soup

Ingredients: Zucchini (3, sliced), spinach (1 cup), onion (1), garlic (2 cloves), vegetable broth (4 cups), olive oil (2 tbsp), lemon juice (1 tbsp), salt, and pepper.

Instructions: Sauté onion and garlic in olive oil. Add zucchini, spinach, and broth, simmer for 15 minutes. Blend until smooth, add lemon juice, salt, and pepper. This soup aids detoxification with zucchini and spinach's high nutrient content.

Warming Sweet Potato and Red Lentil Soup

Ingredients: Sweet potatoes (2, diced), red lentils (1 cup), onion (1), garlic (2 cloves), vegetable broth (4 cups), cumin (1 tsp), olive oil (2 tbsp), salt, and pepper.

Instructions: Sauté onion and garlic in olive oil. Add sweet potatoes, lentils, and broth. Simmer for 25 minutes until lentils are soft. Blend for a smoother texture, and season with cumin, salt, and pepper for a comforting, nourishing meal.

Protein-Rich Quinoa and Vegetable Broth

Ingredients: Quinoa (1/2 cup), carrots (2), celery (2 stalks), zucchini (1), onion (1), vegetable broth (6 cups), olive oil (2 tbsp), thyme (1 tsp), salt, and pepper.

Instructions: Sauté onion, carrots, celery, and zucchini in olive oil. Add quinoa and broth, simmer for 20 minutes until quinoa is cooked. Season with thyme, salt, and pepper. This soup provides a protein boost from the quinoa and a variety of vitamins from the vegetables.

Spinach and Kale Chlorophyll Boosting Soup

Ingredients: Spinach (2 cups), kale (1 cup), garlic (3 cloves), onion (1), vegetable broth (4 cups), olive oil (2 tbsp), lemon juice (1 tbsp), salt, and pepper.

Instructions: Sauté onion and garlic in olive oil. Add spinach, kale, and broth, simmer for 10 minutes. Blend until smooth, season with lemon juice, salt, and pepper. This soup is rich in chlorophyll, helping to cleanse the body and provide essential nutrients.

Chapter 2: Vitality-Enhancing Salads

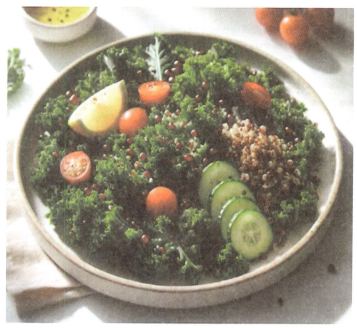

Healing Kale and Quinoa Salad with Lemon Dressing
Ingredients: Kale (2 cups, chopped), cooked quinoa (1 cup), avocado (1), cucumber (1), lemon juice (2 tbsp), olive oil (2 tbsp), salt, and pepper.
Instructions: Massage kale with lemon juice and olive oil until softened. Toss in cooked quinoa, diced avocado, and cucumber. Season with salt and pepper.

Detoxifying Beetroot and Carrot Salad
Ingredients: Beets (2, shredded), carrots (2, shredded), apple cider vinegar (2 tbsp), olive oil (2 tbsp), parsley (1/4 cup, chopped), salt, and pepper.
Instructions: Mix shredded beets and carrots in a bowl. Add apple cider vinegar, olive oil, and parsley. Toss well and season with salt and pepper.

Liver-Cleansing Fennel and Citrus Salad
Ingredients: Fennel bulb (1, thinly sliced), orange (1, segmented), grapefruit (1, segmented), olive oil (2 tbsp), lemon juice (1 tbsp), salt, and pepper.
Instructions: Combine fennel and citrus segments in a bowl. Drizzle with olive oil and lemon juice. Season with salt and pepper.

Antioxidant-Rich Spinach and Berry Salad
Ingredients: Baby spinach (2 cups), mixed berries (1 cup: blueberries, raspberries, strawberries), walnuts (1/4 cup), balsamic vinegar (1 tbsp), olive oil (2 tbsp), salt, and pepper.
Instructions: Toss spinach, berries, and walnuts in a bowl. Drizzle with balsamic vinegar and olive oil, and season with salt and pepper.

Cucumber and Mint Hydrating Salad

Ingredients: Cucumber (2, thinly sliced), fresh mint leaves (1/4 cup), lemon juice (2 tbsp), olive oil (2 tbsp), salt, and pepper.

Instructions: Combine cucumber and mint in a bowl. Drizzle with lemon juice and olive oil, and season with salt and pepper.

Immune-Boosting Arugula and Orange Salad

Ingredients: Arugula (2 cups), orange (1, segmented), red onion (1/4, thinly sliced), olive oil (2 tbsp), apple cider vinegar (1 tbsp), salt, and pepper.

Instructions: Toss arugula, orange, and red onion in a bowl. Drizzle with olive oil and apple cider vinegar, and season with salt and pepper.

Gut-Healing Fermented Vegetable Salad

Ingredients: Sauerkraut (1/2 cup), fermented carrots (1/4 cup), radishes (4, sliced), arugula (1 cup), olive oil (2 tbsp), lemon juice (1 tbsp).

Instructions: Combine arugula, sauerkraut, fermented carrots, and radishes. Drizzle with olive oil and lemon juice, then toss well.

Protein-Packed Lentil and Chickpea Salad

Ingredients: Cooked lentils (1 cup), cooked chickpeas (1 cup), cucumber (1, diced), cherry tomatoes (1 cup, halved), parsley (1/4 cup, chopped), olive oil (2 tbsp), lemon juice (1 tbsp), salt, and pepper.

Instructions: Mix lentils, chickpeas, cucumber, tomatoes, and parsley in a bowl. Drizzle with olive oil and lemon juice, and season with salt and pepper.

Sweet Potato and Black Bean Salad

Ingredients: Sweet potatoes (2, cubed), black beans (1 cup, cooked), red onion (1/2, diced), cilantro (1/4 cup), lime juice (2 tbsp), olive oil (2 tbsp), salt, and pepper.

Instructions: Roast sweet potatoes until tender. Combine with black beans, red onion, and cilantro. Dress with lime juice, olive oil, salt, and pepper.

Liver-Supporting Broccoli and Walnut Salad

Ingredients: Broccoli (2 cups, chopped), walnuts (1/4 cup), red onion (1/4, thinly sliced), apple cider vinegar (2 tbsp), olive oil (2 tbsp), honey (1 tsp), salt, and pepper.

Instructions: Blanch broccoli until bright green. Toss with walnuts, red onion, and a dressing made from vinegar, olive oil, honey, salt, and pepper.

Bone-Strengthening Broccoli and Almond Salad

Ingredients: Broccoli (2 cups, chopped), slivered almonds (1/4 cup), lemon juice (2 tbsp), olive oil (2 tbsp), garlic (1 clove, minced), salt, and pepper.

Instructions: Steam broccoli until tender. Mix with almonds and dress with a lemon juice, olive oil, and garlic mixture. Season with salt and pepper.

Energy-Boosting Quinoa and Avocado Salad

Ingredients: Quinoa (1 cup, cooked), avocado (1, diced), cherry tomatoes (1/2 cup, halved), cucumber (1/2, diced), lemon juice (2 tbsp), olive oil (2 tbsp), salt, and pepper.

Instructions: Combine cooked quinoa with avocado, tomatoes, and cucumber. Dress with lemon juice, olive oil, salt, and pepper.

Probiotic-Rich Sauerkraut Salad with Apple

Ingredients: Sauerkraut (1 cup), apple (1, diced), green onions (2, chopped), olive oil (1 tbsp), caraway seeds (1 tsp), salt, and pepper.

Instructions: Mix sauerkraut with apple and green onions. Drizzle with olive oil and sprinkle with caraway seeds, salt, and pepper.

Anti-Inflammatory Cabbage and Carrot Slaw

Ingredients: Cabbage (2 cups, shredded), carrots (1 cup, grated), apple cider vinegar (2 tbsp), olive oil (2 tbsp), honey (1 tsp), salt, and pepper.

Instructions: Combine cabbage and carrots. Whisk together apple cider vinegar, olive oil, and honey for the dressing, and toss with slaw. Season with salt and pepper.

Detoxifying Seaweed and Cucumber Salad

Ingredients: Wakame seaweed (1/4 cup, soaked), cucumber (1, thinly sliced), sesame seeds (1 tbsp), rice vinegar (2 tbsp), sesame oil (1 tbsp), soy sauce (1 tsp).

Instructions: Soak seaweed and drain. Combine with cucumber and sesame seeds. Dress with rice vinegar, sesame oil, and soy sauce, and toss.

Chapter 3: Nutrient-Dense Smoothies and Bowls

Detoxifying Green Smoothie with Kale and Spinach

Ingredients: Kale (1 cup), spinach (1 cup), cucumber (1/2), lemon juice (1 tbsp), apple (1), water (1 cup), chia seeds (1 tbsp).

Instructions: Blend kale, spinach, cucumber, apple, and water until smooth. Add lemon juice and chia seeds, blend again briefly, and serve.

Protein-Packed Hemp and Chia Smoothie Bowl

Ingredients: Hemp seeds (2 tbsp), chia seeds (1 tbsp), banana (1), almond milk (1 cup), almond butter (1 tbsp), mixed berries (1/2 cup), granola (for topping).

Instructions: Blend banana, almond milk, hemp seeds, chia seeds, and almond butter until smooth. Pour into a bowl, top with mixed berries and granola.

Anti-Inflammatory Turmeric and Ginger Smoothie

Ingredients: Turmeric powder (1 tsp), ginger (1-inch piece), banana (1), coconut milk (1 cup), honey (1 tsp), cinnamon (1/2 tsp).

Instructions: Blend banana, coconut milk, ginger, and turmeric. Add honey and cinnamon, blend again, and serve chilled.

Liver-Cleansing Beet and Carrot Smoothie

Ingredients: Beet (1 small, raw), carrot (1), apple (1), lemon juice (1 tbsp), ginger (1-inch piece), water (1/2 cup).

Instructions: Blend beet, carrot, apple, ginger, and water until smooth. Add lemon juice, blend again, and serve immediately.

Energizing Banana and Almond Butter Smoothie

Ingredients: Banana (1), almond butter (1 tbsp), oats (1/4 cup), almond milk (1 cup), flaxseeds (1 tbsp), honey (1 tsp).

Instructions: Blend banana, almond butter, oats, almond milk, flaxseeds, and honey until smooth. Serve chilled for an energy boost.

Gut-Healing Aloe Vera and Papaya Smoothie

Ingredients: Aloe vera gel (2 tbsp), papaya (1 cup), coconut water (1 cup), lime juice (1 tbsp), mint leaves (for garnish).

Instructions: Blend papaya, coconut water, aloe vera gel, and lime juice until smooth. Garnish with mint leaves and serve.

Antioxidant Berry and Spinach Smoothie

Ingredients: Mixed berries (1 cup), spinach (1 cup), almond milk (1 cup), chia seeds (1 tbsp), honey (1 tsp).

Instructions: Blend berries, spinach, almond milk, and chia seeds until smooth. Add honey, blend again, and serve immediately.

Omega-3 Boosting Flaxseed and Blueberry Smoothie

Ingredients: Blueberries (1 cup), flaxseeds (1 tbsp), banana (1), almond milk (1 cup), oats (1/4 cup), honey (1 tsp).

Instructions: Blend blueberries, banana, almond milk, flaxseeds, and oats until smooth. Add honey, blend again briefly, and serve chilled.

Cleansing Lemon and Ginger Detox Smoothie

Ingredients: Lemon juice (1 tbsp), ginger (1-inch piece), cucumber (1), spinach (1 cup), water (1 cup), honey (1 tsp), ice.

Instructions: Blend lemon juice, ginger, cucumber, spinach, water, and honey until smooth. Serve with ice for a refreshing detox drink.

Bone-Strengthening Almond Milk and Chia Pudding

Ingredients: Almond milk (1 cup), chia seeds (3 tbsp), vanilla extract (1 tsp), honey (1 tsp), berries for topping.

Instructions: Mix almond milk, chia seeds, vanilla, and honey. Let sit in the fridge for 4 hours or overnight. Top with fresh berries before serving.

Heart-Healthy Avocado and Spinach Smoothie

Ingredients: Avocado (1/2), spinach (1 cup), banana (1), almond milk (1 cup), flaxseeds (1 tbsp).

Instructions: Blend avocado, spinach, banana, almond milk, and flaxseeds until smooth. Serve chilled for a heart-boosting smoothie.

Berry and Hemp Seed Smoothie for Vitality

Ingredients: Mixed berries (1 cup), hemp seeds (1 tbsp), banana (1), coconut water (1 cup), chia seeds (1 tsp).

Instructions: Blend berries, hemp seeds, banana, coconut water, and chia seeds until smooth. Serve for a nutrient-packed vitality boost.

Antioxidant-Rich Blueberry and Kale Smoothie Bowl

Ingredients: Blueberries (1/2 cup), kale (1 cup), banana (1), almond milk (1/2 cup), chia seeds (1 tbsp), granola for topping.

Instructions: Blend blueberries, kale, banana, almond milk, and chia seeds until smooth. Pour into a bowl and top with granola for crunch.

Energizing Chia and Coconut Milk Pudding

Ingredients: Coconut milk (1 cup), chia seeds (3 tbsp), maple syrup (1 tsp), shredded coconut for topping.

Instructions: Stir together coconut milk, chia seeds, and maple syrup. Let sit for 4 hours or overnight in the fridge. Top with shredded coconut before serving.

Digestive-Boosting Pineapple and Mint Smoothie

Ingredients: Pineapple (1 cup), mint leaves (1/4 cup), coconut water (1 cup), lime juice (1 tbsp), ice.

Instructions: Blend pineapple, mint, coconut water, lime juice, and ice until smooth. Serve chilled for a refreshing, digestion-enhancing smoothie.

Chapter 4: Everyday Meals for Healing

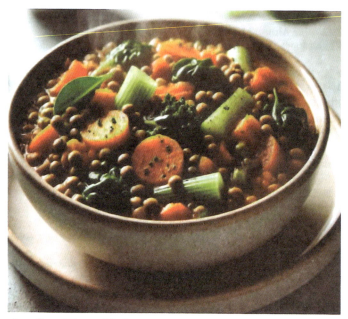

Nourishing Lentil and Vegetable Stew
Ingredients: Green or brown lentils (1 cup), carrots (2), celery (2 stalks), zucchini (1), garlic (3 cloves), onion (1), vegetable broth (4 cups), olive oil (2 tbsp), cumin (1 tsp), salt, and pepper.

Instructions: Sauté onion and garlic in olive oil. Add lentils, chopped vegetables, and broth. Simmer for 30 minutes until lentils are soft. Season with cumin, salt, and pepper.

Gut-Healing Sourdough Bread
Ingredients: Sourdough starter (1 cup), whole wheat flour (3 cups), water (1 1/2 cups), sea salt (2 tsp).

Instructions: Mix sourdough starter, flour, water, and salt until a dough forms. Let rise for 6-8 hours or overnight. Shape into a loaf and bake at 220°C (425°F) for 30-35 minutes.

Roasted Sweet Potato and Chickpea Salad
Ingredients: Sweet potatoes (2, cubed), chickpeas (1 can, drained), spinach (2 cups), olive oil (2 tbsp), paprika (1 tsp), lemon juice (1 tbsp), salt, and pepper.

Instructions: Toss sweet potatoes and chickpeas in olive oil and paprika. Roast at 200°C (400°F) for 25-30 minutes. Serve over spinach, drizzle with lemon juice, and season with salt and pepper.

Protein-Rich Lentil and Quinoa Bowl
Ingredients: Quinoa (1 cup), green lentils (1/2 cup), cucumber (1, chopped), cherry tomatoes (1 cup), olive oil (2 tbsp), lemon juice (1 tbsp), salt, and pepper.

Instructions: Cook quinoa and lentils separately. Combine in a bowl with cucumber and tomatoes. Drizzle with olive oil and lemon juice, season with salt and pepper.

Detoxifying Zucchini Noodles with Pesto

Ingredients: Zucchini (2, spiralized), fresh basil (1 cup), garlic (2 cloves), pine nuts (1/4 cup), olive oil (1/4 cup), lemon juice (1 tbsp), salt, and pepper.

Instructions: Blend basil, garlic, pine nuts, olive oil, and lemon juice into a pesto. Toss zucchini noodles with pesto, and season with salt and pepper.

Fiber-Rich Brown Rice and Veggie Stir Fry

Ingredients: Brown rice (1 cup), broccoli (1 head, chopped), bell peppers (2), carrots (2), garlic (2 cloves), soy sauce (2 tbsp), sesame oil (1 tbsp), olive oil (2 tbsp).

Instructions: Cook brown rice. Sauté garlic and vegetables in olive oil. Add soy sauce and sesame oil, stir in brown rice, and cook for 5 minutes.

Anti-Inflammatory Cauliflower and Turmeric Mash

Ingredients: Cauliflower (1 head), turmeric powder (1 tsp), garlic (2 cloves), olive oil (2 tbsp), coconut milk (1/2 cup), salt, and pepper.

Instructions: Steam cauliflower until soft. Sauté garlic in olive oil with turmeric. Mash cauliflower, stir in garlic and turmeric, add coconut milk, and season with salt and pepper.

Bone-Strengthening Spinach and Almond Stir Fry

Ingredients: Spinach (4 cups), almonds (1/2 cup, sliced), garlic (2 cloves), olive oil (2 tbsp), sesame seeds (1 tbsp), salt, and pepper.

Instructions: Sauté garlic in olive oil until fragrant. Add spinach and cook until wilted. Stir in almonds and sesame seeds, and season with salt and pepper.

Healing Pumpkin and Ginger Mash

Ingredients: Pumpkin (2 cups, cubed), ginger (1-inch piece, grated), coconut oil (1 tbsp), cinnamon (1/2 tsp), salt, and pepper.

Instructions: Steam pumpkin until tender. Mash with coconut oil, ginger, and cinnamon. Season with salt and pepper.

Roasted Carrot and Parsnip Soup

Ingredients: Carrots (4), parsnips (3), garlic (3 cloves), vegetable broth (4 cups), olive oil (2 tbsp), thyme (1 tsp), salt, and pepper.

Instructions: Roast carrots, parsnips, and garlic in olive oil at 400°F (200°C) for 25 minutes. Blend roasted vegetables with broth and thyme, and season with salt and pepper.

Heart-Healthy Grilled Vegetables with Garlic

Ingredients: Zucchini (2), bell peppers (2), eggplant (1), garlic (3 cloves, minced), olive oil (2 tbsp), lemon juice (1 tbsp), salt, and pepper.

Instructions: Slice vegetables and toss with olive oil and garlic. Grill until tender. Drizzle with lemon juice and season with salt and pepper.

Sweet Potato and Lentil Shepherd's Pie

Ingredients: Sweet potatoes (2, mashed), red lentils (1 cup), onion (1), garlic (2 cloves), carrots (2), vegetable broth (2 cups), olive oil (2 tbsp), thyme (1 tsp), salt, and pepper.

Instructions: Sauté onion, garlic, and carrots in olive oil. Add lentils and broth, simmer until soft. Layer lentil mixture in a baking dish, top with mashed sweet potatoes, and bake at 375°F (190°C) for 20 minutes.

Liver-Supporting Beet and Walnut Salad

Ingredients: Beets (2, cooked and sliced), walnuts (1/2 cup), arugula (2 cups), olive oil (2 tbsp), balsamic vinegar (1 tbsp), salt, and pepper.

Instructions: Toss beets, walnuts, and arugula in a bowl. Drizzle with olive oil and balsamic vinegar. Season with salt and pepper.

Omega-3 Packed Chia Seed and Blueberry Bowl

Ingredients: Chia seeds (3 tbsp), almond milk (1 cup), blueberries (1/2 cup), flaxseeds (1 tbsp), honey (1 tsp).

Instructions: Mix chia seeds and almond milk, let sit for 10 minutes to thicken. Top with blueberries, flaxseeds, and honey before serving.

Cleansing Avocado and Spinach Wraps

Ingredients: Avocados (2. sliced), spinach (2 cups), whole wheat tortillas (4), hummus (1/2 cup), lemon juice (1 tbsp), salt, and pepper.

Instructions: Spread hummus on tortillas, top with spinach and avocado slices. Drizzle with lemon juice, season with salt and pepper, and roll up the wraps.

Appendix: Natural Remedies

5-HTP (5-Hydroxytryptophan)
A naturally occurring amino acid called 5-HTP aids in the body's synthesis of serotonin, a neurotransmitter that controls mood and sleep. Serotonin is converted into melatonin, which helps regulate the sleep-wake cycle. Taking 5-HTP in doses of 100 to 300 mg about 30 minutes before bed can help improve sleep quality and support relaxation.

Almond Oil Cuticle Massage
Almond oil is rich in vitamin E and is excellent for keeping cuticles hydrated and preventing nail breakage. Massage a few drops of almond oil into your cuticles every night before bed. This daily habit will improve nail strength and reduce breakage over time, promoting healthier, stronger nails.

Aloe Vera Gel Moisturizer
Aloe vera is widely recognized for its ability to soothe and hydrate the skin. It is particularly beneficial for irritated or inflamed skin due to its anti-inflammatory properties. To use aloe vera as a moisturizer, apply pure aloe vera gel directly onto clean skin after washing. It absorbs quickly into the skin, delivering moisture and helping to reduce redness or irritation. Aloe vera is especially useful for those with sensitive or acne-prone skin. Apply it daily, preferably after cleansing your face in the morning or evening, to keep the skin hydrated and calm.

Aloe Vera Hair Mask
Aloe vera is a natural moisturizer that helps reduce scalp irritation and retain moisture in the hair. Apply fresh aloe vera gel directly to the scalp and hair, leaving it on for 30 minutes before rinsing with warm water. Use this mask once a week to promote scalp health and reduce dryness and irritation.

Aloe Vera Juice
Aloe vera has antifungal properties and supports gut health. Drink 1/4 cup of aloe vera juice diluted in water twice a day. Aloe vera soothes the digestive tract, promotes healing, and helps eliminate toxins that contribute to Candida overgrowth.

Apple Cider Vinegar Drink
Apple cider vinegar is a versatile natural remedy known for its detoxifying properties, and it can also help reduce mucus production during allergy season. By balancing the body's pH levels, apple cider vinegar assists in reducing the severity of allergy symptoms. To make an apple cider vinegar drink, mix one tablespoon of raw, unfiltered apple cider vinegar with a glass of water. Drinking this mixture in the morning can help reduce mucus buildup and clear nasal congestion. Regular consumption of apple cider vinegar also aids in the detoxification process, helping the body eliminate allergens and toxins more efficiently.

Apple Cider Vinegar Toner
Apple cider vinegar is known for its ability to balance the skin's pH and prevent acne. Dilute apple cider vinegar with water at a 1:2 ratio—one part vinegar to two parts water—and apply it to clean skin using a cotton pad. This toner helps remove excess oil, tighten pores, and maintain the skin's natural balance. Apply this toner once a day, preferably in the evening after cleansing. Apple cider vinegar can be especially beneficial for those with oily or acne-prone skin.

Apple Cider Vinegar Tonic
Apple cider vinegar is often recommended for supporting healthy stomach acid production, which is essential for proper digestion. Mixing one tablespoon of apple cider vinegar in a glass of water and drinking it before meals helps to stimulate digestive juices, promoting better breakdown of food and absorption of nutrients. This tonic can be particularly useful for individuals with low stomach acid, a condition that can lead to indigestion, bloating, and nutrient deficiencies. However, it's important to dilute the vinegar with water to prevent irritation of the esophagus and teeth.

Arnica Gel

Arnica gel is widely used for its anti-inflammatory and pain-relieving properties. Apply it directly to sore muscles or bruised areas after physical activity to reduce swelling and pain. It is recommended to use it two to three times a day for the first 48 hours post-activity for best results.

Ashwagandha

Ashwagandha is an adaptogenic herb that helps the body cope with stress and supports hormonal balance. It is particularly useful for reducing cortisol levels, which can interfere with sleep. By reducing the body's stress response, ashwagandha helps promote more restful sleep. The recommended dosage of ashwagandha is between 300 and 500 mg, taken in capsule or powder form before bed.

Ashwagandha Capsules

Ashwagandha helps reduce physical stress and supports muscle strength and recovery. Take one capsule daily, preferably after a meal, to aid in muscle repair and reduce post-exercise fatigue.

Ashwagandha Tea

Ashwagandha is an adaptogenic herb known for its ability to help the body cope with stress. It works by regulating cortisol levels, the hormone most closely associated with stress. You can make ashwagandha tea by boiling one cup of water with one teaspoon of dried ashwagandha root. Allow it to steep for about 10 minutes before drinking. For best results, drink Ashwagandha tea once or twice a day, particularly in the morning and evening, to help manage daily stress and promote relaxation at night.

Astragalus

Astragalus is an adaptogenic herb known for its ability to strengthen the immune system and protect the body from stress. It has been used traditionally in Chinese medicine to prevent colds and respiratory infections. Astragalus can be taken as a tincture or in powdered form and is particularly effective when used preventively during cold and flu season.

B-Complex Vitamins

B-complex vitamins are crucial for maintaining mental health and supporting the nervous system. These vitamins help the body convert food into energy and regulate mood. A B-complex supplement, which includes all eight B vitamins, can be taken daily, with recommended dosages ranging from 50–100 mg of each vitamin per day.

B-Vitamin Complex

B-vitamins are essential for brain health, as they play a critical role in energy production and neurotransmitter function. A deficiency in B-vitamins, particularly B12, can lead to mental fatigue, poor concentration, and memory problems. Taking a B-complex supplement daily ensures that the brain has the necessary nutrients to function optimally. The recommended dosage varies, but a typical B-complex supplement provides a balanced combination of B1, B2, B6, B12, folic acid, and other B-vitamins that support energy production and cognitive clarity. These vitamins are particularly important for individuals who may not be getting sufficient B-vitamins from their diet, such as those following a vegetarian or vegan lifestyle.

Bacopa Monnieri Supplement

Bacopa monnieri is an herb that has been used in traditional medicine for centuries to support memory and cognitive function. It is particularly effective in enhancing memory retention and preventing cognitive decline, making it a valuable supplement for individuals looking to maintain mental clarity as they age. Bacopa works by protecting brain cells from oxidative damage and improving communication between neurons. The recommended dosage for bacopa monnieri supplements is typically 300 mg per day, taken with food. Consistent use of bacopa over several months has been shown to significantly improve memory performance and cognitive processing speed.

Bentonite Clay Face Mask

Bentonite clay is a detoxifying agent that draws out impurities from the skin, making it an excellent choice for those with clogged pores or acne-prone skin. To make a mask, mix bentonite clay with water to form a thick paste. Apply the mask to clean skin and leave it on for 10 to 15 minutes, or until it begins to dry. After rinsing the mask off with warm water, apply a mild moisturizer. This mask can be used once a week to keep the skin clear and free of impurities. Bentonite clay is especially beneficial for deep cleaning the pores and removing toxins from the skin.

Berberine

Berberine is a plant alkaloid found in herbs like goldenseal and Oregon grape root. Take 500 mg of berberine twice daily to help reduce Candida populations. Berberine has antifungal properties and supports the body's ability to maintain microbial balance in the gut.

Bilberry Tea

Bilberry tea is a well-known remedy for improving circulation and protecting the eyes. To prepare this tea, steep one teaspoon of dried bilberry leaves in hot water for about 10 minutes. Drink the tea once or twice a day, particularly in the morning and evening, to benefit from its high content of antioxidants and flavonoids. These compounds are known to enhance blood flow to the eyes and improve vision, especially in low-light conditions. Bilberry is also beneficial for strengthening the tiny blood vessels in the eyes, helping to prevent issues like macular degeneration and cataracts.

Biotin Supplement

Biotin, a B-vitamin, is essential for hair growth and nail health. Taking a daily biotin supplement, as recommended on the product label (typically 2,500–5,000 mcg), can improve the resilience of nails and stimulate hair growth. It's best to incorporate this supplement into your daily routine for long-term benefits.

Black Walnut Extract

Black walnut is known for its antifungal and antimicrobial properties. Take 250 mg of black walnut extract twice a day to combat Candida. Black walnut contains tannins, which create an unfavorable environment for fungi to thrive, making it an effective remedy for fungal infections.

Blueberry Smoothie

Blueberries are rich in antioxidants, particularly anthocyanins, which are known to protect the eyes from oxidative stress. To make a blueberry smoothie, blend a cup of fresh or frozen blueberries with a cup of almond milk, a tablespoon of flaxseed, and a banana for added creaminess. This antioxidant-packed drink supports eye health by protecting against free radical damage and improving circulation to the eyes. Drinking this smoothie once a day can help maintain overall eye health, especially for those exposed to high levels of screen time or environmental pollutants.

Bone Broth Soup

Bone broth has gained recognition as a powerful remedy for gut health due to its high collagen content. Collagen helps to repair and strengthen the lining of the gut, which can become damaged due to factors like poor diet, stress, or chronic use of medications. To make bone broth, slow-cook bones with vegetables and herbs for several hours. The result is a nutrient-dense liquid that supports the healing of the digestive tract. Bone broth can be consumed on its own or used as a base for soups and stews. Regular consumption of bone broth helps to soothe inflammation in the gut and promotes overall digestive health.

Boron Capsules

Boron is another trace mineral that plays a role in bone health by supporting the metabolism of calcium, magnesium, and vitamin D. It also helps maintain the integrity of bones and joints by reducing inflammation and enhancing the body's ability to repair damaged tissues. Boron can be taken in capsule form, with a recommended dosage of 3-6 mg per day. This supplement should be taken with food to maximize absorption.

Boswellia Capsules

Boswellia, also known as Indian frankincense, is an herbal remedy known for reducing inflammation and supporting joint health. Take one to two capsules daily, preferably with meals, to help reduce soreness and enhance mobility after physical activity.

Boswellia Extract

Boswellia, also known as Indian frankincense, is a potent anti-inflammatory herb that has been used for centuries to support joint health. Its active compounds, called boswellic acids, are known to reduce inflammation and pain associated with conditions like arthritis. To support joint health, boswellia extract can be taken in capsule form. The recommended dosage is typically 300-500 mg, taken two to three times daily. It is important to take boswellia with food to enhance absorption and reduce any potential stomach irritation.

Brazil Nuts

Brazil nuts are one of the richest sources of selenium, a vital nutrient for thyroid health. Selenium helps in the conversion of thyroid hormones and protects the thyroid gland from damage caused by oxidative stress. Eating 1-2 Brazil nuts daily can provide the recommended amount of selenium. These nuts make a convenient snack or can be added to meals such as salads or smoothies.

Broccoli Stir-Fry

Cruciferous vegetables like broccoli are beneficial for hormone detoxification, particularly in reducing excess estrogen levels. These vegetables contain compounds that help the liver process and eliminate excess estrogen from the body. Cooking broccoli in a stir-fry is a delicious way to support hormonal balance. Aim to include cruciferous vegetables like broccoli, cauliflower, and Brussels sprouts in your meals at least three times a week for their detoxifying effects.

Butterbur Tincture

Butterbur (*Petasites hybridus*) is a herb traditionally used for treating allergies, particularly those that affect the respiratory system. It works by reducing inflammation in the nasal passages and sinuses, making it especially useful during allergy season. To use butterbur for allergy relief, take a few drops of butterbur tincture under the tongue or mix it with water. This method can help alleviate congestion, sneezing, and nasal discomfort. Butterbur is particularly effective in reducing symptoms without causing drowsiness, which is often a side effect of conventional allergy medications.

Calcium Supplement

Calcium is a key mineral for bone density and strength. It plays a vital role in maintaining bone structure and preventing bone loss, particularly in older adults. Calcium supplements are recommended for those who may not get enough calcium from their diet, particularly individuals who are lactose intolerant or avoid dairy products. The recommended dosage of calcium supplements is 1000-1200 mg per day, taken in divided doses. It is important to take calcium with food to enhance absorption and prevent digestive upset.

Calendula Balm

Calendula is known for its healing and soothing effects on the skin, particularly for conditions such as eczema and dry patches. Using a calendula-infused balm or oil can alleviate irritation and restore moisture to affected areas. Apply a small amount of calendula balm to dry or inflamed areas of the skin as needed, especially in the morning and evening. The anti-inflammatory and antifungal properties of calendula help to heal broken or irritated skin, making it an essential remedy for those with sensitive or problem-prone skin. This balm can be used daily or as needed to manage flare-ups of eczema or dry skin.

Calendula Oil

Calendula has anti-inflammatory properties that promote skin and muscle healing. Apply calendula oil to sore muscles once or twice daily to aid recovery and reduce inflammation.

Calendula Tea

Calendula is a soothing herb with antifungal and anti-inflammatory properties. Brew a tea using one tablespoon of dried calendula flowers in hot water. Drink this once daily to support immune function and reduce fungal infections. Calendula helps heal mucous membranes and supports overall gut health.

California Poppy

California poppy is a natural sedative that is particularly effective for reducing anxiety and promoting deeper sleep. It is commonly used in herbal teas or tinctures. The recommended dose is 1 to 2 grams of dried herb, taken about an hour before bed to help calm the mind and body.

Caprylic Acid

Caprylic acid, found in coconut oil, can also be taken as a supplement to target fungal infections. Take 500 mg of caprylic acid three times a day to combat systemic Candida overgrowth. Caprylic acid breaks down the cell walls of Candida, making it easier for the immune system to eliminate the infection.

Carrot and Spinach Juice

Juicing carrots and spinach provides a nutrient-dense drink packed with beta-carotene and lutein, both of which are essential for maintaining healthy vision. Carrots are high in beta-carotene, a precursor to vitamin A, which is crucial for preventing night blindness and promoting good vision. Spinach, on the other hand, is rich in lutein, an antioxidant that protects the eyes from harmful blue light and UV rays. For optimal benefits, juice two to three fresh carrots and a handful of spinach, and drink it in the morning to kickstart your day with eye-protective nutrients.

Castor Oil Nail Treatment

Castor oil is known for its ability to nourish and strengthen brittle nails. Apply a small amount of castor oil to your nails and cuticles every night before bed. Massage it in gently for a few minutes to stimulate nail growth and strengthen weak nails over time. Regular application will result in healthier, more resilient nails.

Cayenne Pepper and Honey Cough Syrup

Cayenne pepper is known for its ability to stimulate circulation and break up mucus, while honey soothes the throat. To make a **cayenne pepper and honey cough syrup**, mix 1/4 teaspoon of cayenne pepper with 1 tablespoon of honey and a small amount of warm water. Take 1 teaspoon of this syrup every few hours when dealing with a persistent cough or mucus buildup. The cayenne pepper works to clear congestion, while the honey coats and soothes the throat, providing quick relief from coughing fits.

Cayenne Pepper and Lemon Detox Drink

Cayenne pepper is a powerful spice that stimulates metabolism through thermogenesis, the process by which the body burns calories to generate heat. When combined with fresh lemon juice, this detox drink supports digestion and helps detoxify the body. Mix a pinch of cayenne pepper and the juice of half a lemon in a glass of warm water. Drink this mixture first thing in the morning on an empty stomach to kickstart metabolism for the day. This remedy can also be consumed 30 minutes before meals to promote digestion.

Cayenne Pepper Supplement

Cayenne pepper is a powerful circulatory stimulant that helps improve blood flow and lower blood pressure. It works by dilating blood vessels and increasing the body's temperature, which boosts circulation. Cayenne can be taken in supplement form, and a typical dosage is 500 mg, taken once or twice a day with meals. Some individuals may find cayenne to be too strong initially, so it is recommended to start with a lower dose and gradually increase as the body adjusts. This supplement can be particularly effective for individuals with poor circulation or those looking to improve overall cardiovascular function.

Chamomile

Chamomile is another powerful herb that promotes relaxation and reduces anxiety. Its mild sedative properties make it ideal for reducing nervous tension and calming the mind. Chamomile tea is a popular way to consume this herb. Drinking a cup of chamomile tea two to three times a day can help maintain a sense of calm, especially during periods of heightened stress. It's also effective in promoting better sleep if consumed in the evening.

Chamomile Eye Compress

Chamomile is a soothing herb that can be used as an eye compress to relieve redness and irritation. To make a compress, brew two chamomile tea bags and allow them to cool. Once they are no longer hot, place the tea bags over your closed eyes for 10 to 15 minutes. This can be done twice a day, especially after a long day of screen time or if your eyes feel dry and irritated. The anti-inflammatory properties of chamomile help calm redness and reduce swelling around the eyes.

Chamomile Steam Facial

Chamomile is well-known for its calming effects, not only internally but also externally when applied to the skin. A chamomile steam facial helps open pores and cleanse the skin deeply. Boil a pot of water and add a handful of dried chamomile flowers. Lean over the pot with a towel draped over your head to trap the steam, and allow the steam to penetrate your skin for 5 to 10 minutes. This method helps to loosen dirt and impurities while soothing the skin. You can use this steam facial once a week as part of a deeper cleansing routine.

Chamomile Tea

Chamomile is well-known for its calming effects on both the mind and the body, making it an excellent choice for promoting bodily and digestive relaxation. Chamomile tea, made by steeping dried chamomile flowers in hot water, can be consumed before bed to calm the stomach and help prevent issues like acid reflux and indigestion. Chamomile's anti-inflammatory properties soothe the lining of the stomach and intestines, making it useful for those with conditions such as gastritis or IBS. Drinking a cup of chamomile tea in the evening is especially beneficial for individuals whose digestive issues are linked to stress or anxiety.

Chamomile Tea Compress

Chamomile is widely known for its soothing properties, and when applied topically, it can help reduce allergy-related eye discomfort. For those who suffer from puffiness, redness, and itching around the eyes due to seasonal allergies, chamomile tea compresses can provide relief. Steep chamomile tea bags in hot water, then allow them to cool. Once cool, place the tea bags over the eyes to help soothe irritation. Chamomile's anti-inflammatory properties make it an excellent remedy for alleviating the discomfort caused by allergies around the eyes.

Chia Seed Smoothie

Chia seeds are an excellent source of omega-3 fatty acids, which reduce inflammation and support hormonal balance. These fatty acids are essential for hormone production, particularly in regulating mood and energy levels. Adding chia seeds to a smoothie is a simple way to boost your intake of omega-3s. Blend one tablespoon of chia seeds with fruit, greens, and almond milk for a nutrient-dense smoothie that supports overall hormone health.

Chili Pepper Infused Oil

Chili peppers contain capsaicin, a compound that increases thermogenesis and fat burning. By infusing olive oil with chili peppers, you can create a metabolism-boosting cooking oil that enhances the flavor of meals while promoting fat loss. To make chili pepper infused oil, heat olive oil and add fresh or dried chili peppers, allowing them to infuse for several hours. Use this oil in cooking or as a dressing for salads to add a spicy kick while supporting fat burning. Use sparingly, as a little chili oil goes a long way in terms of both flavor and metabolic effect.

Cinnamon Bark Tea

Cinnamon bark contains potent antifungal compounds that can help starve Candida. Brew a tea by simmering one cinnamon stick in hot water for 10 minutes. Drink this once daily to support digestion and reduce Candida overgrowth. Cinnamon is known for its ability to regulate blood sugar levels, which is crucial in managing Candida, as sugar feeds fungal growth.

Cinnamon Tea

Cinnamon helps regulate blood sugar levels, which is crucial for preventing insulin spikes that lead to fat storage. It also reduces sugar cravings, making it easier to manage appetite. To prepare cinnamon tea, simmer cinnamon sticks in water for 10 minutes. Drink this tea in the morning or between meals to help control blood sugar and reduce cravings. Cinnamon tea can be consumed twice a day, particularly before or after meals that contain carbohydrates.

Clove Oil

Clove oil contains eugenol, a potent antifungal compound. Take one to two drops of clove oil mixed with a carrier oil (such as coconut oil) once daily. It can also be added to a warm drink like herbal tea. Clove oil helps inhibit fungal growth and reduce inflammation associated with Candida infections.

Coconut Oil

Coconut oil is rich in caprylic acid, a fatty acid that targets fungal infections. Consume one to two tablespoons of raw, organic coconut oil daily to fight Candida from the inside out. Coconut oil can also be applied topically to areas affected by fungal infections, providing a soothing and antifungal effect on the skin.

Coconut Oil Moisturizer

Coconut oil is an excellent natural moisturizer due to its high content of fatty acids, which help lock in moisture and soften the skin. After showering, when the skin is still slightly damp, apply a thin layer of coconut oil to the body. This helps to seal in moisture and leaves the skin feeling smooth and hydrated. Coconut oil is particularly beneficial for dry skin and can be used daily after bathing. Be cautious with its use on the face, especially for those with acne-prone skin, as it can clog pores for some individuals.

Coconut Oil Supplement

Coconut oil is rich in healthy fats that support the production of hormones in the body. These fats are essential for building the hormones that regulate metabolism, stress, and reproductive health. Using coconut oil in cooking or taking it as a supplement can help ensure you're getting enough healthy fats for optimal hormone production. Try adding one tablespoon of coconut oil to your diet daily, either by cooking with it or adding it to smoothies.

Comfrey Cream

Comfrey cream helps with tissue regeneration and is particularly effective for muscle injuries or strains. Apply it two to three times a day to areas of soreness for muscle recovery, especially after more intense physical exertion.

Comfrey Root Balm

Comfrey root has long been used in traditional medicine for its ability to heal fractures, sprains, and bruises. It contains compounds that promote the regeneration of bone and connective tissue, making it an ideal remedy for joint pain and injuries. Comfrey root balm can be applied topically to the affected area, massaging it gently into the skin. It is best used 2-3 times per day for joint pain, swelling, or to aid in the healing of minor injuries. Comfrey root should not be used on broken skin or open wounds due to the potential for toxicity if absorbed in large amounts.

Cucumber and Mint Water

Hydration plays a critical role in metabolism, and cucumber and mint water is a refreshing way to promote hydration while reducing bloating. Cucumber helps flush out toxins and supports healthy digestion, while mint aids in calming the digestive system. Add cucumber slices and fresh mint leaves to a jug of water and sip throughout the day. Drinking this infusion regularly helps to maintain hydration, which is essential for optimal metabolism and digestion. Aim to consume at least 2 liters of this water daily to stay hydrated and reduce bloating.

Cucumber Eye Compress

Cucumber slices are a classic remedy for reducing puffiness and revitalizing tired skin around the eyes. Cucumber contains antioxidants and has a cooling effect that helps to refresh the delicate skin under the eyes. To use, place chilled cucumber slices over closed eyes and relax for 10 to 15 minutes. This treatment can be done daily, particularly in the morning, to reduce puffiness and improve the appearance of dark circles.

Dandelion Leaf Tea

Dandelion leaf is a natural diuretic that helps the body eliminate excess fluid, reducing the strain on the heart and lowering blood pressure. It also contains potassium, which supports heart function and helps balance electrolytes in the body. Dandelion leaf tea can be consumed once or twice daily to support cardiovascular health. To prepare the tea, steep one teaspoon of dried dandelion leaves in boiling water for 10 minutes. The tea can be consumed on its own or combined with other heart-supporting herbs such as hibiscus or ginger.

Dandelion Root Tea

Dandelion root tea is another powerful natural remedy for managing allergies, particularly because of its support for liver detoxification. The liver plays a crucial role in processing allergens and toxins, and when it is functioning optimally, the body is better equipped to handle allergic reactions. Brew dandelion root tea to help cleanse the liver and enhance its ability to filter out harmful substances from the bloodstream. Drinking this tea regularly can reduce the overall inflammatory response to allergens and support the body's natural detox pathways, making it easier to manage allergy symptoms.

Devil's Claw Capsules

Devil's Claw is effective for relieving muscle and joint pain. Take one or two capsules daily with meals to help reduce inflammation and support recovery after physical exertion.

Echinacea

Echinacea is widely known for its immune-boosting properties. This herb works by stimulating the production of white blood cells, which are essential for fighting off infections. There are several ways to consume echinacea, such as tinctures, teas, or pills. For best results, it is recommended to take echinacea at the onset of cold or flu symptoms to reduce the severity and duration of the illness. Taking echinacea over extended periods is not necessary; instead, it should be used during times of increased risk of infection.

Elderberry

Elderberry is rich in antioxidants and vitamins that support immune function. It is particularly effective in reducing the duration of flu symptoms and can be taken as a syrup, tea, or capsule. Elderberry helps to boost the immune system by increasing cytokine production, which aids in the body's defense against viruses. For preventive purposes, it can be taken daily during cold and flu season.

Elderberry Syrup

Elderberries are rich in antioxidants and have immune-boosting properties, making **elderberry syrup** an excellent preventative remedy during cold and flu season. Take 1 tablespoon of elderberry syrup daily to support immunity and ward off respiratory infections. If symptoms of a cold or flu arise, increase the dose to 1 tablespoon up to three times a day. Elderberry syrup not only strengthens the immune system but also helps reduce the duration and severity of colds and respiratory ailments.

Elderflower Tea

Elderflower (*Sambucus nigra*) is another effective remedy for managing allergy symptoms, especially respiratory congestion. Elderflower tea is known for its ability to relieve nasal congestion and soothe respiratory irritation. Brew elderflower tea to help clear blocked nasal passages and reduce the discomfort associated with seasonal allergies. The herb's anti-inflammatory and antiviral properties also make it beneficial in reducing cold-like symptoms that often accompany allergies. Drinking elderflower tea regularly during allergy season can keep your respiratory system clear and functioning properly.

Epsom Salt Bath

Epsom salts, which are rich in magnesium sulfate, are widely known for their ability to relax muscles and relieve joint pain. Soaking in an Epsom salt bath allows the body to absorb magnesium through the skin, which can help reduce inflammation and ease discomfort. To use Epsom salts for joint health, add 1-2 cups of Epsom salts to a warm bath and soak for 20-30 minutes. This can be done 2-3 times per week to maintain joint flexibility and soothe sore muscles.

Epsom Salt Baths (with Lavender Essential Oil)

Epsom salt is rich in magnesium, which aids in muscle relaxation and recovery. Add 2 cups of Epsom salt and a few drops of lavender essential oil to a warm bath. Soak for 20–30 minutes, ideally after a strenuous workout or at the end of the day to promote deep muscle relaxation.

Eucalyptus

Eucalyptus is commonly used to relieve congestion and support respiratory function. Eucalyptus oil can be added to a diffuser or used in steam inhalations to clear nasal passages and sinuses. It is especially helpful during colds or flu when congestion is a primary symptom.

Eucalyptus Steam Inhalation

Eucalyptus oil is well known for its ability to clear nasal congestion and improve respiratory function. Inhaling eucalyptus vapors can provide immediate relief from allergy-related congestion. To use eucalyptus oil for steam inhalation, add a few drops of the oil to a bowl of steaming water. Cover your head with a towel and lean over the bowl, inhaling the vapors deeply. This method helps open the sinuses and reduce nasal blockage caused by allergies. Eucalyptus also has antimicrobial properties, which can help protect against infections that sometimes arise when the respiratory system is compromised during allergy season.

Evening Primrose Oil

Evening primrose oil is rich in gamma-linolenic acid (GLA), an omega-6 fatty acid that helps balance hormones, particularly for women experiencing PMS or menopause symptoms. GProstaglandins, which are hormone-like substances that control the menstrual cycle, are produced with the help of LA. Take evening primrose oil supplements (usually 500-1000 mg) once daily with meals to help manage symptoms such as breast tenderness, mood swings, and hot flashes.

Eyebright Eye Wash

Eyebright, a herb traditionally used for eye health, can be brewed into a tea and used as a soothing eye wash. To make the solution, steep one teaspoon of dried eyebright in a cup of hot water and let it cool completely. Once cooled, strain the tea and apply it gently to the eyes using a clean cloth or cotton pad. This wash can be used once or twice a day to relieve irritation, dryness, and eye strain, especially after prolonged screen time or exposure to allergens. Eyebright has anti-inflammatory properties that help soothe redness and reduce swelling.

Fennel Seed Chew

Fennel seeds have been used for centuries as a remedy for digestive discomfort. Chewing fennel seeds after meals can help reduce gas and bloating, thanks to the seeds' natural antispasmodic and anti-inflammatory properties. The essential oils in fennel help stimulate the secretion of digestive enzymes, improving overall digestion and reducing the buildup of gas in the intestines. To use this remedy, chew a small amount (about half a teaspoon) of fennel seeds after eating. This simple practice not only freshens the breath but also aids in breaking down food more efficiently, particularly after large or heavy meals.

Fennel Tea Eye Compress

Fennel has natural anti-inflammatory and soothing properties that make it an excellent remedy for eye strain. To make a fennel tea compress, brew a cup of fennel tea and allow it to cool. Once cooled, soak a clean cloth in the tea and apply it over your eyes for 10 to 15 minutes. This compress can be used at the end of the day to relieve eye fatigue, particularly after long hours of work or exposure to bright lights. The soothing properties of fennel help reduce tension in the eye muscles and promote relaxation.

Flaxseed Oil

Flaxseed oil is an excellent source of omega-3 fatty acids, which are essential for maintaining heart health. Omega-3s are known to reduce inflammation in the body, lower blood pressure, and improve cholesterol levels by increasing HDL (good cholesterol) while reducing LDL (bad cholesterol). To reap the benefits of flaxseed oil, it should be taken daily. A typical dosage is one tablespoon of flaxseed oil per day, either consumed directly or added to smoothies, salads, or other cold foods. It is important to store flaxseed oil in the refrigerator, as it can easily go rancid when exposed to heat or light. Avoid using it for cooking, as high temperatures destroy its beneficial properties.

Flaxseed Oil Supplement

Flaxseed oil is an excellent source of omega-3 fatty acids, which are known to help maintain tear production and prevent dry eyes. Taking one to two tablespoons of flaxseed oil daily, either on its own or mixed into smoothies, salads, or other foods, can help improve lubrication in the eyes. Omega-3s are particularly beneficial for individuals suffering from dry eye syndrome, as they help to keep the eyes moist and reduce inflammation that may contribute to dryness and discomfort.

Flaxseed Pudding

Flaxseeds are high in lignans, compounds that help with hormone detoxification, particularly in women. They also provide a good source of fiber, which helps remove excess hormones from the body through the digestive tract. To make flaxseed pudding, mix two tablespoons of ground flaxseeds with half a cup of almond milk and let it sit for a few hours or overnight until it thickens. Consume this fiber-rich pudding in the morning to support hormone balance throughout the day.

Flaxseed Smoothie

Flaxseeds are a rich source of dietary fiber, which helps keep you feeling full for longer periods, thereby suppressing appetite. They also support digestive health and contribute to weight management. To prepare, blend a tablespoon of ground flaxseeds into a smoothie with almond milk, berries, and a handful of leafy greens. This fiber-rich smoothie makes for an ideal breakfast or midday snack, helping to curb hunger and promote digestive regularity.

GABA

GABA (gamma-aminobutyric acid) is a neurotransmitter that helps reduce anxiety and promote relaxation, making it easier to fall asleep. GABA supplements, typically taken in doses of 250 to 500 mg before bed, are particularly useful for those dealing with insomnia or stress-related sleep issues.

Garlic

Garlic's potent antiviral, antibacterial, and antifungal qualities have earned it the moniker "nature's antibiotic." Allicin, the active compound in garlic, is most potent when garlic is consumed raw. Garlic can be finely chopped or crushed and added to food, or taken directly with honey. To maximize its immune-boosting benefits, consume garlic daily, especially during times of illness or heightened exposure to infections.

Garlic and Lemon Detox Soup

Garlic is known for its detoxifying properties and its ability to support digestion, while lemon helps alkalize the body and promote detoxification. Together, these ingredients create a light vegetable broth that supports the body's natural detox processes. To prepare, simmer garlic and fresh lemon slices in a pot of vegetable broth. Enjoy this soup as a light meal or as a starter to aid digestion and promote detoxification. This soup can be consumed 1-2 times a week, especially after periods of indulgence, to help reset the digestive system and support weight loss efforts.

Garlic Capsules

Garlic is a well-known remedy for heart health due to its ability to lower cholesterol and blood pressure. It works by relaxing blood vessels and thinning the blood, which improves circulation and reduces the risk of heart disease. Garlic capsules are an easy and odorless way to incorporate garlic into a daily routine. The recommended dosage is 600 to 1,200 mg of aged garlic extract, taken once daily. For best results, garlic should be taken consistently over time to maintain its heart-healthy effects. It can also be combined with other heart-supporting herbs and supplements to enhance its benefits.

Garlic Infusion

Garlic is one of the most powerful natural antifungal agents. To create a garlic infusion, crush two to three fresh garlic cloves and steep them in a cup of warm water for 10 minutes. Drink this once daily or use it topically on areas affected by Candida to reduce fungal growth. Garlic's active compound, allicin, helps inhibit the spread of Candida and boost the immune system.

Garlic Syrup

Garlic is a potent antimicrobial and immune-boosting food that supports respiratory health. To make **garlic syrup**, chop a few cloves of garlic and mix them with honey in a small jar. Allow the mixture to sit for several hours or overnight to create a syrup. Take 1 teaspoon of this garlic syrup daily to help prevent respiratory infections or 2-3 teaspoons when dealing with colds or flu. Garlic's natural antibacterial and antiviral properties help clear the lungs and reduce the severity of respiratory symptoms.

Ginger

Ginger is another powerful immune-supportive herb. It works by reducing inflammation and boosting circulation, which helps the immune system function more efficiently. Ginger can be consumed fresh in teas or smoothies, or added to meals as a spice. It is particularly helpful in relieving symptoms of colds and flu, such as congestion and sore throat.

Ginger and Honey Tea

Ginger has warming properties and aids in reducing inflammation and muscle pain. To make a soothing tea, steep 1–2 slices of fresh ginger in hot water, add honey for sweetness, and drink it twice daily, especially after workouts to support digestion and reduce muscle discomfort.

Ginger Tea

Ginger is known for its anti-inflammatory and circulatory benefits. It helps to improve blood flow and lower blood pressure, making it a valuable ally for heart health. Ginger can also help reduce cholesterol levels and prevent blood clots, further supporting cardiovascular function. Ginger tea can be consumed one to two times per day to support heart health. To prepare the tea, slice a small piece of fresh ginger root and steep it in boiling water for 10 to 15 minutes. The tea can be sweetened with honey or lemon if desired. Ginger supplements are also available, and a typical dosage is 500 to 1,000 mg per day.

Ginger Tea

Ginger is a potent root that aids digestion, reduces inflammation, and boosts calorie burning. Its thermogenic effect helps the body burn more calories, making it useful for weight loss efforts. To prepare ginger tea, brew several thin slices of fresh ginger in hot water for about 10 minutes. Drink the tea before or after meals to aid digestion and enhance calorie burning. Ginger tea can be consumed up to three times a day, especially before meals, to support metabolism.

Ginkgo Biloba Supplement

Ginkgo biloba is an excellent supplement for enhancing blood circulation, not only throughout the body but specifically to the eyes. The increased blood flow helps supply the optic nerve and retina with the nutrients and oxygen they need to function optimally. Ginkgo biloba can be taken as a daily supplement, typically in doses of 120 to 240 milligrams, depending on the product. It is particularly helpful for people experiencing age-related eye conditions such as glaucoma or macular degeneration, as it helps to support overall vision health and reduce oxidative damage to eye tissues.

Ginkgo Biloba Tea

Ginkgo biloba has long been recognized for its ability to enhance cognitive function, particularly memory and concentration. The leaves of the ginkgo tree contain powerful compounds that improve blood circulation to the brain, thereby increasing oxygen delivery and promoting mental sharpness. To harness the benefits of ginkgo biloba, steep a teaspoon of dried ginkgo biloba leaves in hot water for about 10 minutes. Drinking this tea daily can support cognitive health, especially for individuals who experience memory lapses or difficulty concentrating. The recommended dosage for ginkgo biloba is typically 120–240 mg per day, divided into two or three doses throughout the day, but consuming it in tea form offers a more natural and gentle method of delivery.

Ginseng

Ginseng is known for its ability to reduce stress and boost mental clarity. It helps improve the body's resilience to stress and can enhance cognitive function. Ginseng is available in capsule or tincture form, with a general dosage of 100–200 mg per day.

Ginseng Extract

Ginseng is an adaptogenic herb that boosts mental energy and enhances focus. It has been used for centuries in traditional medicine to improve cognitive performance and combat mental fatigue. Ginseng works by supporting the brain's resistance to stress and enhancing blood circulation to the brain. The recommended dosage for ginseng extract is typically between 100 and 200 mg per day, depending on the form and concentration of the supplement. Taking ginseng in the morning or early afternoon can help sustain mental energy throughout the day, making it a useful remedy for those struggling with concentration during long work hours.

Ginseng Tea

Ginseng is another herb that is often used to enhance energy levels and support weight loss efforts. It helps boost physical endurance and mental clarity, while also improving metabolism and fat oxidation. To prepare, steep ginseng root in hot water for 10 minutes. Drink ginseng tea in the morning or early afternoon to improve energy and metabolism. It can be consumed up to twice a day, but it's best to avoid drinking it late in the day as it may interfere with sleep.

Glycine

Glycine is an amino acid that can help lower the body's core temperature, signaling the brain that it's time to sleep. Taking glycine supplements, typically in doses of 3 grams before bed, has been shown to improve sleep quality. Glycine is also involved in collagen production, which supports the repair of tissues during sleep.

Golden Milk

Golden milk, made with turmeric, is an anti-inflammatory drink that supports gut healing. To prepare golden milk, mix turmeric with warm almond milk, honey, and cinnamon. Turmeric's active compound, curcumin, helps reduce inflammation in the digestive tract, making it an effective remedy for those dealing with conditions such as IBSor inflammatory bowel disease. Drinking golden milk regularly can help soothe the digestive system and promote overall gut health. This drink is best consumed in the evening as part of a calming routine that supports digestion and relaxation.

Golden Milk with Turmeric

Turmeric is a potent anti-inflammatory herb that can help reduce inflammation in the eyes and support overall eye health. To prepare golden milk, mix one teaspoon of turmeric powder with a cup of warm almond milk and a teaspoon of honey. Drinking this beverage before bed can help reduce inflammation throughout the body, including in the eyes, and promote healing. Turmeric's active compound, curcumin, helps protect the eyes from oxidative stress and inflammation, which are common contributors to vision problems.

Grapefruit Salad

Grapefruit is well-known for its fat-burning properties, as it contains compounds that help regulate insulin levels and reduce fat accumulation. Including fresh grapefruit slices in a salad with leafy greens and avocado can further enhance its benefits. The healthy fats from avocado provide additional satiety, while the greens offer essential nutrients. Enjoy this salad for lunch or as a light dinner to support fat burning and maintain energy throughout the day. Eating grapefruit before meals can also reduce calorie intake by promoting a sense of fullness.

Grapefruit Seed Extract

Grapefruit seed extract is a powerful antifungal and antimicrobial remedy. Take 200 mg of grapefruit seed extract twice daily to help eliminate Candida overgrowth. This extract works by disrupting the membranes of Candida cells, preventing them from replicating.

Green Tea

Green tea is rich in antioxidants, particularly catechins, which help fight off infections. Drinking green tea regularly can boost the immune system by enhancing the body's ability to respond to pathogens. Green tea is best consumed without added sugar to maximize its health benefits.

Green Tea Infusion

Green tea is known for its metabolism-boosting properties, making it a natural remedy for supporting weight management. The catechins and antioxidants found in green tea help increase the body's fat-burning potential by improving energy expenditure. To prepare, steep green tea leaves in hot water for 5-10 minutes. Drink 2-3 cups daily to experience its full benefits. Drinking a cup in the morning and another before exercise can be particularly effective for boosting metabolism.

Hawthorn Berry Tincture

Hawthorn berry is renowned for its ability to support cardiovascular health. It has been used for centuries to strengthen the heart and improve blood flow. This herb works by dilating the blood vessels, reducing blood pressure, and increasing the supply of oxygen to the heart. Hawthorn berry tincture can be taken daily to support heart function and regulate blood pressure. It is most effective when taken in small, regular doses. The recommended usage is 20 to 30 drops, taken two to three times a day, diluted in water or juice. When using hawthorn, consistency is essential because the advantages become apparent after a few weeks of consistent use.

Hibiscus Tea

Hibiscus tea is a natural remedy that has been shown to lower blood pressure, making it an excellent choice for those looking to support heart health. Hibiscus works as a diuretic, helping the body eliminate excess fluid, which reduces the workload on the heart. It also contains antioxidants that protect the heart from oxidative stress. Drinking one to two cups of hibiscus tea per day can help maintain healthy blood pressure levels. To prepare the tea, steep one teaspoon of dried hibiscus flowers in boiling water for 5 to 10 minutes. The tea can be consumed hot or cold, depending on preference.

Holy Basil

Holy basil, also known as Tulsi, is an adaptogen that helps reduce stress and balance cortisol levels. It can be consumed as a tea or in supplement form. Drinking 1–2 cups of holy basil tea per day can help manage stress and promote mental clarity. Capsules containing holy basil extract (500 mg) can also be taken daily.

Holy Basil Tea

Holy basil, also known as Tulsi, is a herb that helps lower cortisol levels and manage stress. Drinking holy basil tea daily can help reduce the physical effects of stress on the body, allowing the endocrine system to function more efficiently. To prepare, steep one teaspoon of dried holy basil leaves in hot water for 5-10 minutes. Drink this tea once or twice daily, particularly in the afternoon or evening, to calm the nervous system and regulate cortisol levels.

Honey

Raw honey has natural antibacterial and antiviral properties. It can soothe sore throats and suppress coughs, making it a valuable remedy during colds and flu. Honey can be taken by the spoonful or mixed into teas for immune support.

Honey and Oatmeal Face Scrub

Honey and oatmeal are powerful ingredients for skin care, offering a gentle yet effective exfoliation that also nourishes the skin. To make the scrub, mix 2 tablespoons of oatmeal with 1 tablespoon of honey and add a small amount of water to create a paste. Oatmeal works as a mild exfoliant, removing dead skin cells without causing irritation, while honey provides antibacterial properties and deep moisture. Use this scrub once or twice a week, massaging it into the skin for 1 to 2 minutes before rinsing it off with warm water. This routine helps maintain a smooth, healthy complexion.

Hops

Hops, commonly known for their use in brewing beer, also have sedative properties that can help promote relaxation and sleep. Hops can be taken in the form of herbal tea or supplements. The typical dosage ranges from 300 to 500 mg of dried hops extract, taken about an hour before bed.

Horsetail Tea

Horsetail is a powerful source of silica, a mineral known for promoting strong hair and nails. To prepare, steep 1-2 teaspoons of dried horsetail in a cup of hot water for 10 minutes. Drink this tea once a day to increase your body's silica intake, which helps strengthen hair strands and reduce nail brittleness.

Hot Lemon and Honey Drink

Lemon is rich in vitamin C, which helps boost the immune system, while honey soothes the throat and reduces irritation. To make a **hot lemon and honey drink**, mix the juice of half a lemon with 1-2 teaspoons of honey in a cup of warm water. Drink this mixture 2-3 times a day during respiratory infections or whenever you feel the need to soothe your throat and support your immune system. The combination of lemon and honey also helps thin mucus, making it easier to expel.

Hydration Reminder

Dehydration is a common, yet often overlooked, cause of mental fatigue and cognitive impairment. Even mild dehydration can result in difficulty concentrating, slower cognitive processing, and increased mental fog. It's essential to stay hydrated throughout the day to maintain optimal brain function. A simple way to ensure adequate hydration is to set reminders to drink water regularly. Make it a habit to drink eight glasses of water or more each day if you exercise or spend time in hot conditions. Hydration supports the brain's electrical activity and helps maintain clear, focused thinking.

Kava

Kava is a plant native to the South Pacific that has been used for centuries to reduce anxiety and promote relaxation. It is a natural sedative and can be helpful for those experiencing sleep disturbances due to stress. Kava can be taken in tincture or capsule form, with a typical dose of 100 to 200 mg, taken about 30 to 60 minutes before bed.

Kefir Smoothie

Kefir is another powerful probiotic food that supports the digestive system. Kefir is a fermented milk drink rich in live cultures that help maintain the balance of bacteria in the gut. Blending kefir with fresh fruits and honey creates a delicious smoothie that not only tastes good but also supports digestion. The probiotics in kefir help reduce bloating, improve bowel movements, and enhance the overall efficiency of the digestive system. Kefir smoothies can be enjoyed in the morning or as a snack during the day, particularly for those looking to strengthen their gut microbiome and improve digestive function.

L-Theanine

Green tea contains an amino acid called L-theanine, which helps people relax without making them feel sleepy. It increases levels of calming neurotransmitters in the brain, making it easier to fall asleep. Taking 200 to 400 mg of L-theanine before bed can improve sleep quality, especially when stress or anxiety is a contributing factor to sleeplessness.

Lavender

Lavender has been used for centuries to reduce anxiety, improve mood, and promote restful sleep. Lavender oil can be diffused into the air, applied to the skin (diluted with a carrier oil), or added to a bath to promote relaxation. A few drops of lavender essential oil on the pillow before bedtime can help improve sleep quality, while inhaling lavender throughout the day can reduce feelings of stress and tension.

Lavender Essential Oil (for Massage)

Lavender oil promotes relaxation and helps reduce muscle soreness. Dilute a few drops in a carrier oil and massage into sore areas before bed to calm both the mind and the muscles.

Lavender Oil Hair Treatment

Lavender essential oil, when combined with a carrier oil like coconut oil, can prevent hair thinning and soothe an irritated scalp. Mix 2-3 drops of lavender oil with 1 tablespoon of coconut oil, then massage it into the scalp. Leave it on for 30 minutes before rinsing. Use this treatment once a week to keep your hair strong and your scalp balanced.

Lemon and Sugar Scrub

Lemon is a natural astringent and brightening agent, while sugar serves as an effective exfoliant. To make a body scrub, mix the juice of half a lemon with 1 tablespoon of sugar. Gently scrub the mixture onto the skin, focusing on areas that need exfoliation, such as elbows, knees, and feet. The lemon helps to lighten dark spots and pigmentation, while the sugar sloughs away dead skin cells. Use this scrub once a week for smooth, glowing skin, but avoid using it on the face as lemon can be too harsh for sensitive facial skin.

Lemon Balm

Lemon balm is known for its antiviral and antifungal properties. Drink lemon balm tea twice a day to help reduce fungal infections. Lemon balm's soothing and calming effects also help alleviate stress, which can contribute to Candida overgrowth.

Lemon Balm Tea

Lemon balm is an herb known for its ability to reduce anxiety and promote mental clarity. It is particularly effective for individuals who experience stress-induced brain fog or difficulty focusing due to anxiety. To make lemon balm tea, steep a teaspoon of dried lemon balm leaves in hot water for 5–10 minutes. Drinking this tea during times of stress can help calm the mind and improve cognitive function. Lemon balm's soothing properties make it an excellent remedy for improving mental clarity while also reducing nervous tension.

Licorice Root

Licorice root has antiviral and anti-inflammatory properties that support the immune system. It works especially well for respiratory illnesses like sore throats and bronchitis. Licorice root can be taken as a tea or in supplement form, but it should be used in moderation to avoid side effects.

Licorice Root Tea

Licorice root is a natural remedy known for its ability to support adrenal function and help maintain hormonal balance, particularly in times of stress. Licorice root helps to prolong the activity of cortisol, making it useful for those with adrenal insufficiency or fatigue. Steep one teaspoon of dried licorice root in ten minutes of boiling water to make licorice root tea. Strain the tea and drink it in the morning or early afternoon. Avoid drinking licorice root tea late in the day, as it can increase energy levels and disrupt sleep.

Licorice Root Tincture

Licorice root is a powerful anti-inflammatory herb that can soothe irritated airways and reduce inflammation in the lungs. A **licorice root tincture** is an easy and effective way to utilize this herb. Take 10-20 drops of the tincture diluted in a small glass of water up to three times daily. Licorice also has demulcent properties, meaning it coats the mucous membranes, providing relief from dry coughs and bronchial irritation. However, long-term use of licorice should be avoided in people with high blood pressure or those prone to water retention, as it can have a hypertensive effect when used excessively.

Lutein Salad

Lutein and zeaxanthin are two powerful antioxidants that protect the eyes from blue light damage and support overall eye health. To incorporate these nutrients into your diet, prepare a salad using spinach, kale, and avocados—all of which are high in lutein. Add some olive oil and lemon juice for flavor and to enhance nutrient absorption. Eating a lutein-rich salad regularly, especially at lunchtime, can help reduce the risk of macular degeneration and other age-related eye issues.

Maca Root Powder

Maca root is widely recognized for its ability to balance reproductive hormones, especially in women. It supports overall hormonal health and helps regulate symptoms of menopause and PMS. Maca root powder can easily be incorporated into your daily diet by adding one teaspoon to smoothies, oatmeal, or yogurt. It's best to start with small amounts and gradually increase, taking it in the morning to benefit from its energy-boosting properties without interfering with sleep.

Magnesium

Magnesium is an essential mineral that plays a critical role in regulating the body's stress response. Anxiety and tension might rise when there is a magnesium deficit. Magnesium supplements can help relax muscles, improve sleep quality, and reduce feelings of anxiety. The recommended dosage is 200–400 mg per day, preferably taken in the evening to aid relaxation.

Magnesium Oil

Magnesium plays a critical role in bone health and muscle function. Magnesium oil, when applied topically, helps relax tense muscles and improve joint flexibility. It also aids in the absorption of calcium, which is essential for bone strength. To use magnesium oil, spray it directly onto the skin over affected joints or muscles, and massage gently. The oil should be left on for at least 20 minutes before rinsing off. This can be done once or twice a day, particularly after physical activity or before bed to support muscle relaxation and pain relief.

Magnesium Supplement

Magnesium is an essential mineral that plays a critical role in heart health by regulating blood pressure, supporting normal heart rhythms, and relaxing blood vessels. Many people are deficient in magnesium, which can contribute to high blood pressure and other cardiovascular issues. The recommended daily dosage for magnesium is 300 to 400 mg, taken in the evening, as magnesium can also help promote relaxation and improve sleep quality. Magnesium glycinate or citrate is often preferred, as these forms are easier on the digestive system and more readily absorbed by the body.

Marshmallow Root Tea

Marshmallow root has mucilaginous properties, meaning it creates a soothing coating for irritated mucous membranes, especially in the lungs and throat. To make **marshmallow root tea**, steep 1-2 teaspoons of dried marshmallow root in hot water for 10 minutes. Drink 2-3 cups daily to relieve dry coughs, bronchial irritation, and other respiratory discomforts. The tea's soothing effects can provide much-needed relief for those suffering from conditions such as asthma or chronic bronchitis.

Melatonin

Melatonin is the hormone responsible for regulating the sleep-wake cycle. While the body naturally produces melatonin in response to darkness, some individuals may benefit from melatonin supplements, particularly those who experience difficulty falling asleep. Melatonin supplements are typically taken in doses of 1 to 3 mg, about 30 minutes before bedtime, to help regulate sleep cycles and improve overall sleep quality.

Milk Thistle Supplement

Milk thistle (*Silybum marianum*) is a well-known liver detoxifier that can help reduce the inflammatory response associated with allergies. By supporting liver function, milk thistle ensures that toxins and allergens are processed efficiently, reducing the burden on the immune system. Taking a milk thistle supplement during allergy season can help to cleanse the liver, improve detoxification, and reduce the severity of allergic reactions. The herb's antioxidant properties also help protect liver cells from damage, ensuring that the body remains resilient in the face of allergens.

Mullein Tea

Mullein has been traditionally used to soothe the respiratory system and is especially effective in cases of coughing or bronchial irritation. To prepare **mullein tea**, steep 1-2 teaspoons of dried mullein leaves in a cup of boiling water for 10 minutes. Strain the tea to remove the fine hairs present on the leaves, as these can be irritating if ingested. Mullein acts as an expectorant, helping to loosen mucus and clear the lungs. For optimal results, drink 2-3 cups daily during periods of respiratory distress, especially when dealing with chest congestion or a persistent cough.

Neem Oil

Neem oil has strong antifungal properties and can be used both internally and topically. Take one to two drops of neem oil mixed with water or a carrier oil once daily. Neem's antifungal compounds help target Candida while supporting the body's detoxification processes.

Nettle Tea

Nettle is rich in minerals like iron and calcium, which are essential for strong hair and nails. Brew 1-2 teaspoons of dried nettle leaves in a cup of boiling water for 10 minutes. Drinking this tea daily will help boost your mineral levels, supporting both hair strength and nail health over time.

Olive Leaf Extract

Olive leaf extract is another potent antifungal remedy that supports long-term fungal balance. Take 500 mg of olive leaf extract daily, preferably with food, to inhibit Candida and support immune function. Olive leaf contains oleuropein, which strengthens the body's natural defenses against Candida overgrowth.

Omega-3 Fatty Acids

Omega-3 fatty acids, found in fish oil and flaxseeds, are essential for maintaining mental health and reducing symptoms of depression and anxiety. Omega-3 supplements can be taken daily, with the recommended dosage being 1,000–2,000 mg of EPA and DHA combined. Consuming foods rich in omega-3s, such as fatty fish or flaxseed oil, can also provide similar benefits.

Omega-3 Fish Oil

Omega-3 fatty acids, found in fish oil, are one of the most researched supplements for heart health. Omega-3s reduce inflammation, lower triglyceride levels, and help prevent the formation of blood clots, which can reduce the risk of heart attack and stroke. The recommended dosage for omega-3 fish oil is 1,000 to 2,000 mg of combined EPA and DHA, taken once daily with a meal. Consistency is important when taking omega-3s, as their effects are cumulative over time. Fish oil supplements should be stored in a cool, dark place to prevent them from going rancid.

Omega-3 Smoothie

Omega-3 fatty acids are essential for brain health, as they support the structure and function of brain cells. Omega-3s help maintain the integrity of cell membranes, which are critical for efficient neurotransmitter activity and communication between brain cells. To incorporate omega-3s into your diet, add flaxseeds or chia seeds to a smoothie. These seeds are rich in alpha-linolenic acid (ALA), a plant-based form of omega-3 that can be converted into the active forms EPA and DHA in the body. Blend a tablespoon of flaxseeds or chia seeds with leafy greens, such as spinach or kale, and antioxidant-rich berries like blueberries or raspberries. Drinking this brain-boosting smoothie regularly in the morning can help improve mental performance and protect against cognitive decline.

Onion Poultice

An **onion poultice** is a traditional remedy used to relieve chest congestion and break up mucus in the lungs. To prepare the poultice, sauté chopped onions lightly until they are soft but not browned. Place the warm onions in a cloth or thin towel and apply it directly to the chest for 20-30 minutes. The warmth and properties of the onions help open the airways and make it easier to expel mucus, providing relief from conditions like bronchitis or chest colds. Repeat this treatment once or twice daily when symptoms are at their worst.

Oregano Oil

Oregano oil is a potent antimicrobial agent that can be used to combat bacterial, viral, and fungal infections. It is highly concentrated, so it should be taken in small doses, typically a few drops mixed with water or juice. Oregano oil is particularly effective in treating respiratory infections and supporting overall immune health.

Oregano Oil Capsules

Oregano oil is highly effective against systemic Candida overgrowth. Take one to two capsules of oregano oil daily, ensuring the oil is diluted to avoid irritation. This remedy is best taken with meals to prevent stomach discomfort. Oregano oil contains thymol and carvacrol, which are potent antifungal compounds that work to inhibit fungal growth throughout the body.

Palming Exercise

Palming is a simple yet effective exercise to reduce eye strain and improve focus. To perform this exercise, rub your hands together to generate warmth and then gently place your palms over your closed eyes without applying pressure. Relax in this position for five to ten minutes, allowing your eyes to rest in complete darkness. This technique helps relax the eye muscles, reduces strain, and promotes better focus. Palming can be done two or three times a day, particularly after long periods of reading or screen use.

Papaya Salad

Natural digestive enzymes found in papayas, like papain, help break down proteins and facilitate better digestion. Eating fresh papaya as a light salad can help reduce symptoms of indigestion and bloating. Papaya is also high in fiber and water content, both of which support regular bowel movements. This fruit can be consumed before or after meals as a digestive aid. Adding lime juice and a sprinkle of salt to papaya enhances its flavor while boosting its digestive benefits.

Passionflower

Passionflower is another powerful herb that helps increase the brain's production of GABA, which promotes relaxation and reduces anxiety. Passionflower is commonly taken as a tea or tincture to support deeper sleep. The recommended dosage for sleep support is about 250 to 500 mg of dried extract, which can be taken 30 to 60 minutes before bed.

Pau D'Arco Tea

Pau D'Arco, derived from the bark of the Tabebuia tree, is traditionally used to fight fungal infections. Brew Pau D'Arco bark into a tea by steeping one tablespoon of the bark in hot water for 15 minutes. Drink this twice daily to support the immune system and reduce Candida populations. Pau D'Arco contains lapachol, a compound known for its antifungal properties.

Peppermint Essential Oil

Peppermint essential oil is widely known for its ability to enhance concentration and reduce brain fog. The menthol in peppermint has a stimulating effect on the brain, helping to clear mental fatigue and improve cognitive alertness. To use peppermint oil, apply a few drops to your temples and gently massage it into your skin. This can be particularly effective when you're feeling mentally sluggish or distracted. Alternatively, you can diffuse peppermint oil in your workspace to create an environment conducive to focus and productivity. Peppermint's invigorating properties make it an excellent choice for moments when sharp mental clarity is needed.

Peppermint Oil (for Muscle Rub)

Peppermint oil has a cooling effect that relieves muscle pain and tension. Combine 5–10 drops of peppermint essential oil with a carrier oil like coconut oil, and massage it into sore muscles post-activity to reduce inflammation and provide relief. Use this as needed for muscle tension.

Peppermint Oil Inhalation

Peppermint oil is another effective essential oil for relieving respiratory discomfort and clearing the sinuses. Its menthol content helps to open the airways, making it easier to breathe when allergy symptoms are at their worst. To use peppermint oil, mix it with a carrier oil like coconut oil and rub it on your chest, or add a few drops to a diffuser or bowl of hot water for inhalation. Inhaling peppermint oil vapors can reduce congestion and help soothe irritation in the respiratory tract, providing much-needed relief during peak allergy periods.

Peppermint Oil Scalp Treatment

Peppermint oil is known for its stimulating properties that can help increase hair thickness by activating hair follicles. Mix 2-3 drops of peppermint oil with 1 tablespoon of a carrier oil like jojoba or olive oil. Apply the blend to your hair and let it sit for 20 minutes before washing it off. Use this treatment once a week for best results.

Peppermint Oil Steam

Peppermint oil contains menthol, which is well-known for its ability to clear the sinuses and lungs. To create a **peppermint oil steam inhalation**, add 3-4 drops of peppermint essential oil to a bowl of hot, steaming water. Cover your head with a towel and inhale the vapors deeply for 5-10 minutes. Peppermint helps open the airways and promotes easier breathing, making it a great remedy for sinus congestion and colds. Use this treatment up to twice daily to keep your nasal passages and lungs clear.

Peppermint Tea

Peppermint tea is one of the most effective natural remedies for soothing indigestion and reducing bloating. Peppermint contains menthol, which has a calming effect on the muscles of the digestive tract, helping to alleviate gas and bloating. To prepare peppermint tea, simply brew fresh peppermint leaves in hot water for 5-10 minutes. This tea is best consumed after meals to promote digestion and relieve discomfort from overeating. It can also be used when experiencing symptoms like stomach cramps or mild nausea. Peppermint's cooling properties help relax the GI system, making it an ideal remedy for those dealing with occasional digestive upset.

Probiotic Supplement

Probiotics are essential for restoring gut flora balance and keeping Candida in check. Take a high-quality probiotic supplement daily, preferably one with multiple strains of beneficial bacteria such as Lactobacillus and Bifidobacterium. Probiotics help repopulate the gut with good bacteria, which crowds out harmful pathogens like Candida.

Probiotics

Probiotics support immune health by maintaining the balance of good bacteria in the gut, which is essential for proper immune function. Consuming probiotic-rich foods like yogurt, kefir, and sauerkraut, or taking a probiotic supplement, helps boost the body's natural defenses against pathogens.

Psyllium Husk Drink

Psyllium husk is a fiber-rich supplement that promotes regular bowel movements and supports overall digestive health. When mixed with water or juice, psyllium husk forms a gel-like substance that helps to bulk up stool and move it more easily through the intestines. This makes it an effective remedy for both constipation and diarrhea, as it helps regulate bowel function. Psyllium husk can be taken once a day, preferably in the morning, to support healthy digestion. It's important to drink plenty of water when consuming psyllium to avoid potential digestive discomfort.

Pumpkin Seed Snack

Pumpkin seeds are a natural source of zinc, an essential mineral for both thyroid and reproductive health. Zinc plays a critical role in regulating the production of hormones like thyroid hormone and testosterone. Snack on a handful (about 1 ounce) of raw pumpkin seeds daily or incorporate them into salads or smoothies for a nutrient boost that supports both the thyroid and reproductive systems.

Quercetin Supplement

Quercetin is a flavonoid found in various fruits and vegetables, and it plays a crucial role in managing allergies by stabilizing mast cells, which are responsible for releasing histamine. Histamine is the chemical that triggers allergy symptoms like itching, swelling, and mucus production. Barbara O'Neill recommends increasing intake of foods rich in quercetin, such as apples, onions, and citrus fruits, or taking a quercetin supplement to support the body's natural antihistamine response. By incorporating quercetin into your daily routine, you can reduce the severity of allergic reactions over time.

Reishi Mushroom

Reishi mushrooms are adaptogenic fungi that help modulate the immune system, making it more effective at fighting infections. Reishi can be consumed in powdered form, added to soups, or taken as a supplement. It is especially useful for strengthening the immune system over time.

Rhodiola Rosea

Rhodiola Rosea is another adaptogen that helps the body cope with stress by improving resilience to physical and emotional stressors. It can also help reduce fatigue and improve mood. Rhodiola is typically taken in capsule form, with a recommended dosage of 200–600 mg per day, ideally in the morning to avoid stimulating effects in the evening.

Rhodiola Rosea Capsules

Rhodiola Rosea is another adaptogenic herb known for its ability to reduce fatigue and improve mental performance under stress. It is particularly useful for individuals who experience burnout or exhaustion from prolonged stress. Take 200–400 mg of Rhodiola Rosea in capsule form once or twice daily, preferably in the morning or early afternoon. Rhodiola should not be taken too late in the day, as it may cause difficulty falling asleep due to its energizing effects.

Rhodiola Supplement

Rhodiola is another adaptogen that plays a crucial role in balancing cortisol production and improving energy levels. It is particularly effective in reducing fatigue associated with stress and supporting overall adrenal health. Rhodiola supplements are typically available in capsule form. It's recommended to take one capsule, usually 200–400 mg, in the morning before breakfast. This helps provide energy throughout the day and prevents the body from overproducing cortisol in response to stress.

Rose Water Toner

Rose water is a natural toner that helps tighten pores, hydrate the skin, and refresh the complexion. It is gentle enough to be used daily after cleansing. To use rose water as a toner, spritz it lightly on your face after washing, or apply it with a cotton pad. This simple step helps balance the skin's pH and prepares it for moisturizing. Rose water is suitable for all skin types and can be used in the morning and evening as part of a regular skincare routine.

Rosemary Massage Oil

Rosemary essential oil is known for improving circulation and reducing muscle stiffness. Use rosemary oil diluted in a carrier oil for massage post-activity to increase blood flow and soothe tired muscles. This can be applied once a day, ideally after a warm shower or bath.

Rosemary Oil Inhalation

Rosemary essential oil is another potent natural remedy for mental clarity and focus. The aromatic compounds in rosemary have been shown to stimulate cognitive function and increase alertness. Inhaling rosemary essential oil, either directly from the bottle or through a diffuser, can help improve focus, especially during tasks that require sustained concentration. A simple method is to place a few drops of rosemary essential oil into a diffuser or onto a cloth, and inhale deeply for a few minutes. This practice can be repeated throughout the day to maintain mental sharpness. Research suggests that inhaling rosemary oil can significantly boost memory retention and enhance cognitive performance, making it an ideal remedy for those seeking to improve their focus.

Rosemary Oil Scalp Massage

Rosemary oil has long been used to stimulate hair growth and improve circulation to the scalp. Warm 2-3 tablespoons of rosemary oil slightly, then massage it into the scalp for 10-15 minutes, ensuring full coverage. This massage, done two to three times a week, encourages blood flow to the hair follicles, promoting healthier, thicker hair growth.

Sauerkraut

Sauerkraut, a fermented cabbage dish, is an excellent source of probiotics, which are beneficial bacteria that support gut health. Incorporating sauerkraut into your meals can boost the population of healthy bacteria in your digestive system, aiding in digestion and nutrient absorption. The fermentation process that creates sauerkraut produces lactic acid, which helps break down food in the intestines and promotes regular bowel movements. It's recommended to start with small portions of sauerkraut and gradually increase the amount as your digestive system adjusts to the added probiotics. Homemade or store-bought sauerkraut can be used as a side dish or added to salads and sandwiches for a flavorful boost to digestive health.

Seaweed Salad

Seaweed is an excellent source of iodine, a mineral essential for healthy thyroid function. Incorporating seaweed into meals can naturally support thyroid hormone production, which is critical for metabolism and overall hormonal balance. Add seaweed to salads, soups, or stir-fries a few times per week. A small portion of seaweed, such as nori or wakame, can provide the iodine needed to keep your thyroid healthy.

Silica Powder

Silica is a trace mineral that supports the health of connective tissue, bones, and joints. It helps the body absorb calcium more efficiently and plays a role in collagen production, which is essential for maintaining joint flexibility and skin elasticity. Silica powder can be mixed into water or juice and taken once a day. The typical dosage is 500-1000 mg of silica per day, depending on individual needs. It is recommended to take silica in the morning or with a meal to enhance its effects.

Silica-Rich Hair Rinse

To enhance hair shine and boost silica levels, rinse your hair with a mixture of horsetail tea and apple cider vinegar. Brew a strong cup of horsetail tea and mix it with 2 tablespoons of apple cider vinegar. After shampooing, pour the mixture over your hair and leave it on for a few minutes before rinsing with cool water. This rinse can be used once a week to strengthen hair and improve shine.

Skullcap

Skullcap is a herb traditionally used to calm the nervous system and promote sleep. It is particularly effective in reducing anxiety and nervous tension, which can interfere with sleep. Skullcap can be consumed as a tea or tincture, with a typical dosage of 1 to 2 grams of dried herb taken before bed to support restful sleep.

Skullcap Tea

Skullcap is an excellent herb for calming a hyperactive nervous system. It is particularly useful for people who experience irritability or tension from stress. To make skullcap tea, steep one teaspoon of dried skullcap leaves in a cup of boiling water for 10 minutes. Drink one to two cups daily, especially in the evening, to soothe nerves and prepare for restful sleep.

St. John's Wort

St. John's Wort is an herb commonly used to treat mild depression and anxiety, but it can also help improve sleep. It works by regulating neurotransmitters in the brain that affect mood and sleep cycles. The typical dosage of St. John's Wort for sleep support is 300 to 600 mg, taken in the evening.

St. John's Wort Oil

St. John's Wort oil is beneficial for nerve pain and muscle recovery. Apply it to sore areas twice a day, massaging it in gently. It can be especially useful after heavy exercise to reduce discomfort and promote healing.

St. John's Wort Tincture

St. John's Wort is commonly used to relieve symptoms of mild to moderate depression, making it beneficial for those whose stress has led to emotional imbalance. A tincture is a fast-acting way to use this herb. Take 30-50 drops of St. John's Wort tincture in water up to three times a day. Due to its potential interactions with other medications, it's essential to consult a healthcare provider before use.

Tart Cherry Juice

Natural melatonin sources like tart cherry juice have been demonstrated to increase both the quantity and quality of sleep. Drinking one cup of tart cherry juice an hour before bed may help those struggling with insomnia or short sleep cycles. Tart cherry juice also contains antioxidants that support the body's recovery processes during sleep.

Tea Tree Oil Spot Treatment

Tea tree oil is a natural remedy with potent antibacterial and anti-inflammatory properties, making it ideal for treating acne. To create a spot treatment, dilute tea tree oil with water or a carrier oil (such as coconut or jojoba oil) at a ratio of 1:9—one part tea tree oil to nine parts carrier oil. Dab a small amount of the diluted solution directly onto blemishes using a cotton swab. This treatment helps reduce inflammation and kill bacteria, preventing the spread of acne. Apply once or twice a day as needed, but avoid using it on the entire face, as tea tree oil can be too strong for sensitive areas.

Thyme

Thyme is a natural antiseptic and antimicrobial herb that supports respiratory health. It can help clear mucus and relieve symptoms of colds and coughs. Thyme can be added to teas or used as a seasoning in cooking to provide immune support.

Thyme and Honey Elixir

Thyme is known for its ability to support respiratory health and regulate cortisol levels, particularly during periods of stress. Honey, with its soothing properties, complements thyme's effects, making this elixir an excellent remedy during stressful times. To prepare, steep fresh thyme leaves in hot water for 5 minutes, then strain and add a teaspoon of honey. Drink this warm elixir during the day to calm the mind and support the adrenal glands.

Turmeric

Turmeric contains curcumin, a powerful anti-inflammatory and antioxidant compound. It supports immune health by reducing chronic inflammation in the body, which can weaken the immune system. Turmeric can be added to meals, taken as a supplement, or consumed as a tea. To increase its bioavailability, turmeric should be taken with black pepper.

Turmeric Capsules

Curcumin, a potent anti-inflammatory found in turmeric, relieves stiffness and discomfort in the joints. Curcumin works by inhibiting certain inflammatory enzymes in the body, making it highly effective for conditions like osteoarthritis. Turmeric is best taken in capsule form to ensure consistent dosages. The recommended dosage is 500-1000 mg of curcumin per day, taken in divided doses with meals. For optimal absorption, turmeric capsules should be taken with black pepper extract (piperine) or a source of fat, such as flaxseed oil.

Turmeric Face Mask

Turmeric is known for its anti-inflammatory and brightening properties, making it an effective ingredient for reducing redness and evening out skin tone. To make a turmeric face mask, mix 1 teaspoon of turmeric with 2 tablespoons of yogurt and 1 tablespoon of honey. Apply the mixture to clean skin and leave it on for 10 to 15 minutes before rinsing it off with warm water. The yogurt helps to gently exfoliate the skin while honey moisturizes and turmeric reduces inflammation. Use this mask once a week to keep the skin bright and clear.

Turmeric Golden Milk

Turmeric is known for its powerful anti-inflammatory effects, thanks to its active compound, curcumin. To support muscle recovery, drink turmeric golden milk made from 1 teaspoon of turmeric, a pinch of black pepper (to enhance absorption), and warm almond or coconut milk. This can be consumed once daily, especially in the evening for calming and restorative effects.

Turmeric Latte

Turmeric is well known for its anti-inflammatory properties and its ability to support metabolism. When combined with black pepper, which enhances the absorption of turmeric, it becomes a powerful metabolism-boosting drink. To prepare a turmeric latte, mix 1 teaspoon of turmeric powder with warm almond milk and a dash of black pepper. Drink this in the morning or as a calming evening beverage to help reduce inflammation and support weight management.

Turmeric-Ginger Tea

A combination of turmeric and ginger can help reduce inflammation and detoxify the body, making it harder for Candida to thrive. To prepare the tea, mix one teaspoon of ground turmeric and a slice of fresh ginger in hot water. Drink this twice daily to support detoxification and reduce Candida populations. Both turmeric and ginger possess anti-inflammatory and antifungal properties, supporting the body's natural defenses.

Valerian Root

Valerian root is well-known for its calming properties. It acts as a sedative, helping to alleviate anxiety and promote deep sleep. Valerian root can be taken as a tea, tincture, or in capsule form. For optimal results, it is recommended to take 300–600 mg of valerian extract about 30 minutes to one hour before bedtime. This herb can help individuals who experience difficulty relaxing or suffer from insomnia due to stress.

Vitamin C

Vitamin C is essential for the proper functioning of the immune system. It helps stimulate the production of white blood cells and supports the skin's barrier function against pathogens. Foods rich in vitamin C include citrus fruits, bell peppers, and broccoli. Vitamin C can also be taken as a supplement, especially during cold and flu season.

Vitamin C Smoothie

Vitamin C is known for its immune-boosting properties, and it also acts as a natural antihistamine. By increasing your intake of vitamin C-rich foods, you can help reduce the severity of allergic reactions. A simple way to do this is through a vitamin C smoothie. Blend together citrus fruits like oranges, lemons, and kiwi to create a delicious and refreshing smoothie that can strengthen the immune system and reduce histamine production. The high concentration of vitamin C in these fruits helps reduce inflammation and supports the body in managing allergy symptoms more effectively.

Vitamin D3 Supplement

Vitamin D3 is essential for calcium absorption and bone health. Without adequate levels of vitamin D3, the body cannot properly absorb calcium, leading to weaker bones and an increased risk of fractures. Vitamin D3 supplements are particularly important for individuals who live in areas with limited sunlight or who spend most of their time indoors. The recommended dosage of vitamin D3 is 1000-2000 IU per day, although some individuals may require higher doses depending on their specific needs. Vitamin D3 is best taken with a meal that contains healthy fats to improve absorption.

Warm Water Hydration

Starting the day with a glass of warm water is a simple yet effective way to maintain hydration, which is essential for preventing dry eyes. Hydration supports the production of tears and keeps the eyes moist throughout the day. Drinking a glass of warm water upon waking helps flush out toxins and sets the tone for proper hydration throughout the day. This practice is particularly beneficial for individuals prone to dry eye syndrome or who spend long hours in dry, air-conditioned environments.

Willow Bark Extract

Willow bark is a natural pain reliever that contains salicin, a compound similar to aspirin. It has been used for centuries to reduce inflammation and relieve pain associated with arthritis and joint stiffness. Willow bark extract can be taken in capsule form, with a recommended dosage of 120-240 mg of salicin per day, divided into two or three doses. It is important to take willow bark extract with food to avoid stomach irritation.

Zinc

Zinc is a mineral that plays a crucial role in immune function. It helps the body produce immune cells and protects against respiratory infections. Zinc can be found in foods such as pumpkin seeds, lentils, and spinach, or taken as a supplement during illness to reduce the duration of colds and flu.

Made in the USA
Monee, IL
16 February 2025